Science-Based Approaches to Respond to COVID and Other Public Health Threats

Edited by Erick Guerrero

Published in London, United Kingdom

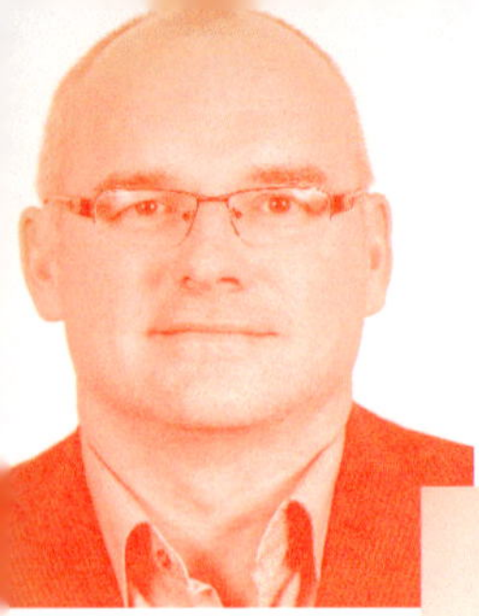
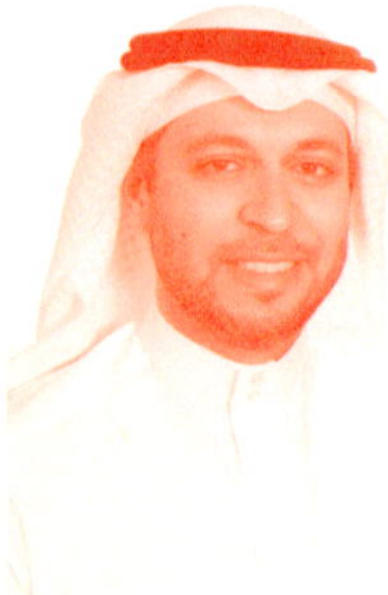
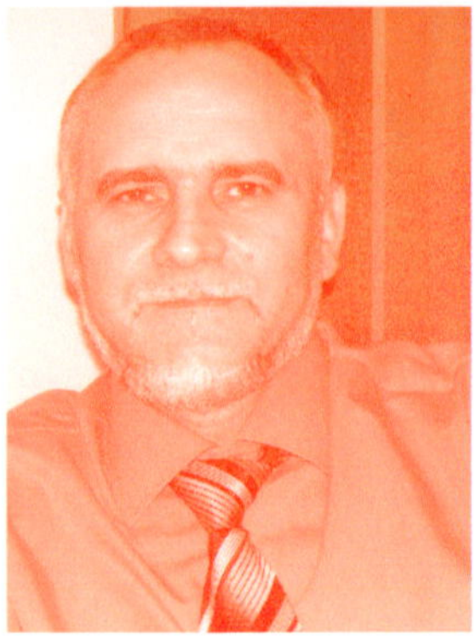
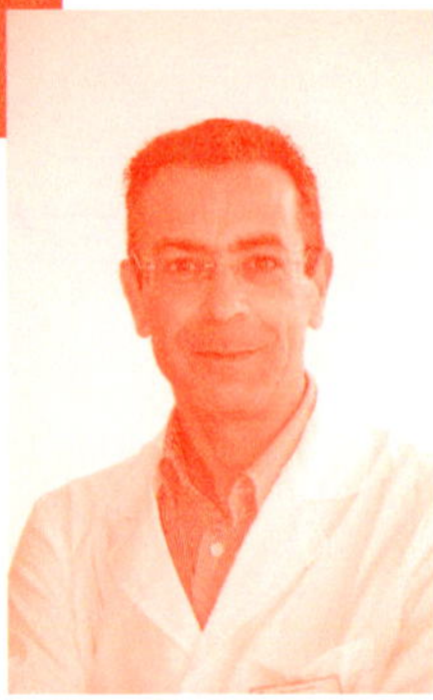
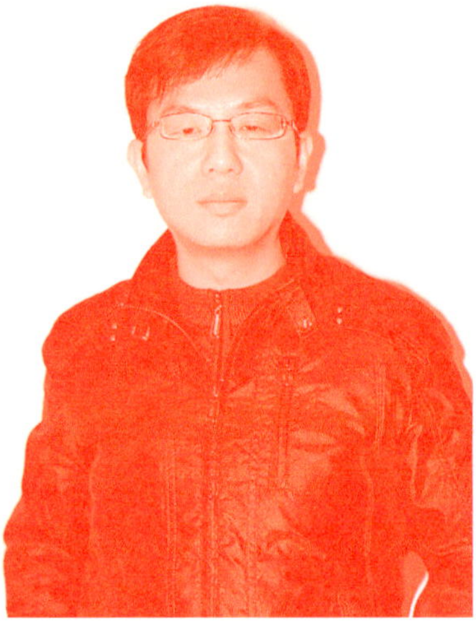
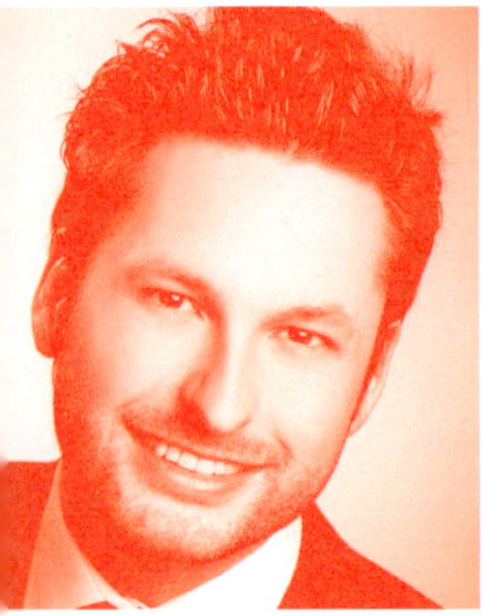
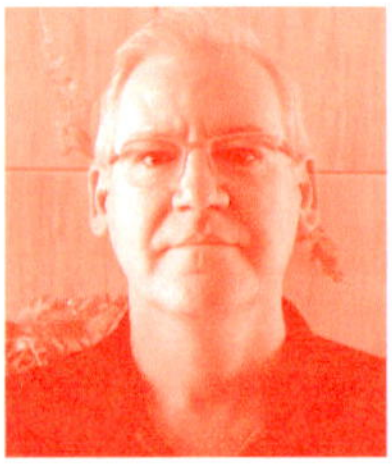

IntechOpen

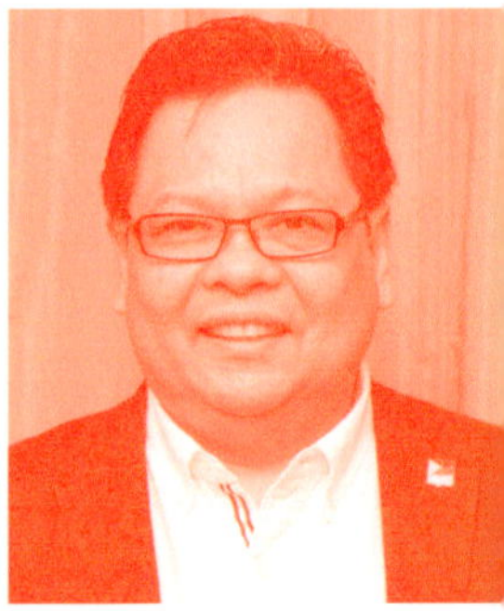
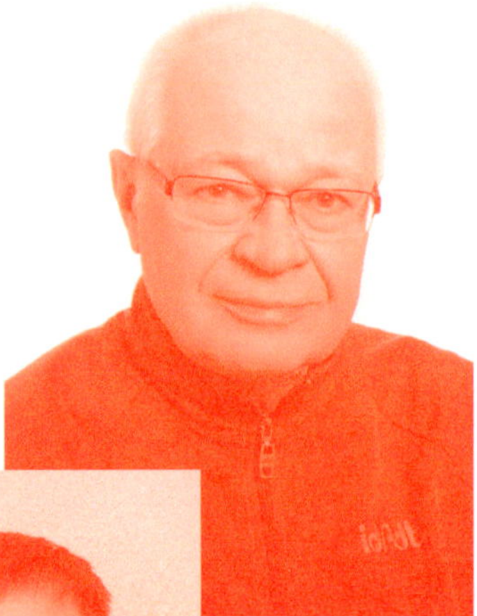
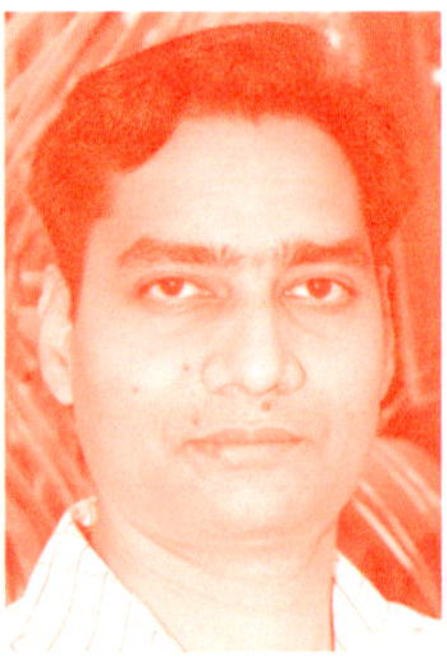
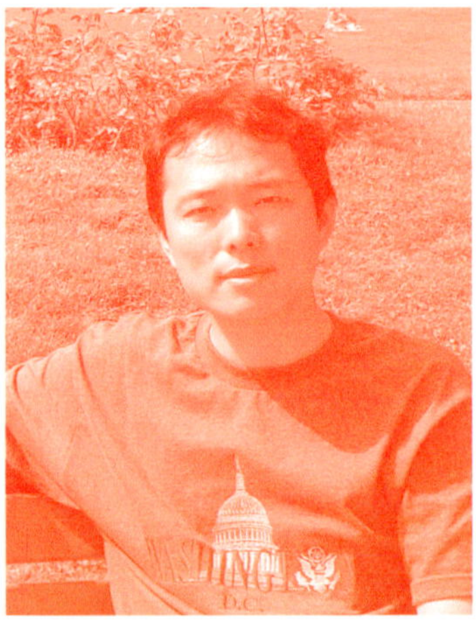
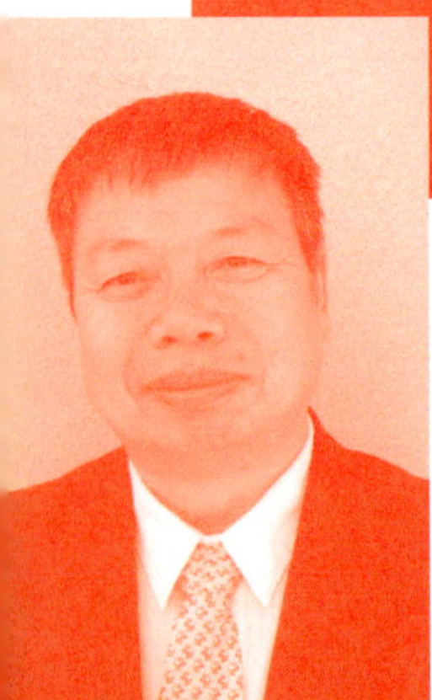
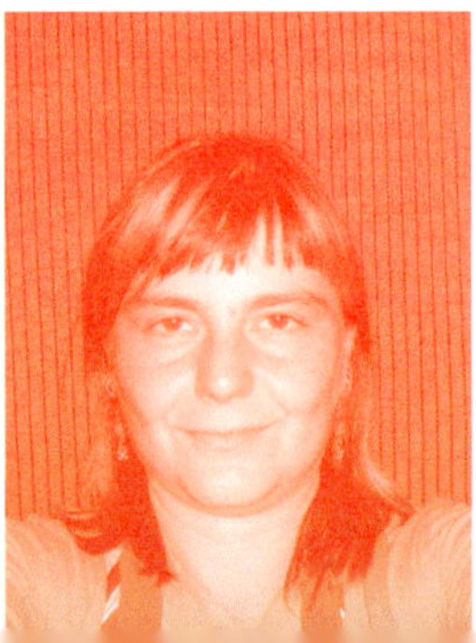

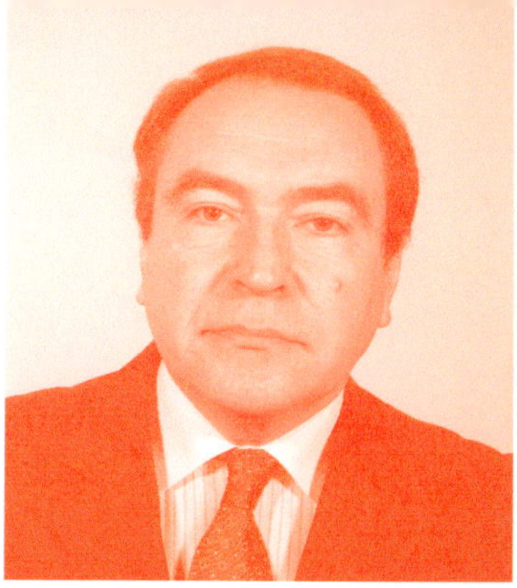
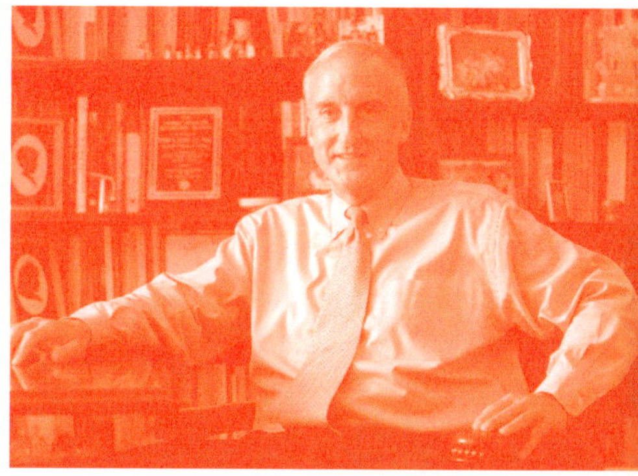
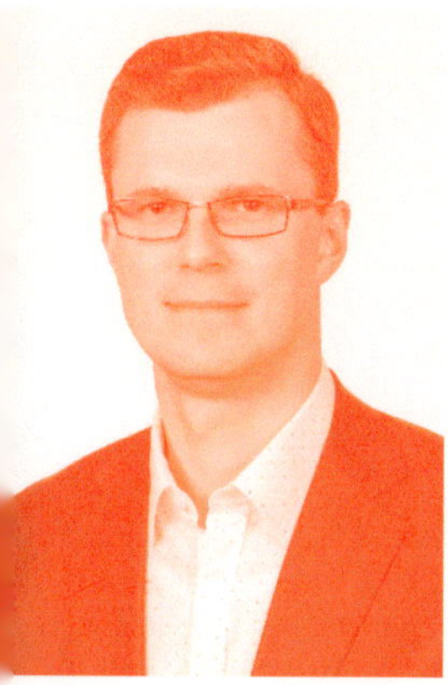
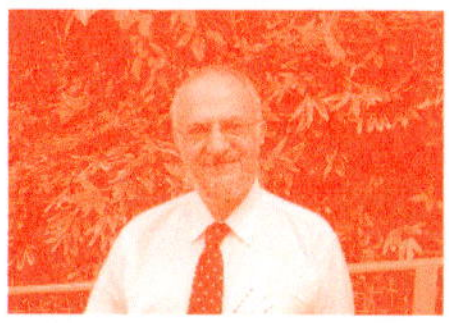
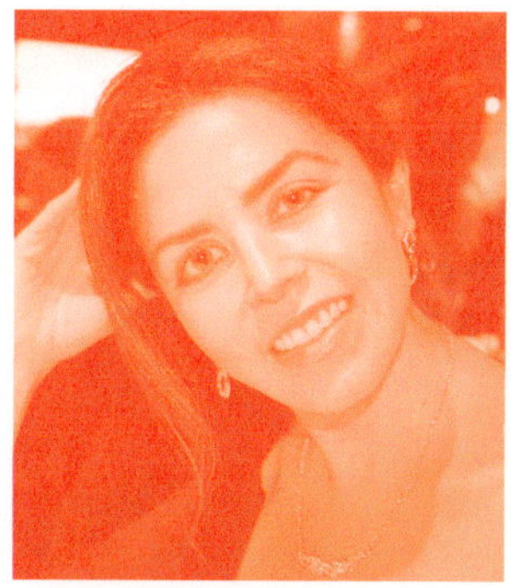

Supporting open minds since 2005

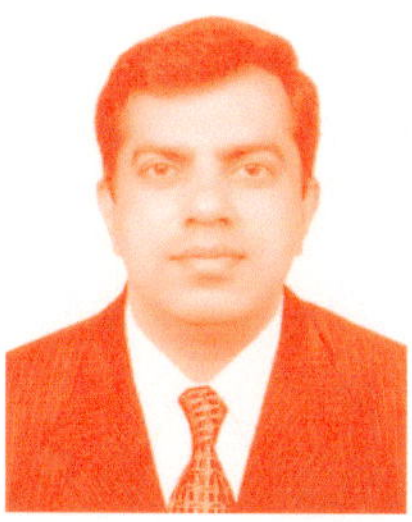
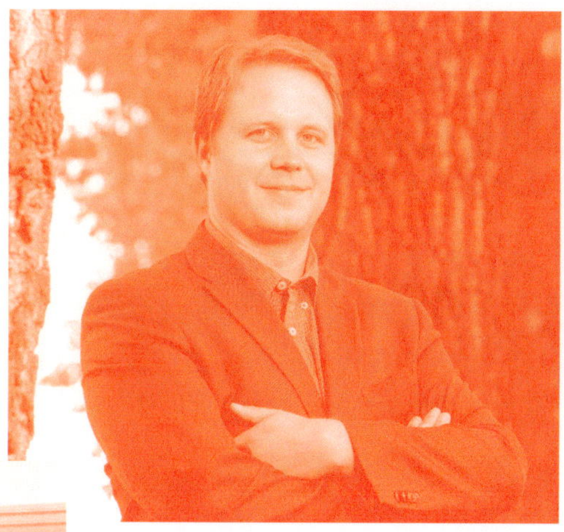
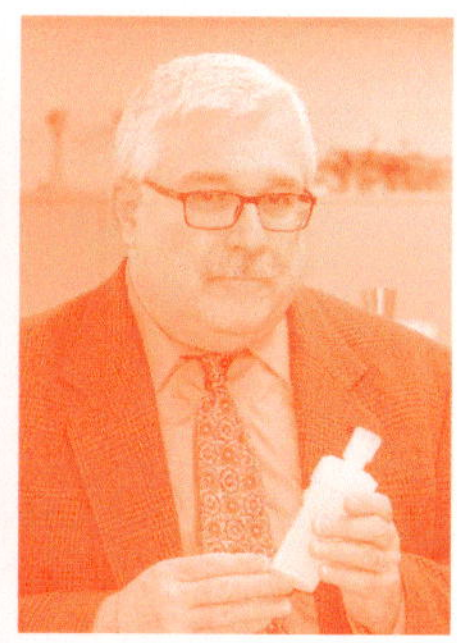
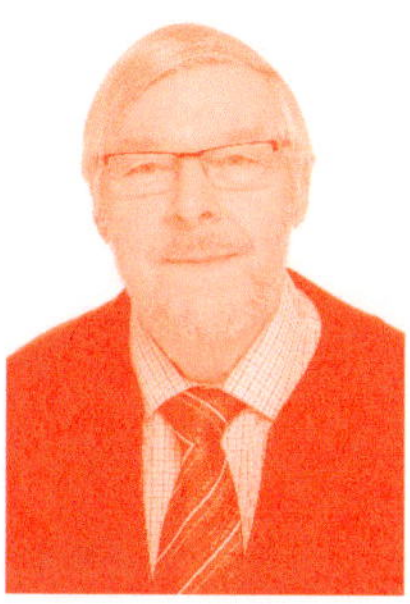
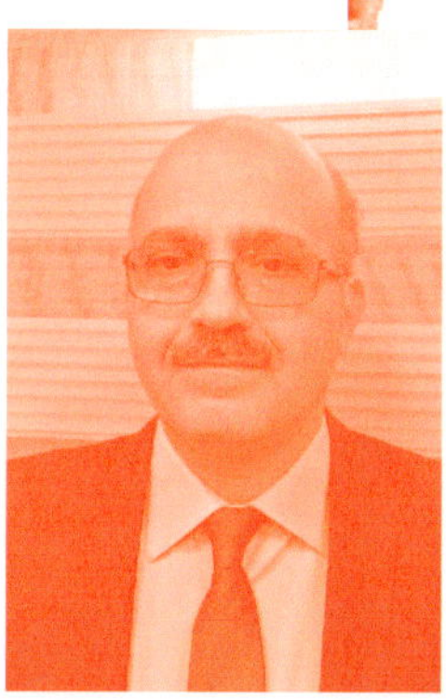
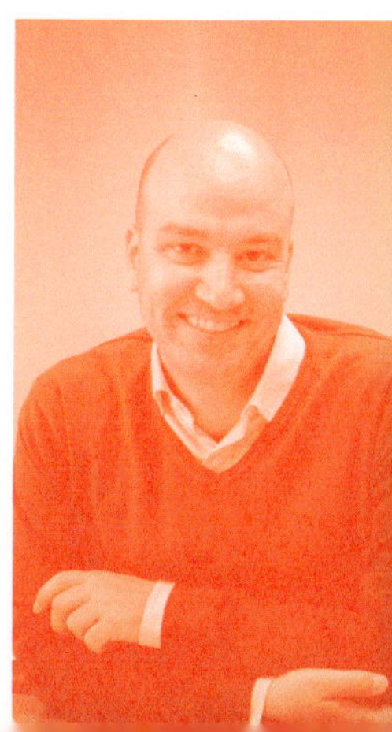
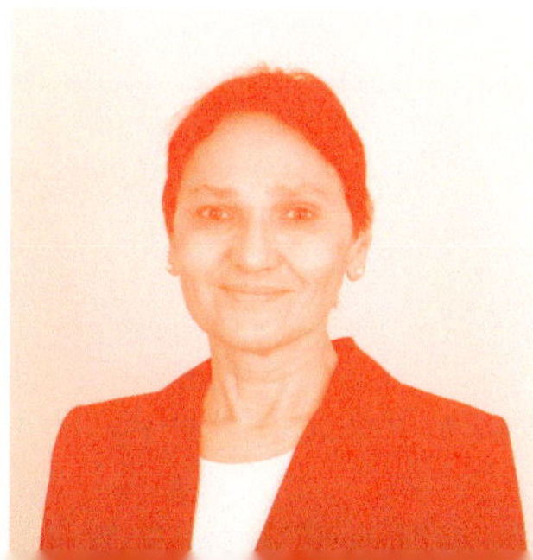

Science-Based Approaches to Respond to COVID and Other Public Health Threats
http://dx.doi.org/10.5772/intechopen.87288
Edited by Erick Guerrero

Contributors
Mirgissa Kaba, Yayehyirad Kitaw, Julius Manjengwa, Alonso Ureta Dumont, Jovanka Trebotich Zúñiga, Peggy Ann A. Honoré, Peter J. Fos, Russel Honore, Ukamaka Gladys Okafor, Hillary Chukwuemeka Asobara, Modinat Aderonke Olaleye, Ebuka Fidelis Umeodinka, Lap Yan Wong, Wai Lim Ling, Dao Shen Tan, Chun Kit Yip, Daniel L. L. Howard, Saptarshi Chatterjee, Nilanjana Dhara, Sumana Saha, Dursun Ali Sirin, Fatih Ozcelik, Arisa Yasui, Muneyoshi Numada, Alessandro Leite Leite Cavalcanti, Isla Camilla Carvalho Laureano, Erick Guerrero, Jemima A. Frimpong, Angelique J. Montgomery, Veronica Serret, Welmoed K. van Deen, Howard Padwa, Rebecca Trotzky-Sirr, Michael Menchine, Daniel L. Howard, Raimi Morufu Olalekan Olalekan, Aziba-anyam Gift Raimi, Teddy Charles Charles Adias

First published in London, United Kingdom, 2021 by IntechOpen
IntechOpen is the global imprint of INTECHOPEN LIMITED, registered in England and Wales, registration number: 11086078, 5 Princes Gate Court, London, SW7 2QJ, United Kingdom
Printed in Croatia

British Library Cataloguing-in-Publication Data
A catalogue record for this book is available from the British Library

Additional hard and PDF copies can be obtained from orders@intechopen.com

Science-Based Approaches to Respond to COVID and Other Public Health Threats
Edited by Erick Guerrero
p. cm.
Print ISBN 978-1-83969-143-0
Online ISBN 978-1-83969-144-7
eBook (PDF) ISBN 978-1-83969-145-4

For EU product safety concerns:
IN TECH d.o.o., Prolaz Marije Krucifikse Kozulić 3, 51000 Rijeka, Croatia, info@intechopen.com or visit our website at intechopen.com.

Meet the editor

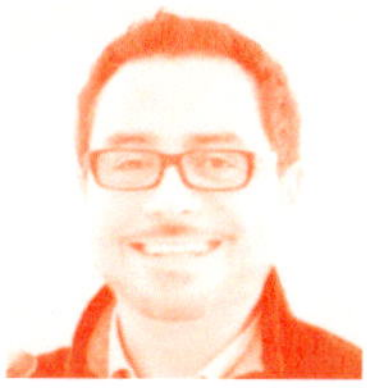

Dr. Erick Guerrero completed his doctoral degree at the University of Chicago in 2009 and received tenure as an associate professor at the University of Southern California in 2016. Dr. Guerrero has a background in clinical psychology and organizational behavior. As a clinician, he has provided counseling for the past twenty-three years. As an organizational researcher, Dr. Guerrero has published more than seventy peer-reviewed manuscripts and three books on racial/ethnic and gender disparities and the implementation of evidence-based practices in healthcare in the United States and Mexico. Funded by the US National Institutes of Health, he is currently co-leading four research studies to respond to COVID-19 and opioid overdose public health crises. Dr. Guerrero is a fellow at Yale University's Innovation to Impact program, and director of the I-LEAD Institute, a research and consulting firm in Silicon Beach, California.

Contents

Preface

As of October 2021, the World Health Organization (WHO) reports close to five million COVID-19-related deaths across the globe. Increasing death rates from other public health threats (e.g., opioid epidemic) also negatively impacted every aspect of human life, especially among vulnerable populations and low-resource regions. As most social, educational, and healthcare systems were not prepared to respond to these public health crises, a diverse group of dedicated and exemplary scientists present in this volume the latest knowledge on ways to respond to COVID-19 and other public health threats and with these efforts improve global health and wellbeing.

This volume provides unique, comprehensive, and science-based approaches to prevent and manage public health threats. Thirteen chapters describe prevention and intervention practices to respond to macro-structural, human process, and micro issues affected by public health threats. For instance, the authors describe how communities may reduce public health risk and generate evidence to inform policy-making and coordination efforts across public and private sectors. Other preventative structural approaches discussed include shelter management approaches to protect individuals before, during, and after a public health crisis, and waste management technologies to prevent the spread of infections.

The book's chapters discuss the human processes necessary to coordinate efforts. For instance, authors describe types of leadership behaviors that best prepare decision-makers to lead amid crisis, and ways in which innovative technologies may help us identify, analyze, and respond to public health threats using public and academic data and computing capacities. Special attention is paid to the role of Artificial Intelligence to anticipate and address the consequences of future public health threats. The book has a special focus on the impact of COVID-19 and other public health crises on vulnerable populations and low-resource regions around the globe.

Public health crises disrupt supply chains and limit efforts to develop pharmacological and other treatment innovations to overcome health threats. In this volume, the authors offer best practices to develop supply chain strategies for emergencies, an issue that has impacted world economies and food supply chains. They also examine the stage of development of the latest medications to treat COVID-19, a shining light in the fight against this pandemic.

This book also addresses public health crises like the opioid overdose epidemic. Authors describe interdisciplinary team approaches to respond to national emergencies and offer recommendations and practices regarding infection prevention and control measures on a wide scale. Overall, this book provides a comprehensive view of science-based approaches to respond to COVID-19 and other public health threats with emphasis on the most vulnerable. The group of committed scientists, whose work is presented in this volume, sought to inform the public and policy-makers about evidence-based practices that may improve the safety and health of all and secure a future for our mother earth.

Erick Guerrero, Ph.D.
Director,
I-Lead Institute,
REHD Corp,
Innovation to Impact Fellow,
Yale University,
USA

Acknowledgments

Support for this work was provided in part by a National Institute of Drug Abuse research grant (R01 DA038608S1) and funding for the editor from the I-Lead Institute. These institutions did not have a role in the writing of the manuscript or in the decision to submit the manuscript for publication.

The editor would like to acknowledge members of the REHD Corp team, Veronica Serret and Tenie Khachikian, who prepared the manuscript for submission. Most importantly, the editor appreciates his wife Emma and his four-year-old daughter, Sophie, for all the support, patience, and love provided during the editing of this volume.

Section 1

Responding to COVID-19 and Its Impact on Disparities and Public Health Services

Chapter 1

Clinical Trials on COVID-19: What is Being Researched in the United States?

Isla Camilla Carvalho Laureano
and Alessandro Leite Cavalcanti

Abstract

The emergence of Coronavirus Disease 2019 (COVID-19) in late 2019 has brought great challenges to public health worldwide and, to date, there is no specific approved therapeutic protocol. Therefore, this chapter will analyze types of intervention for use in patients with COVID-19 developed by American researchers from records made on the Clinical Trials platform. For the search strategy, keywords "COVID-19" in the "Condition or Disease" section and "United States" in the "Country" section were used. No filters were applied. Data were descriptively analyzed. In total, 1,182 studies were obtained, of which 496 met the eligibility criteria. Sample size ranged from 1 to 10,000 participants. Most studies involved the age group of 18–64 years (48.6%). As for design, randomized type (80.5%), parallel (75.6%), open designs (38.7%) and those with therapeutic purpose (88.3%) were more frequent. Most clinical trials used the two-arm trial (67.3%), researched drugs (64.8%), used placebo (55.2%) and were sponsored by pharmaceutical/biotechnology companies (35.4%). Clinical trials developed by American researchers on COVID-19 involve adult and elderly participants, with predominance of randomized, parallel and open design, for therapeutic purposes and mostly evaluated immunosuppressants or combinations of antivirals/immunosuppressants. The drugs and biological products Remdesivir, Baricitinib in combination with Remdesivir, Bamlanivimab and Etesevimab, REGEN-COV and COVID-19 convalescent plasma were also used, authorized for emergency use.

Keywords: Clinical Trial, Evidence-Based Practice, Pharmaceutical Preparations, Vaccines, COVID-19, Coronavirus Infection

1. Introduction

In March 2020, the World Health Organization (WHO) recognized Coronavirus Disease 2019 (COVID-19) as a public health problem and declared the state of pandemic contamination [1]. Since its detection in late 2019, in China, the newly discovered virus, called SARS-CoV-2 [2] spread rapidly around the world with cases, to date, in 223 countries, with more than 127 million infected individuals and nearly 3 million deaths [3]. The region of Americas concentrates almost half of all diagnosed individuals, with the United States being the most affected country, totaling 30 million cases [3].

SARS-CoV-2 belongs to a family of single-stranded, positive-sense and enveloped RNA viruses, known as *Coronaviridae* [4], has high mutation rate and rapid spread, with multiple mutations having appeared and spread during the pandemic [5, 6]. The transmission of the virus occurs through droplets expelled by a person with the disease or through contact with contaminated surfaces [7].

In general, patients with COVID-19 have fever, cough, myalgia, nausea, diarrhea, reduced smell and taste, as well as mild breathlessness [8]. In the most severe cases, patients can develop Acute Respiratory Distress Syndrome (ARDS), heart failure, shock and renal failure [9]. Elderly, obese and individuals with pre-existing conditions, such as diabetes, hypertension, cardiovascular and pulmonary diseases, cancer, chronic kidney disease, among others, have higher risk of progressing to more critical cases of the disease [10]. In addition to symptoms and severity of the disease, the impact of COVID-19 affects all aspects of our lives, generating financial consequences, insecurity and anxiety [11].

Advances have been made in the knowledge of COVID-19 and in the development of safe and effective vaccines [12]. However, there is still no specific pharmacological protocol approved to prevent and/or reduce contamination by the virus, so that there are countless ongoing researches to find an appropriate treatment [13]. The development of vaccines, convalescent plasma therapies, cell-based and monoclonal antibody therapies are some of the treatments studied worldwide. However, the development of new drugs is a long and expensive process, and the current health emergency has led to the use of existing drugs [14].

The pandemic has induced the global scientific community to focus efforts on COVID-19 [15] and clinical trials represent the gold standard for evidence-based practice [16], as they are important methods for assessing intervention modalities, generating impact on current and future clinical practice [17]. However, attention should be paid to clinical trials with inadequate or low-quality designs, and it is important to analyze their designs on clinical trial registration platforms to identify those that provide the best scientific evidence that can reduce the effects of the COVID-19 pandemic [18].

In view of the fact that SARS-CoV-2 is a virus with characteristics never before studied, with several consequences that go beyond contamination, and in the absence of an approved effective therapy, correctly designed clinical trials are essential for evaluating interventions in order to prevent and contain the spread of the disease. Thus, the guiding issue that supported this chapter was: "Which interventions for use in patients with COVID-19 are being evaluated by American researchers?"

2. Methods

The database chosen for this study was the Clinical Trials platform (https://clinicaltrials.gov/), which comprises a web-based resource that provides patients, their family members, health care professionals, researchers, and the public with easy access to information on publicly and privately supported clinical studies on a wide range of diseases and conditions [19]. In the search strategy, keywords "COVID-19" in the "Condition or Disease" section and "United States" in the "Country" section were used.

No filters were applied, so that all registered clinical trials were analyzed. Data were collected in March 2021 by a single previously trained researcher. Studies with suspended, withdrawn and terminated recruitment status, observational and expanded access studies, and those that did not mention COVID-19 diagnosis and those including healthy patients among their eligibility criteria were excluded.

The following information was collected: study location, number of participants, age groups of subjects (0–17, 18–64, >65), allocation (randomized, non-randomized e n/a), intervention model (single group assignment, sequential assignment, crossover assignment, parallel assignment and factorial assignment), masking (blind, double-blind, triple-blind, quadruple-blind and open label), purpose (diagnostic, treatment, prevention, basic science, supportive care, health services research, device feasibility, screening and other), diagnostic criteria for COVID-19 (confirmed, suspect and confirmed or suspect), other eligibility criteria, recruitment status (completed, recruiting, active, not recruiting, not yet recruiting and enrolling by invitation), numbers of arms, type of intervention (dietary supplement, drug, biological, device, diagnostic test, procedure, radiation, behavioral, combination product and other), phase (early phase 1, phase 1, phase 2, phase 3, phase 4, phase 1 and phase 2, phase 2 and phase 3 and n/a), presence of placebo (yes and no), comparison arm (yes and no), and sponsor (university, pharmaceutical/ biotechnology company, research organizations, hospital, health care provider, doctor, united states department of defense and philanthropy).

Types of intervention were classified according to the WHO's Anatomical Therapeutic Chemical Classification System [20]. In cases where they are not included in the WHO's ATC, information present on the companies' websites was used.

Data were tabulated and analyzed using the Microsoft Excel 2016 for Windows software (Microsoft Press, Redmond, WA, USA) and descriptively presented.

3. Results

In total, 5,129 records involving COVID-19 were found and, after the search strategy, 1,182 (23%) corresponded to clinical trials developed in the United States. Of these, eight studies that were suspended, 22 that had been withdrawn, 25 terminated, 325 observational studies, 18 expanded access, 37 that did not include COVID-19 diagnosis and, finally, 251 clinical trials using healthy patients were excluded. At the end, 496 studies met the eligibility criteria and were selected.

The geographic distribution of studies highlights the state of California as the main place for carrying out these surveys (155 studies), followed by Florida (124 studies), Texas (121 e studies), Nova York (115 studies), Illionois (86 studies), Massachusetts (81 studies), Pennsylvania (78 studies), North Carolina (75 studies), Washington and Ohio (73 studies each), Michigan (71 studies), Maryland (70 studies), Georgia (66 studies), Louisiana (64 studies), New Jersey (56 studies), Virginia and Arizona (50 studies each), Minnesota (45 studies), Colorado (39 studies), Alabama (38 studies), Tennessee (35 studies), Missouri (33 studies), Connecticut (30 studies), Utah (29 studies), Oregon (28 studies), South Carolina and Kansas (27 studies), Kentucky (25 studies), New Mexico and Nebraska (22 studies each), Indiana and Iowa (21 studies), Wisconsin and Mississippi (20 studies each), Arkansas (16 studies), Idaho and Rhode Island (14 studies), Oklahoma (11 studies), West Virginia (10 studies), Maine and South Dakota (9 studies each), Hawaii and Montana (7 studies each), Vermont (3 studies), and Alaska and Delaware (1 studies each).

The number of participants ranged from 1 to 10,000 individuals. Most clinical trials analyzed involved adults and older adults, with higher percentage in the age group of 18–64 years (48.6%), while surveys that recruited children and adolescents represented only 2.9%.

Regarding the allocation of participants, only 26 studies (5.2%) were not characterized as randomized. The most frequent intervention model is the parallel (75.6%). Regarding the type of masking, the open study model (38.7%) is the most prevalent, followed by the double-blind model (21.4%), while single-blind studies corresponded to only 4.4%. Studies with therapeutic purposes were carried out in the majority (88.3%) and there is predominance of those who consider proven and positive COVID-19 diagnosis (89.1%) as an inclusion criterion (**Table 1**).

Variables	n	%
Age Groups (in years)*		
0–17	29	2.9
18–64	489	48.6
> 65	487	48.5
Allocation		
Randomized	399	80.5
Non-Randomized	26	5.2
N/a	71	14.3
Intervention Model		
Single Group Assigment	86	17.3
Sequential Assignment	26	5.2
Crossover Assignment	3	0.6
Parallel Assignment	375	75.6
Factorial Assignment	3	1.2
Masking		
Blind	22	4.4
Double-blind	106	21.4
Triple-blind	73	14.7
Quadruple-blind	103	20.8
Open Label	192	38.7
Purpose		
Diagnostic	15	3.0
Treatment	438	88.3
Prevention	12	2.4
Basic Science	2	0.4
Supportive Care	17	3.4
Health Services Research	2	0.4
Device Feasibility	2	0.4
Screening	1	0.2
Other	7	1.4
Diagnostic Criteria for COVID-19		
Confirmed	442	89.1
Suspect	11	2.2
Confirmed or suspect	43	8.7
Recruitment Status		
Completed	66	13.3
Recruiting	295	59.5
Active, not recruiting	68	13.7
Not yet recruiting	50	10.1
Enrolling by invitation	17	3.4

Variables	**n**	**%**
Numbers of Arms		
1	70	14.1
2	334	67.3
3	43	8.7
4	26	5.2
5	7	1.4
6	8	1.6
8	4	0.8
10	1	0.2
12	2	0.4
No information	1	0.2
Type of Intervention*		
Dietary Supplement	16	3.1
Drug	335	64.8
Biological	80	15.5
Device	35	6.7
Diagnostic Test	8	1.5
Procedure	4	0.8
Radiation	4	0.8
Behavioral	4	0.8
Combination Product	3	0.6
Other	28	5.4
Phase		
Early Phase 1	12	2.4
1	45	9.1
2	214	43.2
3	71	14.3
4	26	5.2
1 e 2	35	7.1
2 e 3	26	5.2
N/a	67	13.5
Presence of Placebo		
Yes	274	55.2
No	221	44.6
No information	1	0.2
Comparison Arm		
Yes	121	54.5
No	100	45.0
No information	1	0.5

Variables	n	%
Sponsor*		
University	201	29.4
Pharmaceutical / Biotechnology Company	242	35.4
Research Organizations	65	9.5
Hospital	82	12.0
Health Care Provider	39	5.7
Doctors	36	5.2
United States Department of Defense	6	0.9
Philanthropy	13	1.9

**Some studies involved more than one age group, type of intervention and sponsor; N/a = Not applicable.*

Table 1.
Characteristics of the sample and study design of clinical trials.

Other eligibility criteria used by researchers were the inclusion of individuals with associated risk factors (28 studies), including cancer (4 studies), type 1 or type 2 diabetes mellitus (3 studies) and heart diseases (1 study).

Regarding recruitment status, at the time of data collection, 59.5% of clinical trials were recruiting participants and 13.7% were active, but not recruiting. Regarding the number of arms, most studies use the two-arm test (67.3%). Most clinical trials research a new drug (64.8%), are in phase 2 (43.2%), 55.2% use placebo and 54.5% use comparison arm. As for sponsors, pharmaceutical/biotechnology companies (35.4%) and universities (29.4%) are those that most invest in clinical trials (**Table 1**).

Regarding the identification and classification of drugs, biological interventions, dietary supplements, combined products and some other interventions, 434 clinical trials use interventions in monotherapy and 67 make use of combinations. In monotherapy, most trials assess immunosuppressants (49 studies), followed by COVID-19 Convalescent Plasma (40 studies), antivirals (32 studies), anticancer (30 studies), antithrombotic (24 studies), anti-inflammatory agents (16 studies), antifibrinolytics (14 studies), antimalarials (13 studies), immunostimulants (7 studies), expectorants (6 studies), antibacterials (5 studies), antiparasitic and corticosteroids (4 studies each), antidepressants (3 studies), sex hormones and modulators of the genital system (2 studies) and antiprotozoals (1 study) (**Tables 2** and **4**). Clinical trials using combinations use antivirals /immunosuppressants (9 studies), antimalarials /antibiotics (6 studies), antithrombotic agents (4 studies) and antivirals/corticosteroids (**Tables 3** and **4**).

Interventions and Classes	n*	Interventions and Classes	n*	Interventions and Classes	n*
Antithrombotic Agents	**24**	Interferon	4	AZD7442	2
Heparin	6	CPI-006	2	COVID-19 Therapeutic Biologics - Spike-GM-CSF Protein Lactated Ringer's Injection	2
Enoxaparin	4	Sargramostim	1	Zinc	2
Apixaban	3	**Anticancer**	**30**	IVIG	2
Defibrotide	2	Colchicine	5	Octagam	2
Rivaroxaban	2	Ibrutinib	3	GAMUNEX-C	1

Interventions and Classes	n*	Interventions and Classes	n*	Interventions and Classes	n*
Dipyridamole	2	CYT107	2	Garadacimab	1
Tenecteplase	2	Duvelisib	2	Sodium bicarbonate	1
Acetylsalicylic Acid	1	Ruxolitinib	1	NasoVAX	1
VentaProst	1	Abivertinib	1	NA-831	1
TM5614	1	Pacritinib	1	Ifenprodil	1
Antifibrinolytics	**14**	Decitabine	1	ABBV-2B04	1
Camostat	9	Bempegaldesleukin	1	ABBV-47D11	1
Tranexamic acid	2	Etoposide	1	Ibudilast	1
Ulinastatin	1	Bicalutamide	1	MAS825	1
LYT-100	1	Imatinib	1	BGB-DXP593	1
BLD-2660	1	Upamostat	1	PUL-042	1
Antimalarials	**13**	Nintedanib	1	PurCo	1
Chloroquine or hydroxychloroquine	11	Acalabrutinib	1	Bucillamine	1
Tafenoquine	1	Degarelix	1	Pioglitazone	1
Artesunate	1	Antroquinonol	1	Gimsilumab	1
Antivirals	**24**	Selinexor	1	BI 764198	1
Molnupiravir	4	Zanubrutinib	1	Zilucoplan	1
Favipiravir	3	FT516	1	Lanadelumab	1
Lopinavir/Ritonavir	2	CYNK-001	1	rNAPc2	1
Brequinar	2	**Antiparasitic**	**4**	Aprepitant	1
Silmitasertib	2	Ivermectin	2	Brexanolone	1
Apilimod Dimesylate	1	Niclosamide	1	Pepto Bismol	1
Maraviroc	1	Disulfiram	1	Ruconest	1
Liquid Alpha1-Proteinase Inhibitor	1	**Antiprotozoals**	**1**	Isavuconazonium	1
RBT-9	1	Atovaquone	1	Fostamatinib	1
AT-527	1	**Corticosteroids**	**4**	VIB7734	1
BTL-TML-COVID	1	Dexamethasone	2	Pamrevlumab	1
LAU-7b	1	Ciclesonide	1	CAP-1002	1
Veru-111	1	Prednisone	1	Linagliptin	1
PTC299	1	**Anti-inflammatory**	**16**	CM4620-IE	1
PF-07304814	1	Acebilustat	2	Vadadustat	1
RTB101	1	Ampion	2	Zofin	1
Antibacterials	**5**	N-acetyl glucosamine	1	ADG20	1
Azithromycin	2	Alvelestat	1	GC4419	1
Doxycycline	1	Dociparstat	1	Essential Oil Blend	1
Brilacidin	1	Ensifentrine	1	Fenofibrate	1
Carrimycin	1	Bardoxolone Methyl	1	ATI-450	1
Antidepressants	**3**	Indomethacin	1	Xuanfei Baidu Granules	1
Fluvoxamine	2	EDP1815	1	Emricasan	1

Interventions and Classes	n*	Interventions and Classes	n*	Interventions and Classes	n*
Fluoxetine	1	LSALT peptide	1	ORTD-1	1
Immunosuppressants	**49**	OP-101	1	Metformin	1
Tocilizumab	7	FSD201	1	Umbilical Cord Lining Stem Cells	1
Anakinra	3	RLS-0071	1	BGE-175	1
Cyclosporine	2	ST266	1	Chlorine dioxide	1
Sirolimus	2	**Sex hormones and modulators of the genital system**	**2**	Prazosin	1
Ravulizumab	2	Estradiol	1	Cetylpyridinium Chloride	1
Sarilumab	2	Progesterone	1	Peroxil	1
Leflunomide	2	**Expectorants (mucolytics)**	**6**	Colgate Total Zero	1
Razuprotafib	1	N-acetylcysteine	3	Saline rinse	1
Dapansutrile	1	Pulmozyme	2	Crizanlizumab	1
Abatacept	1	Dornase Alfa	1	AT-001	1
Losmapimod	1	**Outras**	**187**	Hyperpolarized Xe129	1
Apremilast	1	Renin-angiotensin system inhibitors	11	Atorvastatin	1
Olokizumab	1	Mesenchymal stem cells (MSCs)	11	Glycine	1
Infliximab	1	Nitric Oxide	7	Alanine	1
Tociliuzumab	1	Cytotoxic T Lymphocytes	7	Thymalfasin	1
Canakinumab	1	Bamlanivimab	6	TB006	1
Sirukumab	1	Clazakizumab	6	PF-06650833	1
Lenzilumab	1	Chlorhexidine	5	Angiotensin	1
Otilimab	1	Vitamin D	4	Tradipitant	1
Tofacitinib	1	Vitamin C	4	Resistant starch	1
Auxora	1	Mavrilimumab	4	F-652	1
APL-9	1	Povidone Iodine	4	Omega-3	1
CD24Fc	1	Fisetin	3	L-Citrulline	1
TL-895	1	Leronlimab	3	FoTv	1
TD-0903	1	Listerine	3	VisAcT	1
EB05	1	Hydrogen Peroxide	3	Regadenoson	1
ATYR1923	1	Famotidine	2	Sulfur hexafluoride lipid-type A	1
CERC-002	1	Melatonin	2	Lucinactant	1
M5049	1	VIR-7831	2	CBDRA60	1
BMS-986253	1	Nitrogen gas	2	SBI-101	1
GLS-1027	1	NT-I7	2	Zavegepant	1
UTTR1147	1	Betadine	2	Neuromuscular Blocking Agents	1
MSTT1041A	1	Naltrexone	2	*Artemesia annua*	1
TJ003234	1	Human Amniotic Fluid	2	*Nerium oleander*	1

Interventions and Classes	n*	Interventions and Classes	n*	Interventions and Classes	n*
Immunostimulants	7	KB109	2		

*Some studies used several interventions.
The bold entries refer to the drug classes and the total interventions of each class of drugs and biological products according to the WHO's Anatomical Therapeutic Chemical Classification System or information present on the companies' websites.

Table 2.
Monotherapy interventions used in experimental groups of registered clinical trials on COVID-19.

Interventions and Classes	n*
Antithrombotic Agents Combinations	**4**
Heparin + P2Y12	2
Dipyridamole + Acetylsalicylic Acid	1
Enoxaparin + Heparin + Fondapariniux + Argatroban	1
Antimalarials + Antibiotics	**6**
Hydroxychloroquine + Azithromycin	6
Antivirals + Immunosuppressants	**7**
Remdesivir + Tocilizumab	1
Remdesivir + Infliximab	1
Remdesivir + Apremilast	1
Remdesivir + Abatacept	1
Remdesivir + Risankizumab	1
Remdesivir + Apremilast	1
Remdesivir + Lenzilumab	1
Antivirals + Corticosteroids	**2**
Atazanavir + Dexamethasone	1
Remdesivir + Dexamethasone	1
Other Combinations	**41**
Remdesivir + Cenicriviroc	2
Valproate + Quetiapine	1
PurInf (I) + PurInf (II) + PurInf (III)	1
PurPhl + PurClo	1
Colchicine + Rosuvastatin	1
Colchicine + Naltrexone	1
Naltrexone + Ketamine	1
BRII-196 + BRII-198	1
NA-831 + Dexamethasone	1
NA-831 + Atazanavir	1
IVIG + Remdesivir	1
Rintatolimod +Interferon	1
Remdesivir + Interferon	1
Remdesivir + Icatibant	1
Remdesivir + Razuprotafib	1
Remdesivir + anti-CD14	1

Interventions and Classes	**n***
Plasma + Ruxolitinib	1
Bamlanivimab + VIR-7831	1
ABBV-47D11 + ABBV-2B04	1
Mesenchymal Stem Cells + Heparin	1
Metformin + Naltrexone	1
Resveratrol + Vitamin D	1
Nitazoxanide + Vitamin Super B-Complex	1
Vitamin C + Zinc	1
Resveratrol + Zinc	1
Famotidine + N-Acetyl cysteine	1
Chlorine dioxide + Zinc acetate	1
Atovaquone + Azithromycin	1
Camostat Mesilat + Bicalutamide	1
Xylitol + Grapefruit Seed Extract	1
Peroxil + Chlorhexidine	1
Hydroxychloroquine + Azithromycin + Zinc	1
Hydroxychloroquine + Zinc + Doxycycline	1
Hydroxychloroquine + Nitazoxanide + Ribavirin	1
Hydroxychloroquine + Azithromycin + Ritonavir + Lopinavir	1
Bamlanivimab + Remdesivir + VIR-7831 + BRII-196/BRII-198 + AZD7442	1
Chlorine dioxide + Famotidine + Lactoferrin + green tea extract	1
Chlorine dioxide + Zinc acetate + Famotidine + Lactoferrin + green tea extract	1
Hydroxychloroquine + Azithromycin + Vitamin C + Vitamin D + Zinc	1
Ivermectin + Doxycycline Hc + Vitamin C + Vitamin D + Zinc	1

**Some studies used several interventions.*

Table 3.
Combinations of interventions used in experimental groups of registered clinical trials on COVID-19.

Interventions and Classes	**n***
COVID-19 Convalescent Plasma	**40**
Antivirals	**8**
Remdesivir	8
Antivirals + Immunosuppressants	**2**
Remdesivir + Baricitinib	2
Other Combinations	**5**
Bamlanivimab + Etesevimab	2
REGN10933 + REGN10987	3

**Some studies used several interventions.*
The bold entries refer to the drug classes and the total interventions of each class of drugs and biological products according to the WHO's Anatomical Therapeutic Chemical Classification System or information present on the companies' websites.

Table 4.
Monotherapy and combinations of interventions with Emergency Use Authorizations (EUA) issued by U.S. Food and Drug Administration (FDA) used in experimental groups of registered clinical trials on COVID-19.

4. Discussion

Many clinical trials related to the COVID-19 pandemic have emerged in response to society's concerns related to the impacts of the pandemic, and in response to this global emergency. Scientific production on the topic is dynamic and fast, which makes the sharing and synthesis of knowledge important [15]. In this context, the characterization of research efforts can help professionals, researchers, and managers to understand the relevant aspects of the disease.

Considering the serious public health crisis of COVID-19 and the search for discovering safe and effective treatments, high-quality research is needed to evaluate interventions for the prevention of the disease and its treatment. Clinical trials properly designed and conducted make their results valid and can significantly contribute to the effort to improve the effectiveness and efficiency of health interventions [21].

"Clinical Trials" is a robust platform for registering clinical trials, containing detailed information on a large amount of clinical research conducted in 219 countries [22]. According to the Dimensions database, "Clinical Trials" is the leading platform for registering clinical trials on COVID-19, accounting for 58.8% of all registrations [23]. Of the clinical trials registered and found on this platform, a significant number is being developed by American researchers. This research leadership is underpinned by huge public funding, mainly from the National Institutes of Health (NIH), which has already received more than US$ 3.6 billion to fund research on COVID-19 [24], as well as from government agencies, universities and the private sector [25], which demonstrates the urgency of the USA in the face of the severity with which the disease reached the country [18].

Among studies analyzed, the majority of participants are adults and older adults. It is known that COVID-19 is less prevalent in children compared to adults and adolescents and that younger individuals infected with SARS-CoV-2 have less severe symptoms and lower hospitalization and lethality rates [26, 27]. In March 31, 2021, 11.7% of COVID-19 cases in the United States were of children and adolescents up to 17 years of age, corresponding to almost 3 million cases. Of these, for the age group of 0–4 years, there were only 104 deaths (<0.01%) and, for the age group of 5–17 years, only 228 deaths (0.1%) [27]. Therefore, these may be the reasons for choosing the age group of adults and older adults.

The most frequent study design was randomized allocation, the parallel intervention model and the open masking type. The randomization of a clinical trial ensures that, in addition to intervention, there are no systematic differences between study groups, providing impartial results regarding the effect of interventions and reducing biases [18, 28]. Even so, only randomization does not exclude the possibility of systematic differences, because since those involved in a clinical trial are aware of the attributions of interventions, which can influence the result and introduce bias [29]. In our study, masking was not feasible mainly for ethical reasons or because patients are incorporated into healthcare environments, making it difficult to blind the team that manages patient care [30].

There were greater number of clinical trials for therapeutic purposes that evaluate some drug as a type of intervention. These results may be related to the current world scenario and the urgent need for studies analyzing which treatments are shown to be most effective against COVID-19 [18] in an adequate and quick manner. The discovery of an efficient therapy would allow the prophylaxis of health professionals who are on front lines, so that they could get back to work more quickly, in addition to reducing the time spent by critically ill patients in intensive care units, freeing beds [31] and reducing mortality rates. Many studies using a placebo group were also found, and due to the lack of approved available treatment, this procedure is ethically acceptable [18].

In this study, the most frequent sponsors were pharmaceutical/biotechnology companies and universities. However, in the evaluated clinical trials, there was the collaboration of several companies, academic institutions, government agencies, non-profit organizations and individual medical researchers to properly implement resources in the fight against COVID-19 in order to concentrate and accelerate the development and implementation of therapies. This partnership of efforts may reflect the so-called Accelerating COVID-19 Therapeutic Interventions and Vaccines (ACTIV), conducted by NIH and announced in April 2020, in which researchers continue to work intensively to develop new and better treatments [32].

Regarding the classification of many tested drugs, biological interventions, dietary supplements, combined products and some other types of intervention, heterogeneity of classes used can be observed. Most clinical trials have been evaluated immunosuppressants or combinations of antivirals/immunosuppressants, some already with USA issued by the FDA and redirected for the treatment of COVID-19, such as the combination of immunosuppressant Baricitinib – used to treat rheumatological diseases [33] – with antiviral Remdesivir – used to treat patients infected with the Ebola virus, MERS-CoV and SARS-CoV-1 [34], and its use as monotherapy for certain patients hospitalized with COVID-19.

Other authorized drugs that deserve mention are the biological products Bamlanivimab and Etesevimab – neutralizing IgG1 monoclonal antibodies that bind to different but overlapping epitopes in the binding domain to the SARS-CoV-2 spike protein [35] –, REGEN-COV (Casirivimab and Imdevimab) – neutralizing recombinant human IgG1 monoclonal antibodies that target the binding domain to the SARS-CoV-2 spike protein receptor [36] –, and the COVID-19 convalescent plasma – collected from individuals whose plasma contains anti-SARS-CoV-2 antibodies [37].

The COVID-19 pathogenesis begins with the replication of SARS-CoV-2, subsequently followed by an exaggerated immune /inflammatory response to the virus that leads to tissue damage. Regarding this knowledge, it is assumed that antiviral therapies would have greater effect early in the course of the disease, whereas immunosuppressive/anti-inflammatory therapies may be more beneficial in later stages of COVID-19 [33]. The use of these existing drugs helps reducing the cost and time of research; however, further large-scale studies must be carried out to assess the benefits and safety of these drugs.

The findings reported here make it clear that researchers from different fields of medicine have worked together in the development and clinical evaluation of several drugs aimed at treating the numerous medical complications caused by COVID-19. Extensive financial resources, made available by universities and pharmaceutical and biotechnology companies, have been applied in order to allow the conduction of clinical trials with high methodological and scientific rigor for both diagnostic and treatment purposes. Undeniably, the emergency approval of the tested drugs described here by the FDA, while making it possible to save thousands of lives in the American territory, has allowed a better understanding of their effects on individuals affected by COVID-19, which knowledge has been shared and put into practice by managers and medical teams from various countries around the world.

Therefore, during the COVID-19 pandemic and due to all resulting restrictions and difficult circumstances, good scientific practice and data transparency are essential principles that should guide the conduction of clinical trials. The sharing of these results, when properly carried out, helps professionals to make decisions, as well as researchers to identify gaps and more promising interventions, to avoid research waste and to expose patients to unnecessary risks, consequently contributing to the advancement of scientific knowledge.

DOI: http://dx.doi.org/10.5772/intechopen.98494

5. Conclusion

Clinical trials developed by American researchers involving COVID-19 include adult and elderly participants, with predominance of randomized, parallel and open design, those for therapeutic purposes and those that mostly evaluate immunosuppressants or combinations of antivirals/immunosuppressants. The drugs and biological products Remdesivir, Baricitinib in combination with Remdesivir, Bamlanivimab and Etesevimab, REGEN-COV and COVID-19 convalescent plasma were also used, authorized for emergency use.

Conflict of interest

The authors report no conflicts of interest.

Author details

Isla Camilla Carvalho Laureano and Alessandro Leite Cavalcanti*
State University of Paraíba, Campina Grande, Paraíba, Brazil

*Address all correspondence to: alessandrouepb@gmail.com

References

[1] World Health Organization. Archived: WHO Timeline - COVID-19 [Internet]. 2020. Available from: https://www.who.int/news-room/detail/27-04-2020-who-timeline—covid-19 [Accessed: 2021-03-31].

[2] World Health Organization. Naming the coronavirus disease (COVID-19) and the virus that causes it [Internet]. 2021. Available from: https://www.who.int/emergencies/diseases/novel-coronavirus-2019/technical-guidance/naming-the-coronavirus-disease-(covid-2019)-and-the-virus-that-causes-it [Accessed: 2021-03-31].

[3] World Health Organization. Coronavirus disease (COVID-19) pandemic [Internet]. 2021. Available from: https://www.who.int/emergencies/diseases/novel-coronavirus-2019 [Accessed: 2021-03-31].

[4] Coronaviridae Study Group of the International Committee on Taxonomy of Viruses., Gorbalenya AE, Baker SC, Baric RS, Groot RJ, Drosten C, et al. The species Severe acute respiratory syndrome-related coronavirus: classifying 2019-nCoV and naming it SARS-CoV-2. Nat Microbiol. 2020;5: 536–544. DOI: 10.1038/s41564-020-0695-z

[5] Centers for Disease Control and Prevention. About Variants of the Virus that Causes COVID-19 [Internet]. 2021. Available from: https://www.cdc.gov/coronavirus/2019-ncov/transmission/variant.html [Accessed: 2021-03-31].

[6] Koyama T, Platt D, Parida L. Variant analysis of SARS-CoV-2 genomes. Bull World Health Organ. 2020;98:495-504. DOI: 10.2471/BLT.20.253591

[7] Ortiz-Prado E, Simbaña-Rivera K, Gomez-Barreno L, Rubio-Neira M, Guaman LP, Kyriakidis N, et al. Clinical, molecular, and epidemiological characterization of the SARS-CoV-2 virus and the Coronavirus Disease 2019 (COVID-19), a comprehensive literature review. Diagn Microbiol Infect Dis. 2020;98(1):115094. DOI: 10.1016/j.diagmicrobio.2020.115094

[8] Giacomelli A, Pezzati L, Conti F, Bernacchia D, Siano M, Oreni L, et al. Self-reported Olfactory and Taste Disorders in Patients With Severe Acute Respiratory Coronavirus 2 Infection: A Cross-sectional Study. Clin Infect Dis. 2020;71(15):889-890. DOI: 10.1093/cid/ciaa330

[9] Fu L, Wang B, Yuan T, Chen X, Ao Y, Fitzpatrick T, et al. Clinical characteristics of coronavirus disease 2019 (COVID-19) in China: A systematic review and meta-analysis. J Infect. 2020;80(6):656-665. DOI: 10.1016/j.jinf.2020.03.041.

[10] Centers for Disease Control and Prevention. People with Certain Medical Conditions [Internet]. 2021. Available from: https://www.cdc.gov/coronavirus/2019-ncov/need-extra-precautions/people-with-medical-conditions.html [Accessed: 2021-04-01].

[11] Gasparro R, Scandurra C, Maldonato NM, Dolce P, Bochicchio V, Valletta A, et al. Perceived Job Insecurity and Depressive Symptoms among Italian Dentists: The Moderating Role of Fear of COVID-19. Int J Environ Res Public Health. 2020;17(5):5338. DOI: 10.3390/ijerph17155338

[12] World Health Organization. Coronavirus disease (COVID-19): Vaccines [Internet]. 2020. Available from: https://www.who.int/news-room/q-a-detail/coronavirus-disease-(covid-19)-vaccines [Accessed: 2021-04-01].

[13] Dos Santos W.G. Natural history of COVID-19 and current knowledge on treatment therapeutic options. Biomed

Pharmacother. 2020;129:110493. DOI: 10.1016/j.biopha.2020.110493

[14] Chakraborty R, Parvez S. COVID-19: An overview of the current pharmacological interventions, vaccines, and clinical trials. Biochem Pharmacol. 2020;180:114184. DOI: 10.1016/j.bcp.2020.114184

[15] Haghani M, Bliemer MCJ, Goerlandt F, Li J. The scientific literature on Coronaviruses, COVID-19 and its associated safety-related research dimensions: A scientometric analysis and scoping review. Saf Sci. 2020;129:104806. DOI: 10.1016/j.ssci.2020.104806

[16] Spieth PM, Kubasch AS, Penzlin AI, Illigens BM, Barlinn K, Siepmann T. Randomized controlled trials - a matter of design. Neuropsychiatr Dis Treat. 2016;12:1341-1349. DOI: 10.2147/NDT.S101938

[17] Pandis N, Polychronopoulou A, Eliades T. An assessment of quality characteristics of randomised control trials published in dental journals. J Dent. 2010;38(9):713-21. DOI: 10.1016/j.jdent.2010.05.014

[18] Carvalho Laureano IC, Cabral Cavalcanti AF, Cavalcanti AL. Clinical Trials Developed in Brazil on Covid-19: What Is Being Researched?. Shiraz E-Med J. 2020;21(12):e109059. DOI: 10.5812/semj.109059

[19] US National Institutes of Health. ClinicalTrials.gov. ClinicalTrials.gov Background [Internet]. 2018. Available from: https://clinicaltrials.gov/ct2/about-site/background [Accessed: 2021-04-01].

[20] World Health Organization Collaborating Centre for Drug Statistics Methodology. International language for drug utilization research. [Internet]. 2020. Available from: http://www.whocc.no/atcddd/ [Accessed: 2021-04-01].

[21] Umscheid CA, Margolis DJ, Grossman CE. Key concepts of clinical trials: a narrative review. Postgrad Med. 2011;123(5):194-204. DOI: 10.3810/pgm.2011.09.2475

[22] US National Institutes of Health. ClinicalTrials.gov. Trends, charts and maps [Internet]. 2021. Available from: https://clinicaltrials.gov/ct2/resources/trends [Accessed: 2021-04-01].

[23] Dimensions. COVID-19 Report: Publications, Clinical Trials, Funding [Internet]. 2021. Available from: https://reports.dimensions.ai/covid-19/ [Accessed: 2021-04-01].

[24] National Institutes of Health. COVID-19 Research. Funding [Internet]. 2021. Available from: https://covid19.nih.gov/funding [Accessed: 2021-04-01].

[25] Sampat BN, Shadlen KC. The COVID-19 Innovation System. Health Aff (Millwood). 2021;40(3):400-409. DOI: 10.1377/hlthaff.2020.02097

[26] Pierce CA, Preston-Hurlburt P, Dai Y, Aschner CB, Cheshenko N, Galen B, et al. Immune responses to SARS-CoV-2 infection in hospitalized pediatric and adult patients. Sci Transl Med. 2020;12(564):eabd5487. DOI: 10.1126/scitranslmed.abd5487

[27] Centers for Disease Control and Prevention. COVID Data Tracker [Internet]. 2021. Available from: https://covid.cdc.gov/covid-data-tracker/#datatracker-home [Accessed: 2021-04-01].

[28] Kahan BC, Cro S, Doré CJ, Bratton DJ, Rehal S, Maskell NA, et al. Reducing bias in open-label trials where blinded outcome assessment is not feasible: strategies from two randomised trials. Trials. 2014;15:456. DOI: 10.1186/1745-6215-15-456.

[29] Chan AW, Tetzlaff JM, Gotzsche PC, Altman DG, Mann H,

Berlin JA, et al. SPIRIT 2013 explanation and elaboration: guidance for protocols of clinical trials. BMJ. 2013;346:e7586. DOI: 10.1136/bmj.e7586

[30] Gamerman V, Cai T, Elsäßer A. Pragmatic randomized clinical trials: best practices and statistical guidance. Health Serv Outcomes Res Method. 2019;19:23–35. DOI: 10.1007/s10742-018-0192-5

[31] Schlagenhauf P, Grobusch MP, Maier JD, Gautret P. Repurposing antimalarials and other drugs for COVID-19. Travel Med Infect Dis. 2020; 34:101658. DOI: 10.1016/j.tmaid.2020.101658

[32] National Institutes of Health. Accelerating COVID-19 Therapeutic Interventions and Vaccines (ACTIV) [Internet]. 2021. Available from: https://www.nih.gov/research-training/medical-research-initiatives/activ [Accessed: 2021-04-01].

[33] National Institutes of Health. COVID-19 Treatment Guidelines. Therapeutic Management of Adults With COVID-19 [Internet]. 2021. Available from: https://www.covid19treatmentguidelines.nih.gov/therapeutic-management/ [Accessed: 2021-04-01].

[34] Singh AK, Singh A, Singh R, Misra A. Remdesivir in COVID-19: A critical review of pharmacology, pre-clinical and clinical studies. Diabetes Metab Syndr. 2020; 14(4):641-648. DOI: 10.1016/j.dsx.2020.05.018

[35] U.S. Food and Drug Administration. Bamlanivimab and Etesevimab EUA Letter of Authorization February 25 2021[Internet]. 2021. Available from: https://www.fda.gov/media/145801/download [Accessed: 2021-05-13].

[36] U.S. Food and Drug Administration. Regeneron LOA 2.25.2021[Internet]. 2021. Available from: https://www.fda.gov/media/145610/download [Accessed: 2021-05-13].

[37] U.S. Food and Drug Administration. Convalescent Plasma EUA Letter of Authorization March 9, 2021[Internet]. 2021. Available from: https://www.fda.gov/media/141477/download [Accessed: 2021-05-13].

Chapter 2

A Clinical Update on Employing Tocilizumab to Fight COVID-19

Nilanjana Dhara, Sumana Saha and Saptarshi Chatterjee

Abstract

SARS-CoV-2 infection or COVID-19, currently regarded as 'terror' worldwide, has spread uncontrollably as a serious menace. Till date, limited effective medicines or treatments are available. The mortality and morbidity rates have increased considerably, which have been aggravated by acute respiratory distress syndrome (ARDS) and new and old cardiovascular injuries. To control COVID-19, many drugs have been taken into consideration, like ACE2 blockers, anti-inflammatory drugs, antibodies against IL-1 and anti-IL-6, Remdesivir, Dexamethasone, Hydroxychloroquine and vaccines. In this chapter, preference is given to Tocilizumab with the latest status of clinical research update available. Despite several clinical research attempts, some have yielded promising results, others are inconclusive.

Keywords: COVID-19, Tocilizumab, Clinical Studies, Antiviral drugs, Public Health

1. Introduction

Since December 2019, the outbreak of the novel coronavirus (SARS-CoV-2) infection (i.e. COVID-19), from Wuhan, China as a pandemic, has posed a serious threat towards mankind, treatment of which is still unknown [1]. In Jan 30, 2020, the novel coronavirus disease 2019 (COVID-19), was declared as the Sixth public health emergency epidemic by the World Health Organization [WHO] [2]. Till date there is no single drug to control it. Despite Remdesivir being used extensively for the treatment, it is still under clinical trials [3] and not beyond question [4]. The elderly, immune-compromised or people having co-morbidities led to acute respiratory distress syndrome (ARDS), cardiovascular (CV) complications, and multi-organ failure [2, 5]. Common symptoms of the disease include fever, cough, myalgia, malaise, breathlessness and diarrhea [2]. Tocilizumab (a humanized anti-IL-6 receptor antibody) is one of drugs used for the treatment of COVID-19 hospitalized patients [6]. This article summarizes all critical clinical trials to evaluate the efficacy of Tocilizumab.

2. About the molecule

Tocilizumab is an Interleukin-6 Receptor Inhibitor, having a molecular formula of [C6428H9976N1720O2018S42]. Its molecular mass is of [145.0 kDa], CAS number: [375823-41-9]. It is a recombinant humanized monoclonal antibody used in the treatment of inflammatory and autoimmune conditions like Rheumatoid arthritis, multiple myeloma and prostate cancer, nowadays used extensively for COVID-19 treatment [7–11].

3. Tocilizumab as drug

Tocilizumab, an immunosuppressive monoclonal antibody drug having the traditional name Actemra and Atlizumab, has been reported to be effective against COVID-19 in several countries such as China, France, Italy, Switzerland and Qatar Xiaoling [12, 13]. The drug is known to treat patients with hyperinflammatory syndrome and acute respiratory failure [14]. The drug is sold in the European Union (EU) under the trade name RoActemra and in the United States as Actemra [15, 16]. The drug was first approved in 2005 as an orphan drug in Japan, used in the treatment of Castleman's disease [17]. Nowadays, Tocilizumab has acquired license for EU, to be used alone or in combination with DMARDs [disease-modifying anti-rheumatic drugs]. This combined therapy is used in the treatment of rheumatic arthritis in adults, systemic form of juvenile idiopathic arthritis (sJIA) in children above 2 years and with the polyarticular form of juvenile idiopathic arthritis (pJIA) in children more than 2 years of age [17]. This drug displays a long elimination half-life. Several studies were conducted to find out whether the drug is useful or not.

In a single centre study in Brescia [Italy], having an gathering of 100 patients, 8 mg/kg [max 800 mg] of the drug was advised to be given to patients by two consecutive intravenous infusions 12 hr. apart. Significant clinical improvement was observed in this case [18]. In another study by Alattar et al. [19] at Quatar, 25 patients having COVID-19 were administered with Tocilizumab, one to three median doses of the drug individually [4.8 mg/kg]. Tocilizumab was associated with dramatic decline in inflammatory markers, radiological improvement and reduced ventilatory support requirements [19]. In a 61-year-old man with COVID-19 symptoms, with a history of kidney transplantation, 324 mg Tocilizumab was administered via subcutaneous route along with hydroxychloroquine that helped in prevention of the disease and did not require mechanical ventilation [20]. However, contrary reports do exist, that reports that Tocilizumab was not effective for preventing intubation or death in moderately ill hospitalized patients with COVID-19 [21].

4. USFDA approval

The drug Actemra (tocilizumab, Genentech, Inc., South San Francisco, CA) was approved by USFDA to be used for the treatment of Rheumatoid Arthritis (RA), Giant Cell Arthritis (GCA), Polyarticular Juvenile Idiopathic Arthritis (PJIA), Systemic Juvenile Idiopathic Arthritis (SJIA) and Cytokine Release Syndrome (CRS) [22]. However, despite of recommendation of NIH on usage of Tocilizumab for COVID-19 treatment, it has not yet received approval of USFDA.

5. Dosage of tocilizumab for COVID-19 treatment

The use of Tocilizumab is recommended as per the US NIH guidelines only for clinical trial studies [23]. The preference is mainly given to hospitalized patients with increasing oxygen demand with or without elevated markers of systemic inflammation. As per the recommendations, Tocilizumab (single intravenous [IV] dose of tocilizumab 8 mg/kg actual body weight up to 800 mg) in combination with dexamethasone (6 mg daily for up to 10 days) is advised to be administered in certain hospitalized patients experiencing rapid respiratory decompensation due to COVID-19 [24].

6. Storage

This drug should be stored refrigerated at 2 to 8° C (36 to 46 F).

7. Plausible mechanism of tocilizumab against COVID-19

According to a study, by the team of Haiming Wei [25], after the SARS-CoV-2 infection, CD4 + T lymphocytes are activated to become pathogenic T helper cells, generating GM-CSF (Granulo Macrophage Colony Stimulating Factor]. This leads to severe inflammatory storm created by CD14 + CD16+ inflammatory monocytes with elevated expression of IL-6. These excessive immune cells usually invade the pulmonary circulation and cause damage to the immune system, thus leading to functional disability of lungs and mortality. Therefore, drugs like Tocilizumab are administered to prevent the cytokine storm. Tocilizumab has yielded effective results as an IL-6R antagonist.

Excessive stimulation of IL-6 can cause CRS [Cytokine Release Syndrome] in hospitalized patients. The higher the level of CRS, higher is the serum peak concentration of IL-6. IL-6 binds to its receptor IL-6R and a complex is formed. IL-6R then binds to the signal transducer glycoprotein 130 (gp-130) to cause signal transduction. Two types of IL-6R are there, one is the Soluble form (sIL-6R) and the other is Membrane bound form [mIl-6R]. In classical signal transduction pathway, IL-6 binds to mIL-6R [transmembrane integral protein], and forms a complex, which then prohibits the connection of IL-6R with gp130 [integral membrane protein]. Thus no cytokine storm is produced. In the trans-signaling pathway, binding of Tocilizumab to sIl-6R, prevents the binding of IL-6R to gp130 [present on the membrane of monocytes, macrophages, dendritic cells] and thus hinders release of inflammatory storm. JAK/STAT tyrosine kinase system mediates one pathway, while Ras/mitogen-activated protein kinase (MAPK)/ NF-κB-IL-6 pathway mediates the other. Tocilizumab [humanized anti-IL-6R monoclonal antibody], is thus considered a potential drug in COVID-19 treatment [26, 27].

8. Other clinical considerations

Tocilizumab is contraindicated in immunocompromised individuals, those who use biologic immunomodulating drugs, and in patients having alanine aminotransferase >5 times the upper limit of normal; patients with gastrointestinal perforation; those having uncontrolled serious bacterial, fungal, or non-SARS-CoV-2 viral infection; absolute neutrophil count <500 cells/μL; platelet count <50,000 cells/μL. The drug should also be avoided in individuals having a known hypersensitivity to it [28]. It has been recommended to administer Dexamethasone [or an alternative corticosteroid of dosage equal to dexamethasone 6 mg] simultaneously in patients receiving Tocilizumab [9]. A patient's clinical response to dexamethasone is initially accessed before administering Tocilizumab [29]. The combination therapy yields an adverse effect in the form of severe and disseminated strongyloidiasis infestation. Therefore, Ivermectin should be used as a prophylactic treatment [30].

9. Side effects

The common side effects include respiratory tract infections, headache, hypertension, elevation in liver test. Rashes, erythema, oedema, itching can occur at the infection site [31]. Tuberculosis, sepsis and fungal infection are the associated infections that can occur. Hypersensitivity reactions, cancer, reactivation of herpes zoster, gastrointestinal perforation in patients with diverticulitis are also seen in some patients, though not significant [32].

10. Clinical trial status

The process of systemic review was followed and effectiveness of the drug analyzed from the NIH, US National Library of Medicine Clinical Trial Registry (ClinicalTrials.gov). At present (till May 2021), 81 clinical studies could be traced in the name Toclilizumab [until May 2021]. 33 studies have been excluded due to non-relevance. 48 records are included in this study. Some of the studies have yielded promising initial results yet require more time for validation and declared to be effective or safe. Among the 48 trials done on Tocilizumab, 17 are in Recruiting stage, 12 trials have been concluded, 5 have been terminated, 1 has been withdrawn, 5 trials are in not yet recruiting stage and 6 are active but non recruiting. 1 among the 47 trials is in phase 1, 16 trials are in phase 2, 14 are in phase 3 trial. Analyzing the clinical trials from **Table 1**, it is evident that there is attempt to use Toclizumab alone or in combination with other drugs looks promising for the treatment of COVID 19 (**Figure 1**).

11. Comparing tocilizumab with other drugs involved in COVID-19 treatment

Several drugs employed for the treatment of COVID-19 through clinical trials are: Remdesivir, Tocilizumab, Baricitinib, Sarilumab and Hydroxychloroquine. In terms of clinical research output Remdesivir emerges as frontrunner, while Tocilizumab may be considered as a potential drug candidate against COVID-19. Despite the initial attempt of drug repurposing by using Hydroxychloroquine to treat COVID-19, there were limited encouraging results for which, its administration was removed from the line of treatment in various countries. A comparison between Tocilizumab and other drugs involved in the treatment of COVID-19 is presented in **Table 2**.

12. Summarizing prominent publications on tocilizumab related to COVID treatment

Apart from several clinical research outcomes (summarized in **Table 1**) there has been several publications revealing scientific information on the mechanism, application and prospect of the drug candidate Tocilizumab for COVID-19 treatment. There are more than 30 publications found in PubMed (https://pubmed.ncbi.nlm.nih.gov/) in the year 2021 among which few significant ones are summarized in following **Table 3**.

DOI: http://dx.doi.org/10.5772/intechopen.99785

Sl. no.	Clinical trial	Primary objectives	Study type	Status	Study start date	Study completion date	Phase	Observation/ interpretation	Studied by:	Reference	Publication
1	The Use of Tocilizumab in the Management of Patients Who Have Severe COVID-19 With Suspected Pulmonary Hyperinflammation	To assess the therapeutic value of intravenous tocilizumab administered as single 8 mg/Kg dose in patients affected by SARS-CoV2 infection with a pulmonary manifestation causing hypoxia.	Interventional	Recruiting	Apr-20	May-21	Phase 4	Not Available	Hadassah Medical Center	NCT04377750	Nil
2	Tocilizumab to Prevent Clinical Decompensation in Hospitalized, Non-critically Ill Patients With COVID-19 Pneumonitis	To establish proof of concept that tocilizumab is effective in decreasing signs, symptoms, and laboratory evidence of COVID-19 pneumonitis in hospitalized, non-critically ill patients	Interventional	Completed	Apr-20	Jun-20	Phase2	Not Available	University of Chicago	NCT04331795	Nil
3	Low-dose Tocilizumab Versus Standard of Care in Hospitalized Patients With COVID-19 [COVIDOSE-2]	To establish whether low-dose tocilizumab reduces the time to clinical recovery in patients with COVID-19 pneumonitis and hyperinflammation, when compared to a tocilizumab-free	Interventional	Recruiting	Sep-20	Dec-20	Phase 2	Not Available	University of Chicago	NCT04479358	[33]

Sl. no.	Clinical trial	Primary objectives	Study type	Status	Study start date	Study completion date	Phase	Observation/ interpretation	Studied by:	Reference	Publication
		standard of care and to establish whether low-dose tocilizumab is near-equivalent to high-dose tocilizumab (400 mg or 8 mg/kg) in reducing the time to clinical recovery in patients with COVID-19 pneumonitis and hyperinflammation.									
4	Tocilizumab in COVID-19 Pneumonia (TOCIVID-19) (TOCIVID-19)	This study project includes a single-arm phase 2 study and a parallel cohort study, enrolling patients with COVID-19 pneumonia.	Interventional	Active not recruiting	March 19, 2020	December 19, 2022	Phase 2	Not Available	National Cancer Institute, Naples	NCT04317092	[34–36]
5	Study to Evaluate the Efficacy and Safety of Tocilizumab Versus Corticosteroids in Hospitalized COVID-19 Patients With High Risk of Progression	This study aims to compare the efficacy and safety of Methylprednisolone versus Tocilizumab in improving clinical outcomes and reducing the need for ventilator support in COVID-19 patients with moderate COVID-19 disease at risk for	Interventional	Not yet recruiting	April 15, 2020	October 31, 2020	Phase 3	Not Available	University of Malaya	NCT04345445	Nil

Sl. no.	Clinical trial	Primary objectives	Study type	Status	Study start date	Study completion date	Phase	Observation/ interpretation	Studied by:	Reference	Publication
		complications of cytokine storm.									
6	Clinical Efficacy of Heparin and Tocilizumab in Patients With Severe COVID-19 Infection: a Randomized Clinical Trial (HEPMAB)	To study the use of heparin and tocilizumab to potencially reduce inflammation and thrombogenesis in patients with severe COVID-19 infection, improving patients outcomes and survival.	Interventional	Recruiting	November 10, 2020	December 31, 2021	Phase 3	Not Available	Ludhmila Abrahão Hajjar, University of Sao Paulo	NCT04600141	Nil
7	Efficacy of Tocilizumab in Modifying the Inflammatory Parameters of Patients With COVID-19 (COVITOZ-01) (COVITOZ-01)	To study the unicenter, randomized, open-label clinical trial on the efficacy of tocilizumab in modifying the inflammatory parameters of patients with COVID-19.	Interventional	Recruiting	May 4, 2020	August 4, 2020	Phase 2	Not Available	Jose A Perez Molina, Hospital Universitario Ramon y Cajal	NCT04435717	Nil
8	Trial of Tocilizumab for Treatment of Severe COVID-19: ARCHITECTS (ARCHITECTS)	The overall objective is to evaluate the clinical efficacy and safety of tocilizumab relative to placebo among approximately 300	Interventional	Recruiting	June 12, 2020	December 31, 2021	Phase 3	Not Available	Queen's Medical Centre	NCT04412772	Nil

Sl. no.	Clinical trial	Primary objectives	Study type	Status	Study start date	Study completion date	Phase	Observation/ interpretation	Studied by:	Reference	Publication
		hospitalized adult patients who have severe COVID-19									
9	TOCILIZUMAB - An Option for Patients With COVID-19 Associated Cytokine Release Syndrome; A Single Center Experience	To analyze the effectiveness of Tocilizumab in moderate to severe Covid-19 participants on the basis of predefined assessment criteria.	Interventional	Completed	May 12, 2020	June 12, 2020	Phase 4	Not Available	Aijaz Zeeshan Khan Chachar, FMH College of Medicine and Dentistry	NCT04730323	Nil
10	Clinical Trial of Combined Use of Hydroxychloroquine, Azithromycin, and Tocilizumab for the Treatment of COVID-19 (TOCOVID)	To evaluate the use of Tocilizumab in combination with hydroxychloroquine and azithromycin for the treatment of hospitalized adult patients with COVID-19.	Interventional	Recruiting	April 2, 2020	Oct-20	Phase 2	Not Available	Fundació Institut de Recerca de l'Hospital de la Santa Creu i Sant Pau	NCT04332094	Nil
11	Clinical Trial to Evaluate the Effectiveness and Safety of Tocilizumab for Treating Patients With COVID-19 Pneumonia	To evaluate the effectiveness and safety of IV tocilizumab in patients with COVID-19 severe pneumonia who are currently hospitalized or admitted to ICU.	Interventional	Completed	May 22, 2020	December 23, 2020	Phase 2	Not Available	Fundacion SEIMC-GESIDA	NCT04445272	[7]

DOI: http://dx.doi.org/10.5772/intechopen.99785

Sl. no.	Clinical trial	Primary objectives	Study type	Status	Study start date	Study completion date	Phase	Observation/ interpretation	Studied by:	Reference	Publication
12	Tocilizumab for Prevention of Respiratory Failure in Patients With Severe COVID-19 Infection	The purpose of this study is to find out whether the study drug tocilizumab is an effective treatment for COVID-19 infection.	Interventional	Active, not recruiting	May 1, 2020	May 1, 2022	Phase 2	Not Available	Memorial Sloan Kettering Cancer Center	NCT04377659	Nil
13	COVID-19: Salvage Tocilizumab as a Rescue Measure (COVIDSTORM)	To Evaluate the efficacy of Tocilizumab in hospitalized patients in the inflammatory phase of COVID-19.	Interventional	Recruiting	August 14, 2020	December 31, 2021	Phase 3	Not Available	Jarmo Oksi, Turku University Hospital	NCT04577534	Nil
14	Serum IL-6 and Soluble IL-6 Receptor in Severe COVID-19 Pneumonia Treated With Tocilizumab (UHID-COVID19)	To assess the role of interleukin-6 (IL-6) and soluble interleukin 6 receptor (sIL-6R) as predictors of efficacy and safety outcomes in patients with severe coronavirus disease (COVID-19) pneumonia treated with tocilizumab.	Observational	Recruiting	June 16, 2020	May 15, 2021	case only	Not Available	University Hospital for Infectious Diseases, Croatia	NCT04359667	Nil
15	A Study in Patients With COVID-19 and Respiratory Distress Not Requiring Mechanical Ventilation, to Compare Standard-	The study is designed as a randomized, controlled, single-center open-label trial to compare standard-of-care (SOC) treatment	Interventional	Recruiting	June 11, 2020	Feb-21	Phase 2	Not Available	Jonas Sundén-Cullberg, Karolinska University Hospital	NCT04412291	Nil

Sl. no.	Clinical trial	Primary objectives	Study type	Status	Study start date	Study completion date	Phase	Observation/ interpretation	Studied by:	Reference	Publication
	of-care With Anakinra and Tocilizumab Treatment The Immunomodulation-CoV Assessment (ImmCoVA) Study	with SOC + anakinra or SOC + tocilizumab treatment in hospitalized adult subjects who are diagnosed with severe COVID 19.									
16	A Trial Using ANAKINRA, TOCILIZUMAB Alone or in Association With RUXOLITINIB in Severe Stage 2b and 3 of COVID19-associated Disease (INFLAMMACOV)	To use biological drugs currently available for inhibition of IL-1 (anakinra), IL-6 (tocilizumab) or IFNg signaling (ruxolitinib) in the severe forms of COVID19-associated disease.	Interventional	Not yet recruiting	September 1, 2020	November 1, 2022	Phase 3	Not Available	Assistance Publique Hopitaux De Marseille	NCT04424056	Nil
17	Tocilizumab Versus Methylprednisolone in the Cytokine Release Syndrome of Patients With COVID-19	This study compare the efficacy and safety of tocilizumab versus methylprednisolone in the cytokine release syndrome of patients with COVID-19	Interventional	Not yet recruiting	May-20	Aug-20	Phase 2	Not Available	José Raimundo Araujo de Azevedo, Hospital Sao Domingos	NCT04377503	[8, 37–43]
18	Tocilizumab in the Treatment of Coronavirus Induced Disease (COVID-19) (CORON-ACT)	To evaluate whether treatment with TCZ reduces the severity and mortality in	Interventional	Terminated	April 26, 2020	September 27, 2020	Phase 2	Not Available	University Hospital Inselspital, Berne	NCT04335071	[2, 9, 10, 28, 43–53]

Sl. no.	Clinical trial	Primary objectives	Study type	Status	Study start date	Study completion date	Phase	Observation/ interpretation	Studied by:	Reference	Publication
		patients with COVID-19.									
19	A Study to Investigate Intravenous Tocilizumab in Participants With Moderate to Severe COVID-19 Pneumonia (MARIPOSA)	To Investigate Intravenous Tocilizumab in Participants With Moderate to Severe COVID-19 Pneumonia	Interventional	Completed	May 5, 2020	August 12, 2020	Phase 2	Not Available	Hoffmann-La Roche	NCT04363736	Nil
20	Efficacy and Safety of Tocilizumab in the Treatment of SARS-Cov-2 Related Pneumonia (TOSCA)	This is a prospective observational clinical study and it is aimed at verifying tocilizumab efficacy and safety in patients with COVID-19 complicated by acute distress respiratory syndrome (ARDS) and CRS.	Observational	Recruiting	April 1, 2020	March 31, 2021	Observational Model: Cohort	Not Available	Prof. Roberto Giacomelli, University of L'Aquila	NCT04332913	[2, 9, 12, 28, 54–62]
21	Efficacy of Tocilizumab on Patients With COVID-19	To test the effect of Tocilizumab on multi-organ dysfunction in a phase 3 randomized controlled trial among hospitalized patients with COVID-19 infection.	Interventional	Completed	April 20, 2020	August 27, 2020	Phase 3	Tocilizumab provided no benefit in prevention of death (the primary outcome) or reducing the risk of clinical worsening (secondary outcomes).	Stone, John H, M.D., M.P.H, Massachusetts General Hospital	NCT04356937	[21]
22	A Study to Evaluate the Safety and	This study will evaluate the efficacy,	Interventional	Completed	April 3, 2020	July 28, 2020	Phase 3	No difference was noticed between	Hoffmann-La Roche	NCT04320615	Nil

Sl. no.	Clinical trial	Primary objectives	Study type	Status	Study start date	Study completion date	Phase	Observation/ interpretation	Studied by:	Reference	Publication
	Efficacy of Tocilizumab in Patients With Severe COVID-19 Pneumonia (COVACTA)	safety, pharmacodynamics, and pharmacokinetics of tocilizumab (TCZ) compared with a matching placebo in combination with standard of care (SOC) in hospitalized patients with severe COVID-19 pneumonia.						tocilizumab and placebo for clinical status (including death) at Day 28 (the primary outcome), but tocilizumab exhibited a shorter time to recovery and shorter length of ICU stay (secondary outcomes).			
23	Efficacy and Safety of Remdesivir and Tociluzumab for the Management of Severe COVID-19: A Randomized Controlled Trial	To evaluate the efficacy of Remdesivir and Tocilizumab as a treatment for severe Acute Respiratory Distress Syndrome (ARDS) caused by Coronavirus disease 2019 (COVID-19).	Interventional	Completed	August 15, 2020	February 10, 2021	Phase 3	Not Available	Abu Taiub Mohammed Mohiuddin Chowdhury, First Affiliated Hospital Xi'an Jiaotong University	NCT04678739	Nil
24	A Study to Evaluate the Efficacy and Safety of Tocilizumab in Hospitalized Participants With COVID-19 Pneumonia (EMPACTA)	This study (EMPACTA) will a) evaluate the efficacy and safety of tocilizumab (TCZ) compared with a placebo in combination with standard of care (SOC) in	Interventional	Recruiting	May 14, 2020	December 1, 2021	Phase 3	Tocilizumab lowered rates of mechanical ventilation or death by Day 28 but provided no benefit in 28-day mortality.	Genentech, Inc.	NCT04372186	[63]

Sl. no.	Clinical trial	Primary objectives	Study type	Status	Study start date	Study completion date	Phase	Observation/ interpretation	Studied by:	Reference	Publication
		hospitalized participants with COVID-19 pneumonia, and b) include an optional substudy to explore the long-term sequelae of resolved COVID-19 pneumonia.									
25	A Study to Evaluate the Efficacy and Safety of Remdesivir Plus Tocilizumab Compared With Remdesivir Plus Placebo in Hospitalized Participants With Severe COVID-19 Pneumonia (REMDACTA)	This study will evaluate the efficacy and safety of combination therapy with remdesivir plus tocilizumab compared with remdesivir plus placebo in hospitalized patients with COVID-19 pneumonia.	Interventional	Completed	June 16, 2020	March 8, 2021	Phase 3	Not Available	Hoffmann-La Roche	NCT04409262	Nil
26	Safety and Efficacy of Tocilizumab in Moderate to Severe COVID-19 With Inflammatory Markers (TOCIBRAS)	To evaluate the efficacy and safety of Tocilizumab, which rapidly reduces the inflammation process through inhibition of IL-6 in patients with moderate to severe COVID-19 with increased	Interventional	Terminated	May 8, 2020	July 21, 2020	Phase 3	Tocilizumab showed no benefit in this study	Dr Rozana Mesquita Ciconelli, Beneficência Portuguesa de São Paulo	NCT04403685	[64]

Sl. no.	Clinical trial	Primary objectives	Study type	Status	Study start date	Study completion date	Phase	Observation/ interpretation	Studied by:	Reference	Publication
		inflammatory markers.									
27	Anti-il6 Treatment of Serious COVID-19 Disease With Threatening Respiratory Failure (TOCIVID)	To compare the effect of either one of three IL-6 inhibitor administrations, relative to the standard of care, on time to independence from supplementary oxygen therapy, measured in days from baseline to day 28, in patients with severe SARS-CoV-2 pneumonia.	Interventional	Terminated	April 5, 2020	October 8, 2020	Phase 2	Not Available	Marius Henriksen, Frederiksberg University Hospital	NCT04322773	Nil
28	Treatment of COVID-19 Patients With Anti-interleukin Drugs (COV-AID)	To test the safety and effectiveness of individually or simultaneously blocking IL-6 and IL-1 versus standard of care on blood oxygenation and systemic cytokine release syndrome in patients with COVID-19 coronavirus infection and acute hypoxic respiratory failure and systemic	Interventional	Active, not recruiting	April 3, 2020	Mar-21	Phase 3	Not Available	Bart N. Lambrecht, University Hospital, Ghent	NCT04330638	[65]

DOI: http://dx.doi.org/10.5772/intechopen.99785

Sl. no.	Clinical trial	Primary objectives	Study type	Status	Study start date	Study completion date	Phase	Observation/ interpretation	Studied by:	Reference	Publication
		cytokine release syndrome									
29	CORIMUNO-19 - Tocilizumab Trial - TOCI (CORIMUNO-TOCI) (CORIMUNO-TOC)	To determine the therapeutic effect and tolerance of Tocizilumab in patients with moderate, severe pneumonia or critical pneumonia associated with Coronavirus disease 2019 (COVID-19)	Interventional	Active, not recruiting	March 30, 2020	December 31, 2021	Phase 2	In COVID-19 Patients Tocilizumab led to improved ventilator-free survival at Day 14 suggesting possible benefit, but the clinical implications are unclear as there was no difference in survival for tocilizumab vs. usual care through Day 28.	Assistance Publique - Hôpitaux de Paris	NCT04331808	[66]
30	Investigational Treatments for COVID-19 in Tertiary Care Hospital of Pakistan	To study the role of Investigational Therapies Alone or in Combination to Treat Moderate, Severe and Critical COVID-19	Interventional	Completed	April 1, 2020	July 20, 2020	Not applicable	Not Available	sultan mehmood kamran, UNICEF	NCT04492501	[67–73]
31	Tocilizumab in Coronavirus-19 Positive Patients	To determine the impact of adjunctive Tocilizumab (TCZ) to standard of care on the reduction of hyperinflammation-related mortality in COVID-19.	Interventional	Not yet recruiting	July 30, 2020	Jun-21	Phase 3	Not Available	University of Calgary	NCT04423042	[8, 71, 74]

Sl. no.	Clinical trial	Primary objectives	Study type	Status	Study start date	Study completion date	Phase	Observation/ interpretation	Studied by:	Reference	Publication
32	Tocilizumab for the Treatment of Cytokine Release Syndrome in Patients With COVID-19 (SARS-CoV-2 Infection)	TO compare the effect of adding tocilizumab to standard of care versus standard of care alone in treating cytokine release syndrome (CRS) in patients with SARS-CoV-2 infection. CRS is a potentially serious disorder caused by the release of an excessive amount of substance that is made by cells of the immune system (cytokines) as a response to viral infection	Interventional	Withdrawn	April 7, 2020	June 2, 2020	Phase 3	Not Available	Ajay Nooka, Emory University	NCT04361552	Nil
33	Comparison of Tocilizumab Plus Dexamethasone vs. Dexamethasone for Patients With Covid-19 (TOCIDEX)	To determine the therapeutic effect and tolerance of Tocilizumab combined with Dexamethasone in patients with moderate, severe pneumonia or critical pneumonia associated with Coronavirus disease 2019 (COVID-19).	Interventional	Recruiting	July 16, 2020	December 31, 2021	Phase 2	Not Available	Assistance Publique - Hôpitaux de Paris	NCT04476979	Nil

Sl. no.	Clinical trial	Primary objectives	Study type	Status	Study start date	Study completion date	Phase	Observation/ interpretation	Studied by:	Reference	Publication
34	Toclizumam Versus Dexamethasone in Severe Covid-19 Cases	To study randomized controlled trial comparing survival benefit of Tocilizumab therapy with dexamethasone in patients with severe COVID 19	Interventional	Completed	March 1, 2020	August 5, 2020	Not applicable	Not Available	Alaa Rashad, South Valley University	NCT04519385	Nil
35	Tocilizumab for SARS-CoV2 (COVID-19) Severe Pneumonitis	To test the hypothesis that an anti-IL6 treatment can be effective in calming the virus-induced cytokine storm, blocking deterioration of lung function or even promoting a rapid improvement of clinical conditions, preventing naso-tracheal intubation and/or death.	Interventional	Active, not recruiting	March 12, 2020	May-20	Phase 2	Not Available	Armando Gabrielli, Università Politecnica delle Marche	NCT04315480	[75–79]
36	Personalized Immunotherapy for SARS-CoV-2 (COVID-19) Associated With Organ Dysfunction (ESCAPE)	To conduct one trial of personalized immunotherapy in patients with SARS-CoV-2 (COVID-19) associated with organ dysfunction and with laboratory findings of macrophage activation syndrome	Interventional	Completed	April 2, 2020	January 8, 2021	Phase 2	Not Available	Hellenic Institute for the Study of Sepsis	NCT04339712	Nil

Sl. no.	Clinical trial	Primary objectives	Study type	Status	Study start date	Study completion date	Phase	Observation/ interpretation	Studied by:	Reference	Publication
		or immune dysregulation.									
37	Theranostic Implication of Complementary Medicines Against Interleukin Receptors and Gp-130 Proteins	To estimate the relationship of severity of disease with gp-130 and IL-6	Interventional	Completed	July 23, 2020	December 10, 2020	Not Applicable	Not Available	Dr Muhammad Mansoor Hafeez, University of Lahore	NCT04690920	Nil
38	Tocilizumab vs. CRRT in Management of Cytokine Release Syndrome (CRS) in COVID-19 (TACOS)	To study Tocilizumab associated with better clinical outcomes, such as decreased systemic inflammation, improved survival rate, better hemodynamic and improved of respiratory distress.	Observational	Recruiting	February 20, 2020	June 20, 2020	Cohort	Not Available	YIKAI YU, Tongji Hospital	NCT04306705	Nil
39	Tocilizumab for Patients With Cancer and COVID-19 Disease	To enhance access to tocilizumab for patients who cannot participate in the randomized COVACTA trial with specific emphasis on patients with cancer, especially those who belong to high-risk and minority populations and children.	Interventional	Terminated	May 28, 2020	January 14, 2021	Phase 2	Not Available	National Cancer Institute (NCI)	NCT04370834	Nil

Sl. no.	Clinical trial	Primary objectives	Study type	Status	Study start date	Study completion date	Phase	Observation/ interpretation	Studied by:	Reference	Publication
40	Favipiravir Combined With Tocilizumab in the Treatment of Corona Virus Disease 2019	To evaluate the efficacy and safety of favipiravir combined with tocilizumab in the treatment of corona virus disease 2019	Interventional	Recruiting	March 8, 2020	May-20	Not Applicable	Not Available	Guiqiang Wang, Peking University First Hospital	NCT04310228	Nil
41	Tocilizumab in COVID-19 Lahore General Hospital (TC19LGH)	This is intervention single-center study, done at Lahore General Hospital in which 95 beds are allocated for COVID-19 patients including ICUs and HDUs.	Interventional	Recruiting	May 1, 2020	December 30, 2020	Phase 1	Not Available	Dr. M.Irfan Malik, Lahore General Hospital	NCT04560205	[80–83]
42	Comparison of Tocilizumab Versus Tocilizumab/ Infliximab in Patients With COVID-19-associated Cytokine Storm Syndrome	To compare the outcomes of a large cohort of patients with moderate and severe COVID-19 pneumonia treated with tocilizumab in addition to standard management, with those of concomitantly hospitalized patients who received infliximab and tocilizumab in addition to standard management.	Observational	Recruiting	December 1, 2020	June 1, 2021	Cohort	Not Available	Neven Sarhan, Misr International University	NCT04734678	Nil

Sl. no.	Clinical trial	Primary objectives	Study type	Status	Study start date	Study completion date	Phase	Observation/ interpretation	Studied by:	Reference	Publication
43	Assessment of Efficacy and Safety of Tocilizumab Compared to DefeROxamine, Associated With Standards Treatments in COVID-19 (+) Patients Hospitalized In Intensive Care in Tunisia (TRONCHER)	To study the assessment of Efficacy and Safety of Tocilizumab Compared to DefeROxamine, associated with standards treatments in COVID-19 (+) patients, Hospitalized In Intensive care in Tunisia.	Interventional	Not yet recruiting	September 4, 2020	October 4, 2020	Phase 3	Not Available	Dr Jalila Ben Khelil, Abderrahmane Mami Hospital	NCT04361032	Nil
44	Tocilizumab Treatment in Patients With COVID-19	To study the impact of the administration of Tocilizumab on the evolution of the acute respiratory distress syndrome (ARDS) in patients with severe or critical SARS-CoV-2 infection	Interventional	Active, not recruiting	June 1, 2020	August 1, 2021	Phase 2	Not Available	Oscar Gerardo Arrieta Rodríguez, Instituto Nacional de Cancerologia de Mexico	NCT04363853	[1, 2, 5, 54, 77, 84–91]
45	Pharmacokinetics, Pharmacodynamics, and Safety Profile of Understudied Drugs Administered to Children Per Standard of Care (POPS) (POPS or POP02)	To evaluate the PK of understudied drugs currently being administered to children per SOC as prescribed by their treating provider.	Observational	Recruiting	March 5, 2020	April 24, 2024	Prospective	Not Available	Duke University	NCT04278404	[92–142]

Sl. no.	Clinical trial	Primary objectives	Study type	Status	Study start date	Study completion date	Phase	Observation/ interpretation	Studied by:	Reference	Publication
46	Efficacy of Early Administration of Tocilizumab in COVID-19 Patients	To study early administration of Tocilizumab compared to late administration of Tocilizumab can reduce the number of patients with COVID-19 pneumonia who require mechanical ventilation.	Interventional	Terminated	March 31, 2020	June 6, 2020	Phase 2	Not Available	Azienda Unità Sanitaria Locale Reggio Emilia	NCT04346355	[143]
47	Comparative Therapeutic Efficacy and Safety of Different Antiviral and Anti Inflammatory Drugs in COVID-19 Patients.	To study the comparison of the outcomes of a large cohort of moderate and severe COVID-19 patients received different Antiviral and Anti Inflammatory Drugs.	Interventional	Recruiting	October 1, 2020	April 5, 2021	Phase 4	Not Available	Ahmed Essam, October 6 University	NCT04779047	Nil
48	Anti-IL6 and Corticosteroid Monotherapy vs. Combination in COVID-19	To evaluate the safety and efficacy of anti-IL6 alone vs. anti-IL6 corticosteroid combination in patients with COVID-19 pneumonia	Observational	Recruiting	July 22, 2020	July 22, 2021	Other	Not Available	King Faisal Specialist Hospital & Research Center	NCT04486521	[144]

Table 1.
Update of the status of clinical trials for the use of tocilizumab in the treatment of COVID-19.

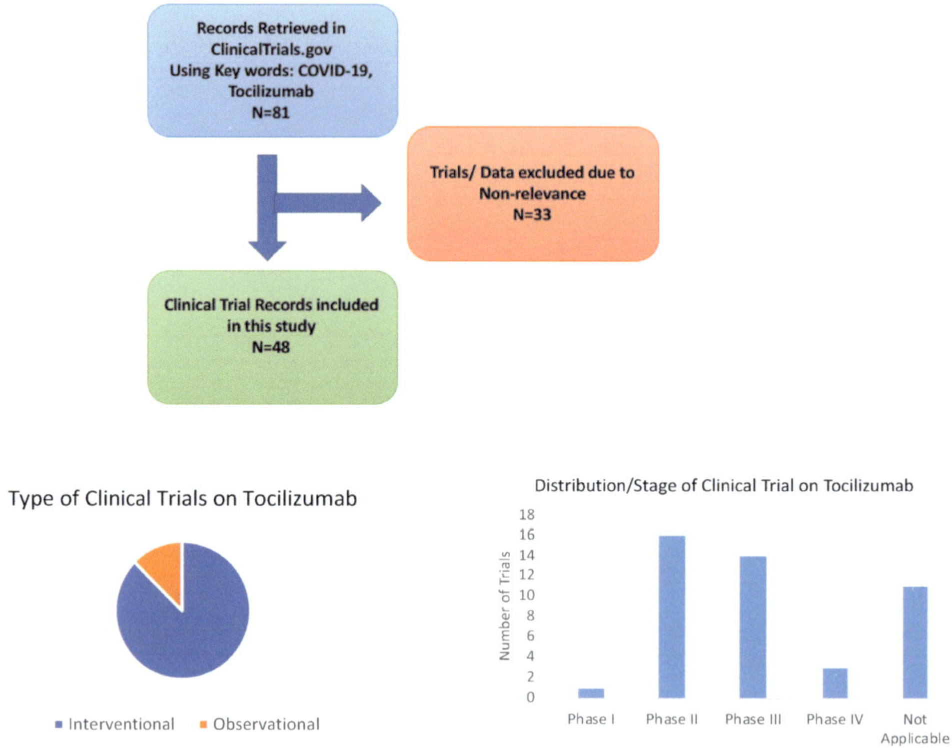

Figure 1.
Status of clinical trials and stage: tocilizumab.

Sl. no.	Name of the drug	Mechanism of action	Clinical trial status	Significant findings	References
1	Tocilizumab	Tocilizumab has rendered effective results as an IL-6R antagonist, to prevent the cytokine storm.	At present, 87 clinical studies could be traced in the name Tocilizumab. Out of which, 1 is in early phase 1; 3 are in phase1; 33 are in phase 2; 24 are in phase 3; and 4 are in phase 4.	Although Tocilizumab is approved by the USFDA (Not for COVID-19 treatment), still its positive effects cannot be predicted in all patients. Among some hospitalized patients with severe or critical COVID-19,a shorter time to recovery and shorter length of ICU stay was seen in those who received this drug. It still it cannot be referred to as an anti-viral drug	—

Sl. no.	Name of the drug	Mechanism of action	Clinical trial status	Significant findings	References
				and may only be effective in patients having inflammation and lung damage caused by the coronavirus.	
2	Remdesivir	The drug inhibits the synthesis of viral RNA by delayed chain termination method.	At present, 110 clinical studies could be traced in the name Remdesivir. Of which 1 study is in early phase 1; 9 are in phase 1; 35 are in phase 2; 41 are in phase 3; 3 are in phase 4.	The USFDA approved drug Remdesivir has been used alone or in combination with other drugs to curb the severity of COVID-19. However it still needs to be administered to a large mass to predict the significant outcomes.	[3, 4]
3	Baricitinib	Baricitinib is an inhibitor of JAK-1 and JAK-2, which dampens the proinflammatory cytokine signaling. It also inhibits AP2-associated protein kinase [AAK-1].	At present, 20 studies could be traced in the name of Baricitinib. Out of which, 10 are in phase2; 11 are in phase 3; and 1 is in phase 4	The USFDA approved drug appears to be relatively safe and well tolerated when used for rheumatoid arthritis. Nowadays they are used for COVID-19 treatment, combined with Remdesivir. Mortality rates have been significantly lowered.	[145, 146]
4	Sarilumab	Sarilumab is a human recombinant IgG1 antibody that binds to both forms of IL-6R, inhibiting the IL-6 mediated signaling.	At present, 17 clinical studies could be traced in the name Sarilumab, out of which 1 is in phase1; 6 are in phase 2; 1 is in phase 2,3; 3 are in phase 1 and 1 is in phase 4.	The drug has been already approved by USFDA for treatment of patients with COVID-19.No benefit of Sarilumab with respect to time to clinical improvement or mortality was observed in case of this drug.	[147]

Sl. no.	Name of the drug	Mechanism of action	Clinical trial status	Significant findings	References
5	Hydroxychloroquine	The drug increases endosomal pH, interferes with the glycosylation of cellular receptors of SARS-COV and blocks viral infection.	At present, 281 clinical studies could be traced in the name Hydroxychloroquine. Out of which 5 studies are in early phase 1; 14 are in phase 1; 88 are in phase 2; 116 are in phase 3; 24 are in phase 4.	The drug has not been approved by FDA for treatment of COVID-19 patients. No significant observation can be noted, as trials are still ongoing.	

Table 2.
Comparing tocilizumab with other drugs employed for COVID-19 treatment.

Sl. no.	Year of publication	Title of publication	Significant observation	Reference
1	2020	Tocilizumab in patients hospitalized with Covid-19 Pneumonia	This trial consisted of more than 25% of the patients who were older than 65 years of age, more than 75% having at least one coexisting disease condition, and greater than 80% were in a minority racial or ethnic group. Scientists found that the possibility of progression to mechanical ventilation or death by day 28 was considerably lower among patients who received tocilizumab plus standard care in comparison to those who received placebo plus standard care.	[148]
2	2020	Tocilizumab in patients with severe COVID-19: a retrospective cohort study	This trial consisted of 1351 patients who were admitted to the recruiting centres. 544 (40%) patients with severe pneumonia were also taken into consideration. There were 359 (66%) male patients, with a median age of 67 years. Tocilizumab [administered intravenously or subcutaneously] plus standard care could reduce the mortality rate or curb the usage of mechanical ventilation in severe COVID-19 patients compared to those who received only standard care as per shown in this study.	[149]
3	2020	Impact of tocilizumab administration on mortality in severe COVID-19.	In this trial 84 patients were administered with tocilizumab and 190 patients were not treated with tocilizumab. Scientists could not predict or conclude any favorable outcome from this trial.	[150]

Sl. no.	Year of publication	Title of publication	Significant observation	Reference
4	2020	Why Tocilizumab could an effective treatment for severe COVID-19?	The IL-6 antagonist, Tocilizumab is highly recommended by scientists to curb the mortality of severe COVID-19. Scientists hope this drug could be beneficial in curbing the severity of COVID-19 pandemic. This study analyses the beneficial effects of this drug.	[151]
5	2020	Effective treatment of severe COVID-19 patients with Tocilizumab.	The average age of the subjects in this study were 56.8 ± 16.5 y and ranged from 25 to 88 years. Out of them in 21 patients, improvement of the rate of deterioration of COVID-19 patients was observed by scientists, which suggested that this drug could be effective enough to treat patients with COVID-19.	[152]
6	2020	Hydroxychloroquine and tocilizumab therapy in COVID-19 patients- An observational study.	In this retrospective observational cohort study consisting of 2512 patients hospitalized COVID-19 patients, within a 13- hospital network, scientists could not predict any favorable outcome. On the contrary, the use of Tocilizumab alone yielded effective results, that is, it helped in reducing the death rate.	[153]
7	2020	Time to Reassess Tocilizumab's Role in COVID-19 Pneumonia.	The efficacy of the drug was unclear from this study compared to other observational studies.	[154]
8	2021	Tocilizumab in COVID-19: some clarity amid controversy.	The recovery trial showed some evidence regarding the use of Tocilizumab in COVID-19 patients. Scientists found that only 31% of the population receiving Tocilizumab showed promises of recovery as compared to those receiving placebo. Still, this drug therapy needs to be combined with other drugs for better outcomes.	[155]
9	2021	Effectiveness of Tocilizumab in patients hospitalized with COVID-19.	Scientists found that Tocilizumab may be effective in diminishing the health hazards of patients with moderate to severe COVID-19 – associated pneumonia and elevated CRP level. Yet it needs to be administered to a large mass to fathom its efficacy.	[156]
10	2021	Tocilizumab in hospitalized patients with severe Covid-19 Pneumonia.	Scientists could not gather any significant clinical status or predict any lowering of mortality rate in comparison to placebo at 28 days.	[157]

Table 3.
Prominent publications reporting the treatment of COVID-19 using Tocilizumab.

13. Conclusion

Although the drug Tocilizumab has shown to reduce mortality and morbidity, still it cannot be referred to as an anti-COVID drug and may only be effective in patients having inflammation and lung damage caused by the coronavirus. Moreover the sensitivity of the drug limits its usage to a specific age and certain patients. Moreover, Tocilizumab is not-yet approved by the USFDA. This drug brings a ray of hope, as it's very much effective in mitigating immune damage, lung functional injuries and arterial oxygen saturation. Scientists therefore hope that this drug could be beneficial to a large mass of population in diminishing the adverse effects of the pandemic.

Conflict of interest

The authors declare that they neither have any conflict of interest nor is involved directly or indirectly with any clinical trials of any of the drugs mentioned in the chapter.

Author details

Nilanjana Dhara, Sumana Saha and Saptarshi Chatterjee*
Department of Microbiology, School of Life Science and Biotechnology, Adamas University, West Bengal, India

*Address all correspondence to: saptarshi.chatterjee@adamasuniversity.ac.in; saptarshi.gcc09@gmail.com

References

[1] Lu, H., Stratton, C. W., & Tang, Y. W. (2020). Outbreak of pneumonia of unknown etiology in Wuhan, China: The mystery and the miracle. Journal of medical virology, 92(4), 401–402. https://doi.org/10.1002/jmv.25678

[2] Chen, N., Zhou, M., Dong, X., Qu, J., Gong, F., Han, Y., Qiu, Y., Wang, J., Liu, Y., Wei, Y., Xia, J., Yu, T., Zhang, X., & Zhang, L. (2020). Epidemiological and clinical characteristics of 99 cases of 2019 novel coronavirus pneumonia in Wuhan, China: a descriptive study. Lancet (London, England), 395(10223), 507–513. https://doi.org/10.1016/S0140-6736(20)30211-7

[3] Chatterjee S. (2021). Remdesivir: Critical Clinical Appraisal for COVID 19 Treatment. Drug research, 71(3), 138–148. https://doi.org/10.1055/a-1288-4078

[4] Chatterjee S. (2021). Status of Remdesivir: Not Yet Beyond Question!. Archives of medical research, 52(1), 102–103. https://doi.org/10.1016/j.arcmed.2020.09.004

[5] Wang, D., Hu, B., Hu, C., Zhu, F., Liu, X., Zhang, J., Wang, B., Xiang, H., Cheng, Z., Xiong, Y., Zhao, Y., Li, Y., Wang, X., & Peng, Z. (2020). Clinical Characteristics of 138 Hospitalized Patients With 2019 Novel Coronavirus-Infected Pneumonia in Wuhan, China. JAMA, 323(11), 1061–1069. https://doi.org/10.1001/jama.2020.1585

[6] Frey N., Grange S., Woodworth T. Relationship between serum concentrations of the interleukin-6 receptor inhibitor tocilizumab and C-reactive protein reduction in RA patients: 6 months' data from a phase 3 study. Arthritis Rheum. 2007;56:148–149.

[7] Maude, S. L., Barrett, D., Teachey, D. T., & Grupp, S. A. (2014). Managing cytokine release syndrome associated with novel T cell-engaging therapies. Cancer journal (Sudbury, Mass.), 20(2), 119–122. https://doi.org/10.1097/PPO.0000000000000035

[8] Zhang, C., Wu, Z., Li, J. W., Zhao, H., & Wang, G. Q. (2020). Cytokine release syndrome in severe COVID-19: interleukin-6 receptor antagonist tocilizumab may be the key to reduce mortality. International journal of antimicrobial agents, 55(5), 105954. https://doi.org/10.1016/j.ijantimicag.2020.105954

[9] Le, R. Q., Li, L., Yuan, W., Shord, S. S., Nie, L., Habtemariam, B. A., Przepiorka, D., Farrell, A. T., & Pazdur, R. (2018). FDA Approval Summary: Tocilizumab for Treatment of Chimeric Antigen Receptor T Cell-Induced Severe or Life-Threatening Cytokine Release Syndrome. The oncologist, 23(8), 943–947. https://doi.org/10.1634/theoncologist.2018-0028

[10] Richter, A., Listing, J., Schneider, M., Klopsch, T., Kapelle, A., Kaufmann, J., Zink, A., & Strangfeld, A. (2016). Impact of treatment with biologic DMARDs on the risk of sepsis or mortality after serious infection in patients with rheumatoid arthritis. Annals of the rheumatic diseases, 75(9), 1667–1673. https://doi.org/10.1136/annrheumdis-2015-207838

[11] Stone, J. H., Tuckwell, K., Dimonaco, S., Klearman, M., Aringer, M., Blockmans, D., Brouwer, E., Cid, M. C., Dasgupta, B., Rech, J., Salvarani, C., Schett, G., Schulze-Koops, H., Spiera, R., Unizony, S. H., & Collinson, N. (2017). Trial of Tocilizumab in Giant-Cell Arteritis. The New England journal of medicine, 377(4), 317–328. https://doi.org/10.1056/NEJMoa1613849

[12] Xu, X., Han, M., Li, T., Sun, W., Wang, D., Fu, B., Zhou, Y., Zheng, X., Yang, Y., Li, X., Zhang, X., Pan, A., & Wei, H. (2020). Effective treatment of

severe COVID-19 patients with tocilizumab. Proceedings of the National Academy of Sciences of the United States of America, 117(20), 10970–10975. https://doi.org/10.1073/pnas.2005615117

[13] Michot, J. M., Albiges, L., Chaput, N., Saada, V., Pommeret, F., Griscelli, F., Balleyguier, C., Besse, B., Marabelle, A., Netzer, F., Merad, M., Robert, C., Barlesi, F., Gachot, B., & Stoclin, A. (2020). Tocilizumab, an anti-IL-6 receptor antibody, to treat COVID-19-related respiratory failure: a case report. Annals of oncology: official journal of the European Society for Medical Oncology, 31(7), 961–964. https://doi.org/10.1016/j.annonc.2020.03.300

[14] Toniati, P., Piva, S., Cattalini, M., Garrafa, E., Regola, F., Castelli, F., Franceschini, F., Airò, P., Bazzani, C., Beindorf, E. A., Berlendis, M., Bezzi, M., Bossini, N., Castellano, M., Cattaneo, S., Cavazzana, I., Contessi, G. B., Crippa, M., Delbarba, A., De Peri, E., ... Latronico, N. (2020). Tocilizumab for the treatment of severe COVID-19 pneumonia with hyperinflammatory syndrome and acute respiratory failure: A single center study of 100 patients in Brescia, Italy. Autoimmunity reviews, 19(7), 102568. https://doi.org/10.1016/j.autrev.2020.102568

[15] Assessment Report For RoActemra [Internet] 1st ed. London: European Medicines Agency; 2009. [accessed 2017January3]. http://www.ema.europa.eu/docs/en_GB/document_library/EPAR_-_Public_assessment_report/human/000955/WC500054888.pdf

[16] RoACTEMRA [Internet] F Hoffmann-La Roche Ltd; c2017 [accessed 2017January2]. http://www.roche.com/products/product-details.htm?productId=30d444d8-7658-469e-9fce-f4de549c00c4

[17] Venkiteshwaran A. (2009). Tocilizumab. mAbs, 1(5), 432–438. https://doi.org/10.4161/mabs.1.5.9497

[18] Luo, P., Liu, Y., Qiu, L., Liu, X., Liu, D., & Li, J. (2020). Tocilizumab treatment in COVID-19: A single center experience. Journal of medical virology, 92(7), 814–818. https://doi.org/10.1002/jmv.25801

[19] Alattar, R., Ibrahim, T., Shaar, S. H., Abdalla, S., Shukri, K., Daghfal, J. N., Khatib, M. Y., Aboukamar, M., Abukhattab, M., Alsoub, H. A., Almaslamani, M. A., & Omrani, A. S. (2020). Tocilizumab for the treatment of severe coronavirus disease 2019. Journal of medical virology, 92(10), 2042–2049. https://doi.org/10.1002/jmv.25964

[20] Fontana, F., Alfano, G., Mori, G., Amurri, A., Tei, L., Ballestri, M., Leonelli, M., Facchini, F., Damiano, F., Magistroni, R., & Cappelli, G. (2020). COVID-19 pneumonia in a kidney transplant recipient successfully treated with tocilizumab and hydroxychloroquine. American journal of transplantation: official journal of the American Society of Transplantation and the American Society of Transplant Surgeons, 20(7), 1902–1906. https://doi.org/10.1111/ajt.15935

[21] Stone, J. H., Frigault, M. J., Serling-Boyd, N. J., Fernandes, A. D., Harvey, L., Foulkes, A. S., Horick, N. K., Healy, B. C., Shah, R., Bensaci, A. M., Woolley, A. E., Nikiforow, S., Lin, N., Sagar, M., Schrager, H., Huckins, D. S., Axelrod, M., Pincus, M. D., Fleisher, J., Sacks, C. A., ... BACC Bay Tocilizumab Trial Investigators (2020). Efficacy of Tocilizumab in Patients Hospitalized with Covid-19. The New England journal of medicine, 383(24), 2333–2344. https://doi.org/10.1056/NEJMoa2028836

[22] https://www.accessdata.fda.gov/drugsatfda_docs/label/2017/125276s114lbl.pdf

[23] Bhimraj, A., Morgan, R. L., Shumaker, A. H., Lavergne, V., Baden,

L., Cheng, V. C., Edwards, K. M., Gandhi, R., Muller, W. J., O'Horo, J. C., Shoham, S., Murad, M. H., Mustafa, R. A., Sultan, S., & Falck-Ytter, Y. (2020). Infectious Diseases Society of America Guidelines on the Treatment and Management of Patients with COVID-19. Clinical infectious diseases: an official publication of the Infectious Diseases Society of America, ciaa478. Advance online publication. https://doi.org/10.1093/cid/ciaa478

[24] https://www.covid19treatmentguidelines.nih.gov/immunomodulators/interleukin-6-inhibitors/

[25] Yonggang Zhou, Binqing Fu, Xiaohu Zheng, Dongsheng Wang, Changcheng Zhao, Yingjie Qi, Rui Sun, Zhigang Tian, Xiaoling Xu, Haiming Wei, Pathogenic T-cells and inflammatory monocytes incite inflammatory storms in severe COVID-19 patients, National Science Review, 7:6 2020,998–1002, https://doi.org/10.1093/nsr/nwaa041

[26] Tanaka, T., Narazaki, M., & Kishimoto, T. (2016). Immunotherapeutic implications of IL-6 blockade for cytokine storm. Immunotherapy, 8(8), 959–970. https://doi.org/10.2217/imt-2016-0020

[27] Braun, G. S., Nagayama, Y., Maruta, Y., Heymann, F., van Roeyen, C. R., Klinkhammer, B. M., Boor, P., Villa, L., Salant, D. J., Raffetseder, U., Rose-John, S., Ostendorf, T., & Floege, J. (2016). IL-6 Trans-Signaling Drives Murine Crescentic GN. Journal of the American Society of Nephrology: JASN, 27(1), 132–142. https://doi.org/10.1681/ASN.2014111147

[28] Huang, C., Wang, Y., Li, X., Ren, L., Zhao, J., Hu, Y., Zhang, L., Fan, G., Xu, J., Gu, X., Cheng, Z., Yu, T., Xia, J., Wei, Y., Wu, W., Xie, X., Yin, W., Li, H., Liu, M., Xiao, Y., ... Cao, B. (2020). Clinical features of patients infected with 2019 novel coronavirus in Wuhan, China. Lancet (London, England), 395(10223), 497–506. https://doi.org/10.1016/S0140-6736(20)30183-5

[29] Rosas, I. O., Bräu, N., Waters, M., Go, R. C., Hunter, B. D., Bhagani, S., Skiest, D., Aziz, M. S., Cooper, N., Douglas, I. S., Savic, S., Youngstein, T., Del Sorbo, L., Cubillo Gracian, A., De La Zerda, D. J., Ustianowski, A., Bao, M., Dimonaco, S., Graham, E., Matharu, B., ... Malhotra, A. (2021). Tocilizumab in Hospitalized Patients with Severe Covid-19 Pneumonia. The New England journal of medicine, 384(16), 1503–1516. https://doi.org/10.1056/NEJMoa2028700

[30] Lier, A. J., Tuan, J. J., Davis, M. W., Paulson, N., McManus, D., Campbell, S., Peaper, D. R., & Topal, J. E. (2020). Case Report: Disseminated Strongyloidiasis in a Patient with COVID-19. The American journal of tropical medicine and hygiene, 103(4), 1590–1592. https://doi.org/10.4269/ajtmh.20-0699

[31] Oldfield, V., Dhillon, S., & Plosker, G. L. (2009). Tocilizumab: a review of its use in the management of rheumatoid arthritis. Drugs, 69(5), 609–632. https://doi.org/10.2165/00003495-200969050-00007

[32] Sebba A. (2008). Tocilizumab: the first interleukin-6-receptor inhibitor. American journal of health-system pharmacy: AJHP: official journal of the American Society of Health-System Pharmacists, 65(15), 1413–1418. https://doi.org/10.2146/ajhp070449

[33] Strohbehn, G. W., Reid, P. D., & Ratain, M. J. (2020). Applied Clinical Pharmacology in a Crisis: Interleukin-6 Axis Blockade and COVID-19. Clinical pharmacology and therapeutics, 108(3), 425–427. https://doi.org/10.1002/cpt.1931

[34] Perrone, F., Piccirillo, M. C., Ascierto, P. A., Salvarani, C., Parrella, R., Marata, A. M., Popoli, P., Ferraris,

L., Marrocco-Trischitta, M. M., Ripamonti, D., Binda, F., Bonfanti, P., Squillace, N., Castelli, F., Muiesan, M. L., Lichtner, M., Calzetti, C., Salerno, N. D., Atripaldi, L., Cascella, M., ... TOCIVID-19 investigators, Italy (2020). Tocilizumab for patients with COVID-19 pneumonia. The single-arm TOCIVID-19 prospective trial. Journal of translational medicine, 18(1), 405. https://doi.org/10.1186/s12967-020-02573-9

[35] Chiodini, P., Arenare, L., Piccirillo, M. C., Perrone, F., & Gallo, C. (2020). A phase 2, open label, multicenter, single arm study of tocilizumab on the efficacy and tolerability of tocilizumab in the treatment of patients with COVID-19 pneumonia (TOCIVID-19 trial): Statistical analysis plan. Contemporary clinical trials communications, 20, 100665. https://doi.org/10.1016/j.conctc.2020.100665

[36] Piccirillo, M. C., Ascierto, P., Atripaldi, L., Cascella, M., Costantini, M., Dolci, G., Facciolongo, N., Fraganza, F., Marata, A., Massari, M., Montesarchio, V., Mussini, C., Negri, E. A., Parrella, R., Popoli, P., Botti, G., Arenare, L., Chiodini, P., Gallo, C., Salvarani, C., ... Perrone, F. (2020). TOCIVID-19 - A multicenter study on the efficacy and tolerability of tocilizumab in the treatment of patients with COVID-19 pneumonia. Study protocol. Contemporary clinical trials, 98, 106165. https://doi.org/10.1016/j.cct.2020.106165

[37] Guan, W. J., Ni, Z. Y., Hu, Y., Liang, W. H., Ou, C. Q., He, J. X., Liu, L., Shan, H., Lei, C. L., Hui, D., Du, B., Li, L. J., Zeng, G., Yuen, K. Y., Chen, R. C., Tang, C. L., Wang, T., Chen, P. Y., Xiang, J., Li, S. Y., ... China Medical Treatment Expert Group for Covid-19 (2020). Clinical Characteristics of Coronavirus Disease 2019 in China. The New England journal of medicine, 382 (18), 1708–1720. https://doi.org/10.1056/NEJMoa2002032

[38] Grasselli, G., Zangrillo, A., Zanella, A., Antonelli, M., Cabrini, L., Castelli, A., Cereda, D., Coluccello, A., Foti, G., Fumagalli, R., Iotti, G., Latronico, N., Lorini, L., Merler, S., Natalini, G., Piatti, A., Ranieri, M. V., Scandroglio, A. M., Storti, E., Cecconi, M., ... COVID-19 Lombardy ICU Network (2020). Baseline Characteristics and Outcomes of 1591 Patients Infected With SARS-CoV-2 Admitted to ICUs of the Lombardy Region, Italy. JAMA, 323 (16), 1574–1581. https://doi.org/10.1001/jama.2020.5394

[39] Mehta, P., McAuley, D. F., Brown, M., Sanchez, E., Tattersall, R. S., Manson, J. J., & HLH Across Speciality Collaboration, UK (2020). COVID-19: consider cytokine storm syndromes and immunosuppression. Lancet (London, England), 395(10229), 1033–1034. https://doi.org/10.1016/S0140-6736(20)30628-0

[40] Ye, Q., Wang, B., & Mao, J. (2020). The pathogenesis and treatment of the `Cytokine Storm' in COVID-19. The Journal of infection, 80(6), 607–613. https://doi.org/10.1016/j.jinf.2020.03.037

[41] Cao, B., Wang, Y., Wen, D., Liu, W., Wang, J., Fan, G., Ruan, L., Song, B., Cai, Y., Wei, M., Li, X., Xia, J., Chen, N., Xiang, J., Yu, T., Bai, T., Xie, X., Zhang, L., Li, C., Yuan, Y., ... Wang, C. (2020). A Trial of Lopinavir-Ritonavir in Adults Hospitalized with Severe Covid-19. The New England journal of medicine, 382(19), 1787–1799. https://doi.org/10.1056/NEJMoa2001282

[42] Grein, J., Ohmagari, N., Shin, D., Diaz, G., Asperges, E., Castagna, A., Feldt, T., Green, G., Green, M. L., Lescure, F. X., Nicastri, E., Oda, R., Yo, K., Quiros-Roldan, E., Studemeister, A., Redinski, J., Ahmed, S., Bernett, J., Chelliah, D., Chen, D., ... Flanigan, T. (2020). Compassionate Use of Remdesivir for Patients with Severe Covid-19. The New England journal of medicine, 382(24), 2327–2336. https://doi.org/10.1056/NEJMoa2007016

[43] Wu, C., Chen, X., Cai, Y., Xia, J., Zhou, X., Xu, S., Huang, H., Zhang, L., Zhou, X., Du, C., Zhang, Y., Song, J., Wang, S., Chao, Y., Yang, Z., Xu, J., Zhou, X., Chen, D., Xiong, W., Xu, L., ... Song, Y. (2020). Risk Factors Associated With Acute Respiratory Distress Syndrome and Death in Patients With Coronavirus Disease 2019 Pneumonia in Wuhan, China. JAMA internal medicine, 180(7), 934–943. https://doi.org/10.1001/jamainternmed.2020.0994

[44] Zhou, F., Yu, T., Du, R., Fan, G., Liu, Y., Liu, Z., Xiang, J., Wang, Y., Song, B., Gu, X., Guan, L., Wei, Y., Li, H., Wu, X., Xu, J., Tu, S., Zhang, Y., Chen, H., & Cao, B. (2020). Clinical course and risk factors for mortality of adult inpatients with COVID-19 in Wuhan, China: a retrospective cohort study. Lancet (London, England), 395 (10229), 1054–1062. https://doi.org/10.1016/S0140-6736(20)30566-3

[45] Morrondo, C. D., Zarza, L. P., Gil, J. G., Pinto Tasende, J. A., Diez, P. D., & López, J. M. (2016). Benefit of Tocilizumab Therapy for Adult-Onset Still Disease Complicated With Acute Respiratory Distress Syndrome. Journal of clinical rheumatology: practical reports on rheumatic & musculoskeletal diseases, 22(5), 291–293. https://doi.org/10.1097/RHU.0000000000000374

[46] Shakoory, B., Carcillo, J. A., Chatham, W. W., Amdur, R. L., Zhao, H., Dinarello, C. A., Cron, R. Q., & Opal, S. M. (2016). Interleukin-1 Receptor Blockade Is Associated With Reduced Mortality in Sepsis Patients With Features of Macrophage Activation Syndrome: Reanalysis of a Prior Phase III Trial. Critical care medicine, 44(2), 275–281. https://doi.org/10.1097/CCM.0000000000001402

[47] Neuenschwander, B., Capkun-Niggli, G., Branson, M., & Spiegelhalter, D. J. (2010). Summarizing historical information on controls in clinical trials. Clinical trials (London, England), 7(1), 5–18. https://doi.org/10.1177/1740774509356002

[48] Jones, G., Sebba, A., Gu, J., Lowenstein, M. B., Calvo, A., Gomez-Reino, J. J., Siri, D. A., Tomsic, M., Alecock, E., Woodworth, T., & Genovese, M. C. (2010). Comparison of tocilizumab monotherapy versus methotrexate monotherapy in patients with moderate to severe rheumatoid arthritis: the AMBITION study. Annals of the rheumatic diseases, 69(1), 88–96. https://doi.org/10.1136/ard.2008.105197

[49] Stone, J. H., Tuckwell, K., Dimonaco, S., Klearman, M., Aringer, M., Blockmans, D., Brouwer, E., Cid, M. C., Dasgupta, B., Rech, J., Salvarani, C., Schett, G., Schulze-Koops, H., Spiera, R., Unizony, S. H., & Collinson, N. (2017). Trial of Tocilizumab in Giant-Cell Arteritis. The New England journal of medicine, 377(4), 317–328. https://doi.org/10.1056/NEJMoa1613849

[50] Villiger, P. M., Adler, S., Kuchen, S., Wermelinger, F., Dan, D., Fiege, V., Bütikofer, L., Seitz, M., & Reichenbach, S. (2016). Tocilizumab for induction and maintenance of remission in giant cell arteritis: a phase 2, randomised, double-blind, placebo-controlled trial. Lancet (London, England), 387(10031), 1921–1927. https://doi.org/10.1016/S0140-6736(16)00560-2

[51] Yang, S., Cao, P., Du, P., Wu, Z., Zhuang, Z., Yang, L., Yu, X., Zhou, Q., Feng, X., Wang, X., Li, W., Liu, E., Chen, J., Chen, Y., & He, D. (2020). Early estimation of the case fatality rate of COVID-19 in mainland China: a data-driven analysis. Annals of translational medicine, 8(4), 128. https://doi.org/10.21037/atm.2020.02.66

[52] Khanna, D., Denton, C. P., Jahreis, A., van Laar, J. M., Frech, T. M., Anderson, M. E., Baron, M., Chung, L., Fierlbeck, G., Lakshminarayanan, S., Allanore, Y., Pope, J. E., Riemekasten,

G., Steen, V., Müller-Ladner, U., Lafyatis, R., Stifano, G., Spotswood, H., Chen-Harris, H., Dziadek, S., ... Furst, D. E. (2016). Safety and efficacy of subcutaneous tocilizumab in adults with systemic sclerosis (faSScinate): a phase 2, randomised, controlled trial. Lancet (London, England), 387(10038), 2630–2640. https://doi.org/10.1016/S0140-6736(16)00232-4

[53] Ruan, Q., Yang, K., Wang, W., Jiang, L., & Song, J. (2020). Clinical predictors of mortality due to COVID-19 based on an analysis of data of 150 patients from Wuhan, China. Intensive care medicine, 46(5), 846–848. https://doi.org/10.1007/s00134-020-05991-x

[54] Yang, X., Yu, Y., Xu, J., Shu, H., Xia, J., Liu, H., Wu, Y., Zhang, L., Yu, Z., Fang, M., Yu, T., Wang, Y., Pan, S., Zou, X., Yuan, S., & Shang, Y. (2020). Clinical course and outcomes of critically ill patients with SARS-CoV-2 pneumonia in Wuhan, China: a single-centered, retrospective, observational study. The Lancet. Respiratory medicine, 8(5), 475–481. https://doi.org/10.1016/S2213-2600(20)30079-5

[55] Hays, P., Costello, C., & Asudani, D. (2019). Clinical care of chimeric antigen receptor T-cell patients and managing immune-related adverse effects in the ambulatory and hospitalized setting: a review. Future oncology (London, England), 15(36), 4235–4246. https://doi.org/10.2217/fon-2019-0467

[56] Hunter, C. A., & Jones, S. A. (2015). IL-6 as a keystone cytokine in health and disease. Nature immunology, 16(5), 448–457. https://doi.org/10.1038/ni.3153

[57] Pathan, N., Hemingway, C. A., Alizadeh, A. A., Stephens, A. C., Boldrick, J. C., Oragui, E. E., McCabe, C., Welch, S. B., Whitney, A., O'Gara, P., Nadel, S., Relman, D. A., Harding, S. E., & Levin, M. (2004). Role of interleukin 6 in myocardial dysfunction of meningococcal septic shock. Lancet (London, England), 363(9404), 203–209. https://doi.org/10.1016/S0140-6736(03)15326-3

[58] Salehi, S., Abedi, A., Balakrishnan, S., & Gholamrezanezhad, A. (2020). Coronavirus Disease 2019 (COVID-19): A Systematic Review of Imaging Findings in 919 Patients. AJR. American journal of roentgenology, 215(1), 87–93. https://doi.org/10.2214/AJR.20.23034

[59] Shimabukuro-Vornhagen, A., Gödel, P., Subklewe, M., Stemmler, H. J., Schlößer, H. A., Schlaak, M., Kochanek, M., Böll, B., & von Bergwelt-Baildon, M. S. (2018). Cytokine release syndrome. Journal for immunotherapy of cancer, 6(1), 56. https://doi.org/10.1186/s40425-018-0343-9

[60] van der Stegen, S. J., Davies, D. M., Wilkie, S., Foster, J., Sosabowski, J. K., Burnet, J., Whilding, L. M., Petrovic, R. M., Ghaem-Maghami, S., Mather, S., Jeannon, J. P., Parente-Pereira, A. C., & Maher, J. (2013). Preclinical in vivo modeling of cytokine release syndrome induced by ErbB-retargeted human T cells: identifying a window of therapeutic opportunity?. Journal of immunology (Baltimore, Md.: 1950), 191(9), 4589–4598. https://doi.org/10.4049/jimmunol.1301523

[61] Winkler, U., Jensen, M., Manzke, O., Schulz, H., Diehl, V., & Engert, A. (1999). Cytokine-release syndrome in patients with B-cell chronic lymphocytic leukemia and high lymphocyte counts after treatment with an anti-CD20 monoclonal antibody (rituximab, IDEC-C2B8). Blood, 94(7), 2217–2224.

[62] Xu, Z., Shi, L., Wang, Y., Zhang, J., Huang, L., Zhang, C., Liu, S., Zhao, P., Liu, H., Zhu, L., Tai, Y., Bai, C., Gao, T., Song, J., Xia, P., Dong, J., Zhao, J., & Wang, F. S. (2020). Pathological findings of COVID-19 associated with acute respiratory distress syndrome. The Lancet. Respiratory medicine, 8(4),

420–422. https://doi.org/10.1016/S2213-2600(20)30076-X

[63] Salama, C., Han, J., Yau, L., Reiss, W. G., Kramer, B., Neidhart, J. D., Criner, G. J., Kaplan-Lewis, E., Baden, R., Pandit, L., Cameron, M. L., Garcia-Diaz, J., Chávez, V., Mekebeb-Reuter, M., Lima de Menezes, F., Shah, R., González-Lara, M. F., Assman, B., Freedman, J., & Mohan, S. V. (2021). Tocilizumab in Patients Hospitalized with Covid-19 Pneumonia. The New England journal of medicine, 384(1), 20–30. https://doi.org/10.1056/NEJMoa2030340

[64] Veiga, V. C., Prats, J., Farias, D., Rosa, R. G., Dourado, L. K., Zampieri, F. G., Machado, F. R., Lopes, R. D., Berwanger, O., Azevedo, L., Avezum, Á., Lisboa, T. C., Rojas, S., Coelho, J. C., Leite, R. T., Carvalho, J. C., Andrade, L., Sandes, A. F., Pintão, M., Castro, C. G., Jr, ... Coalition covid-19 Brazil VI Investigators (2021). Effect of tocilizumab on clinical outcomes at 15 days in patients with severe or critical coronavirus disease 2019: randomised controlled trial. BMJ (Clinical research ed.), 372, n84. https://doi.org/10.1136/bmj.n84

[65] Maes, B., Bosteels, C., De Leeuw, E., Declercq, J., Van Damme, K., Delporte, A., Demeyere, B., Vermeersch, S., Vuylsteke, M., Willaert, J., Bollé, L., Vanbiervliet, Y., Decuypere, J., Libeer, F., Vandecasteele, S., Peene, I., & Lambrecht, B. (2020). Treatment of severely ill COVID-19 patients with anti-interleukin drugs (COV-AID): A structured summary of a study protocol for a randomised controlled trial. Trials, 21(1), 468. https://doi.org/10.1186/s13063-020-04453-5

[66] Hermine, O., Mariette, X., Tharaux, P. L., Resche-Rigon, M., Porcher, R., Ravaud, P., & CORIMUNO-19 Collaborative Group (2021). Effect of Tocilizumab vs Usual Care in Adults Hospitalized With COVID-19 and Moderate or Severe Pneumonia: A Randomized Clinical Trial. JAMA internal medicine, 181(1), 32–40. https://doi.org/10.1001/jamainternmed.2020.6820

[67] Knaup, H., Stahl, K., Schmidt, B., Idowu, T. O., Busch, M., Wiesner, O., Welte, T., Haller, H., Kielstein, J. T., Hoeper, M. M., & David, S. (2018). Early therapeutic plasma exchange in septic shock: a prospective open-label nonrandomized pilot study focusing on safety, hemodynamics, vascular barrier function, and biologic markers. Critical care (London, England), 22(1), 285. https://doi.org/10.1186/s13054-018-2220-9

[68] Keith, P., Day, M., Perkins, L., Moyer, L., Hewitt, K., & Wells, A. (2020). A novel treatment approach to the novel coronavirus: an argument for the use of therapeutic plasma exchange for fulminant COVID-19. Critical care (London, England), 24(1), 128. https://doi.org/10.1186/s13054-020-2836-4

[69] Shi, H., Zhou, C., He, P., Huang, S., Duan, Y., Wang, X., Lin, K., Zhou, C., Zhang, X., & Zha, Y. (2020). Successful treatment with plasma exchange followed by intravenous immunoglobulin in a critically ill patient with COVID-19. International journal of antimicrobial agents, 56(2), 105974. https://doi.org/10.1016/j.ijantimicag.2020.105974

[70] Chen, L., Xiong, J., Bao, L., & Shi, Y. (2020). Convalescent plasma as a potential therapy for COVID-19. The Lancet. Infectious diseases, 20(4), 398–400. https://doi.org/10.1016/S1473-3099(20)30141-9

[71] Xu, X., Han, M., Li, T., Sun, W., Wang, D., Fu, B., Zhou, Y., Zheng, X., Yang, Y., Li, X., Zhang, X., Pan, A., & Wei, H. (2020). Effective treatment of severe COVID-19 patients with tocilizumab. Proceedings of the National Academy of Sciences of the United States of America, 117(20),

10970–10975. https://doi.org/10.1073/pnas.2005615117

[72] Beigel, J. H., Tomashek, K. M., Dodd, L. E., Mehta, A. K., Zingman, B. S., Kalil, A. C., Hohmann, E., Chu, H. Y., Luetkemeyer, A., Kline, S., Lopez de Castilla, D., Finberg, R. W., Dierberg, K., Tapson, V., Hsieh, L., Patterson, T. F., Paredes, R., Sweeney, D. A., Short, W. R., Touloumi, G., ... ACTT-1 Study Group Members (2020). Remdesivir for the Treatment of Covid-19 - Final Report. The New England journal of medicine, 383(19), 1813–1826. https://doi.org/10.1056/NEJMoa2007764

[73] Leng, Z., Zhu, R., Hou, W., Feng, Y., Yang, Y., Han, Q., Shan, G., Meng, F., Du, D., Wang, S., Fan, J., Wang, W., Deng, L., Shi, H., Li, H., Hu, Z., Zhang, F., Gao, J., Liu, H., Li, X., ... Zhao, R. C. (2020). Transplantation of ACE2- Mesenchymal Stem Cells Improves the Outcome of Patients with COVID-19 Pneumonia. Aging and disease, 11(2), 216–228. https://doi.org/10.14336/AD.2020.0228

[74] Alzghari, S. K., & Acuña, V. S. (2020). Supportive Treatment with Tocilizumab for COVID-19: A Systematic Review. Journal of clinical virology: the official publication of the Pan American Society for Clinical Virology, 127, 104380. https://doi.org/10.1016/j.jcv.2020.104380

[75] Tian, S., Hu, W., Niu, L., Liu, H., Xu, H., & Xiao, S. Y. (2020). Pulmonary Pathology of Early-Phase 2019 Novel Coronavirus (COVID-19) Pneumonia in Two Patients With Lung Cancer. Journal of thoracic oncology: official publication of the International Association for the Study of Lung Cancer, 15(5), 700–704. https://doi.org/10.1016/j.jtho.2020.02.010

[76] Ashour, H. M., Elkhatib, W. F., Rahman, M. M., & Elshabrawy, H. A. (2020). Insights into the Recent 2019 Novel Coronavirus (SARS-CoV-2) in Light of Past Human Coronavirus Outbreaks. Pathogens (Basel, Switzerland), 9(3), 186. https://doi.org/10.3390/pathogens9030186

[77] Channappanavar, R., & Perlman, S. (2017). Pathogenic human coronavirus infections: causes and consequences of cytokine storm and immunopathology. Seminars in immunopathology, 39(5), 529–539. https://doi.org/10.1007/s00281-017-0629-x

[78] Zumla, A., Ippolito, G., Ntoumi, F., Seyfert-Margolies, V., Nagu, T. J., Cirillo, D., Chakaya, J. M., Marais, B., & Maeurer, M. (2020). Host-directed therapies and holistic care for tuberculosis. The Lancet. Respiratory medicine, 8(4), 337–340. https://doi.org/10.1016/S2213-2600(20)30078-3

[79] Sabbatinelli, J., Giuliani, A., Matacchione, G., Latini, S., Laprovitera, N., Pomponio, G., Ferrarini, A., Svegliati Baroni, S., Pavani, M., Moretti, M., Gabrielli, A., Procopio, A. D., Ferracin, M., Bonafè, M., & Olivieri, F. (2021). Decreased serum levels of the inflammaging marker miR-146a are associated with clinical non-response to tocilizumab in COVID-19 patients. Mechanisms of ageing and development, 193, 111413. https://doi.org/10.1016/j.mad.2020.111413

[80] Wichmann, D., Sperhake, J. P., Lütgehetmann, M., Steurer, S., Edler, C., Heinemann, A., Heinrich, F., Mushumba, H., Kniep, I., Schröder, A. S., Burdelski, C., de Heer, G., Nierhaus, A., Frings, D., Pfefferle, S., Becker, H., Bredereke-Wiedling, H., de Weerth, A., Paschen, H. R., Sheikhzadeh-Eggers, S., ... Kluge, S. (2020). Autopsy Findings and Venous Thromboembolism in Patients With COVID-19: A Prospective Cohort Study. Annals of internal medicine, 173(4), 268–277. https://doi.org/10.7326/M20-2003

[81] Ramos-Casals, M., Brito-Zerón, P., López-Guillermo, A., Khamashta, M. A., & Bosch, X. (2014). Adult

haemophagocytic syndrome. Lancet (London, England), 383(9927), 1503–1516. https://doi.org/10.1016/S0140-6736(13)61048-X

[82] Radbel, J., Narayanan, N., & Bhatt, P. J. (2020). Use of Tocilizumab for COVID-19-Induced Cytokine Release Syndrome: A Cautionary Case Report. Chest, 158(1), e15–e19. https://doi.org/10.1016/j.chest.2020.04.024

[83] Liu, B., Li, M., Zhou, Z., Guan, X., & Xiang, Y. (2020). Can we use interleukin-6 (IL-6) blockade for coronavirus disease 2019 (COVID-19)-induced cytokine release syndrome (CRS)?. Journal of autoimmunity, 111, 102452. https://doi.org/10.1016/j.jaut.2020.102452

[84] Hui, D. S., I Azhar, E., Madani, T. A., Ntoumi, F., Kock, R., Dar, O., Ippolito, G., Mchugh, T. D., Memish, Z. A., Drosten, C., Zumla, A., & Petersen, E. (2020). The continuing 2019-nCoV epidemic threat of novel coronaviruses to global health - The latest 2019 novel coronavirus outbreak in Wuhan, China. International journal of infectious diseases: IJID: official publication of the International Society for Infectious Diseases, 91, 264–266. https://doi.org/10.1016/j.ijid.2020.01.009

[85] Paules, C. I., Marston, H. D., & Fauci, A. S. (2020). Coronavirus Infections-More Than Just the Common Cold. JAMA, 323(8), 707–708. https://doi.org/10.1001/jama.2020.0757

[86] Hu, X., Deng, Y., Wang, J., Li, H., Li, M., & Lu, Z. (2004). Short term outcome and risk factors for mortality in adults with critical severe acute respiratory syndrome (SARS). Journal of Huazhong University of Science and Technology. Medical sciences = Hua zhong ke ji da xue xue bao. Yi xue Ying De wen ban = Huazhong keji daxue xuebao. Yixue Yingdewen ban, 24(5), 514–517. https://doi.org/10.1007/BF02831124

[87] Schmitt, J., Boutonnet, M., Goutorbe, P., Raynaud, L., Carfantan, C., Luft, A., Pasquier, P., Meaudre, E., & Bordes, J. (2020). Acute respiratory distress syndrome in the forward environment. Retrospective analysis of acute respiratory distress syndrome cases among French Army war casualties. The journal of trauma and acute care surgery, 89(2S Suppl 2), S207–S212. https://doi.org/10.1097/TA.0000000000002633

[88] Ferguson, N. D., Fan, E., Camporota, L., Antonelli, M., Anzueto, A., Beale, R., Brochard, L., Brower, R., Esteban, A., Gattinoni, L., Rhodes, A., Slutsky, A. S., Vincent, J. L., Rubenfeld, G. D., Thompson, B. T., & Ranieri, V. M. (2012). The Berlin definition of ARDS: an expanded rationale, justification, and supplementary material. Intensive care medicine, 38 (10), 1573–1582. https://doi.org/10.1007/s00134-012-2682-1

[89] Bhatraju, P. K., Ghassemieh, B. J., Nichols, M., Kim, R., Jerome, K. R., Nalla, A. K., Greninger, A. L., Pipavath, S., Wurfel, M. M., Evans, L., Kritek, P. A., West, T. E., Luks, A., Gerbino, A., Dale, C. R., Goldman, J. D., O'Mahony, S., & Mikacenic, C. (2020). Covid-19 in Critically Ill Patients in the Seattle Region - Case Series. The New England journal of medicine, 382(21), 2012–2022. https://doi.org/10.1056/NEJMoa2004500

[90] Wu, Z., & McGoogan, J. M. (2020). Characteristics of and Important Lessons From the Coronavirus Disease 2019 (COVID-19) Outbreak in China: Summary of a Report of 72 314 Cases From the Chinese Center for Disease Control and Prevention. JAMA, 323(13), 1239–1242. https://doi.org/10.1001/jama.2020.2648

[91] Wang, W., Tang, J., & Wei, F. (2020). Updated understanding of the outbreak of 2019 novel coronavirus (2019-nCoV) in Wuhan, China. Journal

of medical virology, 92(4), 441–447. https://doi.org/10.1002/jmv.25689

[92] Benjamin, D. K., Jr, Smith, P. B., Murphy, M. D., Roberts, R., Mathis, L., Avant, D., Califf, R. M., & Li, J. S. (2006). Peer-reviewed publication of clinical trials completed for pediatric exclusivity. JAMA, 296(10), 1266–1273. https://doi.org/10.1001/jama.296.10.1266

[93] Phan, H., Leder, M., Fishley, M., Moeller, M., & Nahata, M. (2010). Off-label and unlicensed medication use and associated adverse drug events in a pediatric emergency department. Pediatric emergency care, 26(6), 424–430. https://doi.org/10.1097/PEC.0b013e3181e057e1

[94] Long, D., Koren, G., & James, A. (1987). Ethics of drug studies in infants: how many samples are required for accurate estimation of pharmacokinetic parameters in neonates?. The Journal of pediatrics, 111(6 Pt 1), 918–921. https://doi.org/10.1016/s0022-3476(87)80219-6

[95] European Union. Ethical considerations for clinical trials on medicinal products conducted with the paediatric population. (2008). European journal of health law, 15(2), 223–250. https://doi.org/10.1163/157180908x333228

[96] Wade, K. C., Wu, D., Kaufman, D. A., Ward, R. M., Benjamin, D. K., Jr, Sullivan, J. E., Ramey, N., Jayaraman, B., Hoppu, K., Adamson, P. C., Gastonguay, M. R., Barrett, J. S., & National Institute of Child Health and Development Pediatric Pharmacology Research Unit Network (2008). Population pharmacokinetics of fluconazole in young infants. Antimicrobial agents and chemotherapy, 52(11), 4043–4049. https://doi.org/10.1128/AAC.00569-08

[97] de Hoog, M., Schoemaker, R. C., Mouton, J. W., & van den Anker, J. N. (2000). Vancomycin population pharmacokinetics in neonates. Clinical pharmacology and therapeutics, 67(4), 360–367. https://doi.org/10.1067/mcp.2000.105353

[98] García, B., Barcia, E., Pérez, F., & Molina, I. T. (2006). Population pharmacokinetics of gentamicin in premature newborns. The Journal of antimicrobial chemotherapy, 58(2), 372–379. https://doi.org/10.1093/jac/dkl244

[99] Capparelli, E., Hochwald, C., Rasmussen, M., Parham, A., Bradley, J., & Moya, F. (2005). Population pharmacokinetics of cefepime in the neonate. Antimicrobial agents and chemotherapy, 49(7), 2760–2766. https://doi.org/10.1128/AAC.49.7.2760-2766.2005

[100] Pullen, J., Stolk, L. M., Nieman, F. H., Degraeuwe, P. L., van Tiel, F. H., & Zimmermann, L. J. (2006). Population pharmacokinetics and dosing of amoxicillin in (pre)term neonates. Therapeutic drug monitoring, 28(2), 226–231. https://doi.org/10.1097/01.ftd.0000198648.39751.11

[101] Tremoulet, A., Le, J., Poindexter, B., Sullivan, J. E., Laughon, M., Delmore, P., Salgado, A., Ian-U Chong, S., Melloni, C., Gao, J., Benjamin, D. K., Jr, Capparelli, E. V., Cohen-Wolkowiez, M., & Administrative Core Committee of the Best Pharmaceuticals for Children Act-Pediatric Trials Network (2014). Characterization of the population pharmacokinetics of ampicillin in neonates using an opportunistic study design. Antimicrobial agents and chemotherapy, 58(6), 3013–3020. https://doi.org/10.1128/AAC.02374-13

[102] Hornik, C. P., Benjamin, D. K., Jr, Smith, P. B., Pencina, M. J., Tremoulet, A. H., Capparelli, E. V., Ericson, J. E., Clark, R. H., Cohen-Wolkowiez, M., & Best Pharmaceuticals for Children Act—Pediatric Trials Network (2016).

Electronic Health Records and Pharmacokinetic Modeling to Assess the Relationship between Ampicillin Exposure and Seizure Risk in Neonates. The Journal of pediatrics, 178, 125–129. e1. https://doi.org/10.1016/j.jpeds.2016.07.011

[103] Le, J., Poindexter, B., Sullivan, J. E., Laughon, M., Delmore, P., Blackford, M., Yogev, R., James, L. P., Melloni, C., Harper, B., Mitchell, J., Benjamin, D. K., Jr, Boakye-Agyeman, F., & Cohen-Wolkowiez, M. (2018). Comparative Analysis of Ampicillin Plasma and Dried Blood Spot Pharmacokinetics in Neonates. Therapeutic drug monitoring, 40(1), 103–108. https://doi.org/10.1097/FTD.0000000000000466

[104] Gonzalez, D., Melloni, C., Yogev, R., Poindexter, B. B., Mendley, S. R., Delmore, P., Sullivan, J. E., Autmizguine, J., Lewandowski, A., Harper, B., Watt, K. M., Lewis, K. C., Capparelli, E. V., Benjamin, D. K., Jr, Cohen-Wolkowiez, M., & Best Pharmaceuticals for Children Act – Pediatric Trials Network Administrative Core Committee (2014). Use of opportunistic clinical data and a population pharmacokinetic model to support dosing of clindamycin for premature infants to adolescents. Clinical pharmacology and therapeutics, 96(4), 429–437. https://doi.org/10.1038/clpt.2014.134

[105] Gonzalez, D., Delmore, P., Bloom, B. T., Cotten, C. M., Poindexter, B. B., McGowan, E., Shattuck, K., Bradford, K. K., Smith, P. B., Cohen-Wolkowiez, M., Morris, M., Yin, W., Benjamin, D. K., Jr, & Laughon, M. M. (2016). Clindamycin Pharmacokinetics and Safety in Preterm and Term Infants. Antimicrobial agents and chemotherapy, 60(5), 2888–2894. https://doi.org/10.1128/AAC.03086-15

[106] Gonzalez, D., Melloni, C., Poindexter, B. B., Yogev, R., Atz, A. M., Sullivan, J. E., Mendley, S. R., Delmore, P., Delinsky, A., Zimmerman, K., Lewandowski, A., Harper, B., Lewis, K. C., Benjamin, D. K., Jr, Cohen-Wolkowiez, M., & Best Pharmaceuticals for Children Act–Pediatric Trials Network Administrative Core Committee (2015). Simultaneous determination of trimethoprim and sulfamethoxazole in dried plasma and urine spots. Bioanalysis, 7(9), 1137–1149. https://doi.org/10.4155/bio.15.38

[107] Autmizguine, J., Melloni, C., Hornik, C. P., Dallefeld, S., Harper, B., Yogev, R., Sullivan, J. E., Atz, A. M., Al-Uzri, A., Mendley, S., Poindexter, B., Mitchell, J., Lewandowski, A., Delmore, P., Cohen-Wolkowiez, M., Gonzalez, D., & the Pediatric Trials Network Steering Committee (2017). Population Pharmacokinetics of Trimethoprim-Sulfamethoxazole in Infants and Children. Antimicrobial agents and chemotherapy, 62(1), e01813-17. https://doi.org/10.1128/AAC.01813-17

[108] Dallefeld, S. H., Atz, A. M., Yogev, R., Sullivan, J. E., Al-Uzri, A., Mendley, S. R., Laughon, M., Hornik, C. P., Melloni, C., Harper, B., Lewandowski, A., Mitchell, J., Wu, H., Green, T. P., & Cohen-Wolkowiez, M. (2018). A pharmacokinetic model for amiodarone in infants developed from an opportunistic sampling trial and published literature data. Journal of pharmacokinetics and pharmacodynamics, 45(3), 419–430. https://doi.org/10.1007/s10928-018-9576-y

[109] Hornik, C. P., Gonzalez, D., van den Anker, J., Atz, A. M., Yogev, R., Poindexter, B. B., Ng, K. C., Delmore, P., Harper, B. L., Melloni, C., Lewandowski, A., Gelber, C., Cohen-Wolkowiez, M., Lee, J. H., & Pediatric Trial Network Steering Committee (2018). Population Pharmacokinetics of Intramuscular and Intravenous Ketamine in Children. Journal of clinical pharmacology, 58(8), 1092–1104. https://doi.org/10.1002/jcph.1116

[110] Drolet, B. A., Boakye-Agyeman, F., Harper, B., Holland, K., Lewandowski, A., Stefanko, N., Melloni, C., & Pediatric Trials Network Steering Committee (See Acknowledgments for a listing of committee members.) (2020). Systemic timolol exposure following topical application to infantile hemangiomas. Journal of the American Academy of Dermatology, 82(3), 733–736. https://doi.org/10.1016/j.jaad.2019.02.029

[111] Hornik, C. P., Yogev, R., Mourani, P. M., Watt, K. M., Sullivan, J. E., Atz, A. M., Speicher, D., Al-Uzri, A., Adu-Darko, M., Payne, E. H., Gelber, C. E., Lin, S., Harper, B., Melloni, C., Cohen-Wolkowiez, M., Gonzalez, D., & Best Pharmaceuticals for Children Act-Pediatric Trials Network Steering Committee (2019). Population Pharmacokinetics of Milrinone in Infants, Children, and Adolescents. Journal of clinical pharmacology, 59 (12), 1606–1619. https://doi.org/10.1002/jcph.1499

[112] Cohen-Wolkowiez, M., Ouellet, D., Smith, P. B., James, L. P., Ross, A., Sullivan, J. E., Walsh, M. C., Zadell, A., Newman, N., White, N. R., Kashuba, A. D., & Benjamin, D. K., Jr (2012). Population pharmacokinetics of metronidazole evaluated using scavenged samples from preterm infants. Antimicrobial agents and chemotherapy, 56(4), 1828–1837. https://doi.org/10.1128/AAC.06071-11

[113] Cohen-Wolkowiez, M., Benjamin, D. K., Jr, Ross, A., James, L. P., Sullivan, J. E., Walsh, M. C., Zadell, A., Newman, N., White, N. R., Kashuba, A. D., & Ouellet, D. (2012). Population pharmacokinetics of piperacillin using scavenged samples from preterm infants. Therapeutic drug monitoring, 34(3), 312–319. https://doi.org/10.1097/FTD.0b013e3182587665

[114] Biomarkers Definitions Working Group. (2001). Biomarkers and surrogate endpoints: preferred definitions and conceptual framework. Clinical pharmacology and therapeutics, 69(3), 89–95. https://doi.org/10.1067/mcp.2001.113989

[115] Kearns, G. L., & Artman, M. (2015). Functional Biomarkers: an Approach to Bridge Pharmacokinetics and Pharmacodynamics in Pediatric Clinical Trials. Current pharmaceutical design, 21 (39), 5636–5642. https://doi.org/10.2174/1381612821666150901105337

[116] Husain, A., Loehle, J. A., & Hein, D. W. (2007). Clinical pharmacogenetics in pediatric patients. Pharmacogenomics, 8(10), 1403–1411. https://doi.org/10.2217/14622416.8.10.1403

[117] Zheng, H., Webber, S., Zeevi, A., Schuetz, E., Zhang, J., Lamba, J., Bowman, P., & Burckart, G. J. (2002). The MDR1 polymorphisms at exons 21 and 26 predict steroid weaning in pediatric heart transplant patients. Human immunology, 63(9), 765–770. https://doi.org/10.1016/s0198-8859(02)00426-3

[118] Watson, R. S., Crow, S. S., Hartman, M. E., Lacroix, J., & Odetola, F. O. (2017). Epidemiology and Outcomes of Pediatric Multiple Organ Dysfunction Syndrome. Pediatric critical care medicine: a journal of the Society of Critical Care Medicine and the World Federation of Pediatric Intensive and Critical Care Societies, 18 (3_suppl Suppl 1), S4–S16. https://doi.org/10.1097/PCC.0000000000001047

[119] Typpo, K. V., Petersen, N. J., Hallman, D. M., Markovitz, B. P., & Mariscalco, M. M. (2009). Day 1 multiple organ dysfunction syndrome is associated with poor functional outcome and mortality in the pediatric intensive care unit. Pediatric critical care medicine: a journal of the Society of Critical Care Medicine and the World Federation of Pediatric Intensive and Critical Care Societies, 10(5), 562–570.

https://doi.org/10.1097/PCC.0b013e3181a64be1

[120] Wang, L., McGregor, T. L., Jones, D. P., Bridges, B. C., Fleming, G. M., Shirey-Rice, J., McLemore, M. F., Chen, L., Weitkamp, A., Byrne, D. W., & Van Driest, S. L. (2017). Electronic health record-based predictive models for acute kidney injury screening in pediatric inpatients. Pediatric research, 82(3), 465–473. https://doi.org/10.1038/pr.2017.116

[121] Kaddourah, A., Basu, R. K., Bagshaw, S. M., Goldstein, S. L., & AWARE Investigators (2017). Epidemiology of Acute Kidney Injury in Critically Ill Children and Young Adults. The New England journal of medicine, 376(1), 11–20. https://doi.org/10.1056/NEJMoa1611391

[122] Ricci, Z., & Goldstein, S. L. (2016). Pediatric Continuous Renal Replacement Therapy. Contributions to nephrology, 187, 121–130. https://doi.org/10.1159/000442370

[123] Hayes, L. W., Oster, R. A., Tofil, N. M., & Tolwani, A. J. (2009). Outcomes of critically ill children requiring continuous renal replacement therapy. Journal of critical care, 24(3), 394–400. https://doi.org/10.1016/j.jcrc.2008.12.017

[124] Nolin, T. D., Aronoff, G. R., Fissell, W. H., Jain, L., Madabushi, R., Reynolds, K., Zhang, L., Huang, S. M., Mehrotra, R., Flessner, M. F., Leypoldt, J. K., Witcher, J. W., Zineh, I., Archdeacon, P., Roy-Chaudhury, P., Goldstein, S. L., & Kidney Health Initiative (2015). Pharmacokinetic assessment in patients receiving continuous RRT: perspectives from the Kidney Health Initiative. Clinical journal of the American Society of Nephrology: CJASN, 10(1), 159–164. https://doi.org/10.2215/CJN.05630614

[125] Buck M. L. (2003). Pharmacokinetic changes during extracorporeal membrane oxygenation: implications for drug therapy of neonates. Clinical pharmacokinetics, 42 (5), 403–417. https://doi.org/10.2165/00003088-200342050-00001

[126] Watt, K., Li, J. S., Benjamin, D. K., Jr, & Cohen-Wolkowiez, M. (2011). Pediatric cardiovascular drug dosing in critically ill children and extracorporeal membrane oxygenation. Journal of cardiovascular pharmacology, 58(2), 126–132. https://doi.org/10.1097/FJC.0b013e318213aac2

[127] Goldstein, S. L., & Nolin, T. D. (2014). Lack of drug dosing guidelines for critically ill patients receiving continuous renal replacement therapy. Clinical pharmacology and therapeutics, 96(2), 159–161. https://doi.org/10.1038/clpt.2014.102

[128] Lewis, S. J., & Mueller, B. A. (2014). Antibiotic dosing in critically ill patients receiving CRRT: underdosing is overprevalent. Seminars in dialysis, 27(5), 441–445. https://doi.org/10.1111/sdi.12203

[129] Centers for Disease Control and Prevention (CDC) (2006). Improved national prevalence estimates for 18 selected major birth defects–United States, 1999-2001. MMWR. Morbidity and mortality weekly report, 54(51), 1301–1305.

[130] Pritchard, M., Reeves, R. H., Dierssen, M., Patterson, D., & Gardiner, K. J. (2008). Down syndrome and the genes of human chromosome 21: current knowledge and future potentials. Report on the Expert workshop on the biology of chromosome 21 genes: towards gene-phenotype correlations in Down syndrome. Washington D.C., September 28-October 1, 2007. Cytogenetic and genome research, 121(1), 67–77. https://doi.org/10.1159/000124384

[131] Padmakumar, B., Evans Jones, L. G., & Sills, J. A. (2002). Is arthritis more common in children with Down syndrome?. Rheumatology (Oxford,

England), 41(10), 1191–1193. https://doi.org/10.1093/rheumatology/41.10.1191

[132] Garré, M. L., Relling, M. V., Kalwinsky, D., Dodge, R., Crom, W. R., Abromowitch, M., Pui, C. H., & Evans, W. E. (1987). Pharmacokinetics and toxicity of methotrexate in children with Down syndrome and acute lymphocytic leukemia. The Journal of pediatrics, 111(4), 606–612. https://doi.org/10.1016/s0022-3476(87)80131-2

[133] Peeters, M. A., Rethore, M. O., & Lejeune, J. (1995). In vivo folic acid supplementation partially corrects in vitro methotrexate toxicity in patients with Down syndrome. British journal of haematology, 89(3), 678–680. https://doi.org/10.1111/j.1365-2141.1995.tb08390.x

[134] Jones, J. T., Talib, N., Lovell, D., & Becker, M. L. (2019). Clinical Features and Treatment of Down Syndrome Arthropathy: Experience from Two US Tertiary Hospitals. Paediatric drugs, 21 (1), 33–39. https://doi.org/10.1007/s40272-018-0322-0

[135] Foley, C. M., Deely, D. A., MacDermott, E. J., & Killeen, O. G. (2019). Arthropathy of Down syndrome: an under-diagnosed inflammatory joint disease that warrants a name change. RMD open, 5(1), e000890. https://doi.org/10.1136/rmdopen-2018-000890

[136] Blatt, J., Albo, V., Prin, W., Orlando, S., & Wollman, M. (1986). Excessive chemotherapy-related myelotoxicity in children with Down syndrome and acute lymphoblastic leukaemia. Lancet (London, England), 2 (8512), 914. https://doi.org/10.1016/s0140-6736(86)90429-0

[137] Taub, J. W., & Ge, Y. (2005). Down syndrome, drug metabolism and chromosome 21. Pediatric blood & cancer, 44(1), 33–39. https://doi.org/10.1002/pbc.20092

[138] Uffmann, M., Rasche, M., Zimmermann, M., von Neuhoff, C., Creutzig, U., Dworzak, M., Scheffers, L., Hasle, H., Zwaan, C. M., Reinhardt, D., & Klusmann, J. H. (2017). Therapy reduction in patients with Down syndrome and myeloid leukemia: the international ML-DS 2006 trial. Blood, 129(25), 3314–3321. https://doi.org/10.1182/blood-2017-01-765057

[139] Taub, J. W., Huang, X., Matherly, L. H., Stout, M. L., Buck, S. A., Massey, G. V., Becton, D. L., Chang, M. N., Weinstein, H. J., & Ravindranath, Y. (1999). Expression of chromosome 21-localized genes in acute myeloid leukemia: differences between Down syndrome and non-Down syndrome blast cells and relationship to in vitro sensitivity to cytosine arabinoside and daunorubicin. Blood, 94(4), 1393–1400.

[140] Ogden, C. L., Carroll, M. D., Curtin, L. R., McDowell, M. A., Tabak, C. J., & Flegal, K. M. (2006). Prevalence of overweight and obesity in the United States, 1999-2004. JAMA, 295(13), 1549–1555. https://doi.org/10.1001/jama.295.13.1549

[141] Sherwin, J., Heath, T., & Watt, K. (2016). Pharmacokinetics and Dosing of Anti-infective Drugs in Patients on Extracorporeal Membrane Oxygenation: A Review of the Current Literature. Clinical therapeutics, 38(9), 1976–1994. https://doi.org/10.1016/j.clinthera.2016.07.169

[142] Srinivasan, V., Nadkarni, V. M., Helfaer, M. A., Carey, S. M., Berg, R. A., & American Heart Association National Registry of Cardiopulmonary Resuscitation Investigators (2010). Childhood obesity and survival after in-hospital pediatric cardiopulmonary resuscitation. Pediatrics, 125(3), e481–e488. https://doi.org/10.1542/peds.2009-1324

[143] Salvarani, C., Dolci, G., Massari, M., Merlo, D. F., Cavuto, S., Savoldi, L., Bruzzi, P., Boni, F., Braglia, L., Turrà, C., Ballerini, P. F., Sciascia, R., Zammarchi, L., Para, O., Scotton, P. G., Inojosa, W. O., Ravagnani, V., Salerno, N. D., Sainaghi, P. P., Brignone, A., ... RCT-TCZ-COVID-19 Study Group (2021). Effect of Tocilizumab vs Standard Care on Clinical Worsening in Patients Hospitalized With COVID-19 Pneumonia: A Randomized Clinical Trial. JAMA internal medicine, 181(1), 24–31. https://doi.org/10.1001/jamainternmed.2020.6615

[144] Walkey, A. J., Kumar, V. K., Harhay, M. O., Bolesta, S., Bansal, V., Gajic, O., & Kashyap, R. (2020). The Viral Infection and Respiratory Illness Universal Study (VIRUS): An International Registry of Coronavirus 2019-Related Critical Illness. Critical care explorations, 2(4), e0113. https://doi.org/10.1097/CCE.0000000000000113

[145] Kalil, A. C., Patterson, T. F., Mehta, A. K., Tomashek, K. M., Wolfe, C. R., Ghazaryan, V., Marconi, V. C., Ruiz-Palacios, G. M., Hsieh, L., Kline, S., Tapson, V., Iovine, N. M., Jain, M. K., Sweeney, D. A., El Sahly, H. M., Branche, A. R., Regalado Pineda, J., Lye, D. C., Sandkovsky, U., Luetkemeyer, A. F., ... ACTT-2 Study Group Members (2021). Baricitinib plus Remdesivir for Hospitalized Adults with Covid-19. The New England journal of medicine, 384 (9), 795–807. https://doi.org/10.1056/NEJMoa2031994

[146] Azzi, Y., Bartash, R., Scalea, J., Loarte-Campos, P., & Akalin, E. (2021). COVID-19 and Solid Organ Transplantation: A Review Article. Transplantation, 105(1), 37–55. https://doi.org/10.1097/TP.0000000000003523

[147] Lescure FX, Honda H, Fowler RA, Lazar JS, Shi G, Wung P, Patel N, Hagino O; Sarilumab COVID-19 Global Study Group. Sarilumab in patients admitted to hospital with severe or critical COVID-19: a randomised, double-blind, placebo-controlled, phase 3 trial. Lancet Respir Med. 2021 May;9 (5):522-532. doi: 10.1016/S2213-2600(21)00099-0.

[148] Salama, C., & Mohan, S. V. (2021). Tocilizumab in Patients Hospitalized with Covid-19 Pneumonia. Reply. The New England journal of medicine, 384 (15), 1473–1474. https://doi.org/10.1056/NEJMc2100217

[149] Guaraldi, G., Meschiari, M., Cozzi-Lepri, A., Milic, J., Tonelli, R., Menozzi, M., Franceschini, E., Cuomo, G., Orlando, G., Borghi, V., Santoro, A., Di Gaetano, M., Puzzolante, C., Carli, F., Bedini, A., Corradi, L., Fantini, R., Castaniere, I., Tabbì, L., Girardis, M., ... Mussini, C. (2020). Tocilizumab in patients with severe COVID-19: a retrospective cohort study. The Lancet. Rheumatology, 2(8), e474–e484. https://doi.org/10.1016/S2665-9913(20)30173-9

[150] Tsai, A., Diawara, O., Nahass, R. G., & Brunetti, L. (2020). Impact of tocilizumab administration on mortality in severe COVID-19. Scientific reports, 10(1), 19131. https://doi.org/10.1038/s41598-020-76187-y

[151] Fu, B., Xu, X., & Wei, H. (2020). Why tocilizumab could be an effective treatment for severe COVID-19?. Journal of translational medicine, 18(1), 164. https://doi.org/10.1186/s12967-020-02339-3

[152] Xu, X., Han, M., Li, T., Sun, W., Wang, D., Fu, B., Zhou, Y., Zheng, X., Yang, Y., Li, X., Zhang, X., Pan, A., & Wei, H. (2020). Effective treatment of severe COVID-19 patients with tocilizumab. Proceedings of the National Academy of Sciences of the United States of America, 117(20), 10970–10975. https://doi.org/10.1073/pnas.2005615117

[153] Dong, E., Du, H., & Gardner, L. (2020). An interactive web-based dashboard to track COVID-19 in real time. The Lancet. Infectious diseases, 20(5), 533–534. https://doi.org/10.1016/S1473-3099(20)30120-1

[154] Parr J. B. (2021). Time to Reassess Tocilizumab's Role in COVID-19 Pneumonia. JAMA internal medicine, 181(1), 12–15. https://doi.org/10.1001/jamainternmed.2020.6557

[155] Gupta, S., & Leaf, D. E. (2021). Tocilizumab in COVID-19: some clarity amid controversy. Lancet (London, England), 397(10285), 1599–1601. https://doi.org/10.1016/S0140-6736(21)00712-1

[156] Mariette, X., Hermine, O., Tharaux, P. L., Resche-Rigon, M., Steg, P. G., Porcher, R., & Ravaud, P. (2021). Effectiveness of Tocilizumab in Patients Hospitalized With COVID-19: A Follow-up of the CORIMUNO-TOCI-1 Randomized Clinical Trial. JAMA internal medicine, e212209. Advance online publication. https://doi.org/10.1001/jamainternmed.2021.2209

[157] Rosas, I. O., Bräu, N., Waters, M., Go, R. C., Hunter, B. D., Bhagani, S., Skiest, D., Aziz, M. S., Cooper, N., Douglas, I. S., Savic, S., Youngstein, T., Del Sorbo, L., Cubillo Gracian, A., De La Zerda, D. J., Ustianowski, A., Bao, M., Dimonaco, S., Graham, E., Matharu, B., ... Malhotra, A. (2021). Tocilizumab in Hospitalized Patients with Severe Covid-19 Pneumonia. The New England journal of medicine, 384(16), 1503–1516. https://doi.org/10.1056/NEJMoa2028700

Chapter 3

Racial Health Disparities in Coronavirus Deaths

Daniel L. Howard

Abstract

Preliminary racial data on the coronavirus pandemic indicates that African Americans are much more likely to experience infections, hospitalizations, and death from the virus in comparison to other racial groups. While this appears to be an alarming health outcome regarding African Americans, it is, in fact, not surprising, nor even new information, considering the historical context of racial health disparities and the marginal health of African Americans in the United States. The leading causes of death for African Americans generally and historically reflects the leading causes of death for the entire United States population. More research, and obviously data, is needed to fully understand the factors that cause the overall racial health disparities, in general, and racial disparities in coronavirus cases and deaths, in particular. In the case of the coronavirus pandemic, the racial disparities in deaths reflect racial differences in the way that African Americans live, work, and exist as a result of their 'second-class citizenship' with respect to their lower socioeconomic status in comparison to other racial groups. From a health policy perspective, challenges exist to reversing the current trend in coronavirus deaths among African Americans due to a myriad of historic, consistent, and pervasive societally-induced deficits within African American life. The proposed chapter will rely on systematic review of the extant literature on racial health disparities to identify multiple factors that may affect African American deaths due to the current coronavirus pandemic. The chapter will also rely on this framework to inform evidence-based approaches to improve public health for African Americans.

Keywords: African Americans, race, health disparities, health equity, social determinants of health, coronavirus, COVID-19

1. Introduction

Preliminary racial data on the coronavirus pandemic indicates that African Americans are much more likely to experience infections, hospitalizations, and death from the virus in comparison to other racial groups. Of the 25,152,433 cases of COVID-19 infections and 419,827 deaths due to this infection in the United States as of January 26, 2021 (**Table 1**), the percentage of African Americans (12.2%) and Hispanics (20.8%) experience coronavirus infections (**Table 2**) near their representative percentages in the general population (13.4% and 18.5%, respectively) (**Table 3**). In addition, African Americans, Hispanics, and American Indians are among the highest proportion of individuals with laboratory-confirmed COVID-related hospitalizations per 100,000 population (564, 524.2, and 645.7, respectively) compared to whites (261.9) (**Table 4**). Finally, a higher percentage of African Americans (15.6%), specifically and uniquely,

Confirmed cases	25,152,433
Deaths	419,827

CDC/Updated: Jan 26 2021 12:16 PM.

Table 1.
Coronavirus confirmed infections and total deaths in the United States.

Race/Ethnicity	Percentage	Count
Hispanic/Latino	20.8	1,998,031
American Indian/Alaska Native, Non-Hispanic	1.3	126,045
Asian, Non-Hispanic	3.6	344,630
Black, Non-Hispanic	12.2	1,171,902
Native Hawaiian/Other Pacific Islander, Non-Hispanic	0.4	35,183
White, Non-Hispanic	55.8	5,353,940
Multiple/Other, Non-Hispanic	6	571,110

CDC/Updated: Jan 26 2021 12:16 PM. Data from 18,807,907 cases. Race/Ethnicity was available for 9,600,841 (51%) cases.

Table 2.
Percent of coronavirus infections by racial groups (as of January 26, 2021).

Self-Identified Race	*Percent of Population*
Non-Hispanic white	60.1%
Hispanic and Latino (of any race)	18.5%
Black or African American	13.4%
Asian	5.9%
Two or more races	2.8%
Native Americans and Alaska Natives	1.3%
Native Hawaiians and Other Pacific Islanders	0.2%

US Census Bureau April 1 2020 Estimates (web). United States Census Bureau. April 2020. Retrieved January 26, 2021.

Table 3.
2019 U.S. Census Bureau estimates.

Overall	380.3
White	261.9
Black	564
Hispanic/Latino	524.2
Asian/Pacific Islander	214.6
American Indian/Alaskan Native	645.7

COVID-NET: COVID-19 Associated Hospitalization Surveillance Network, Centers for Disease Control and Prevention. WEBSITE. Accessed January 26, 2021.

Table 4.
Percent of laboratory-confirmed Covid diagnosis hospitalizations per 100,000 by racial groups (as of January 16, 2021).

Race/Ethnicity	Percentage	Count
Hispanic/Latino	13.1	30,338
American Indian/Alaska Native, Non-Hispanic	1	2,349
Asian, Non-Hispanic	4.3	9,847
Black, Non-Hispanic	15.6	36,207
Native Hawaiian/Other Pacific Islander, Non-Hispanic	0.2	532
White, Non-Hispanic	61.5	142,411
Multiple/Other, Non-Hispanic	4.2	9,686

CDC/Updated: Jan 26 2021 12:16 PM. Data from 298,564 deaths. Race/Ethnicity was available for 231,370 (77%) deaths.

Table 5.
Percent of coronavirus deaths by racial groups.

experience death from this infection at a much higher percentage than they are represented in the general population (**Table 5**).

While this appears to be an alarming health outcome regarding African Americans, it is, in fact, not surprising, nor even new information, considering the historical context of racial health disparities and the marginal health of African Americans in the United States. In a co-authored article entitled, "The Color Line and the Health of African Americans" [1], I noted that one of the first examinations of African American health was in the W.E.B. DuBois classic study of the Philadelphia Black population of the late 1880s, *The Philadelphia Negro*, which revealed that the death rate of Philadelphia Blacks was higher in comparison to other populations [1, 2]. In fact, other early examinations of Black health status noted historically that African Americans have greater morbidity and mortality than other Americans [3–5]. And, many studies since have consistently shown that African Americans live sicker and die younger than other racial groups [6].

The leading causes of death for African Americans generally and historically reflects the leading causes of death for the entire United States population [6]. In 2017, these included diseases of the heart, cancer, stroke, homicide (specific to Blacks only), and unintentional injuries [7]. Moreover, the health status of African Americans identifies a higher prevalence of cardiovascular diseases, cancer, hypertension, diabetes, obesity, and sexually transmitted infections, i.e., HIV infections, when compared with whites [6, 7]. The projected deaths from coronavirus in 2020, with estimates in the hundreds of thousands to millions and its predominance among African Americans, will undoubtedly catapult it into the top five of leading causes of death for African Americans [8].

As a result of this pervasive deficit in health status and health outcome among African Americans, a "Task Force on Black and Minority Health" was established in 1984 by the U.S. Department of Health and Human Services that resulted in the landmark "Heckler Report" in 1985 [9, 10]. This report by Secretary Heckler marked the first convening of a group of health experts by the U.S. government to conduct a comprehensive study of racial and ethnic minority health and elevated minority health to a national stage [10]. The term 'racial health disparity' was coined shortly thereafter [11, 12], which is defined as differences in the incidence, prevalence, mortality and burden of diseases and other adverse health conditions that exist among specific populations in the United States [13]. In 2000, Congress passed The Minority Health and Health Disparities Research and Education Act (Public Law 106–525) to address "the significant disparity in the overall rate of disease incidence, prevalence, morbidity, mortality or survival rates." The Act created the National *Center* on Minority Health and Health and Health Disparities at the National Institutes of Health (NIH). This Center was re-designated as one of twenty-one [14] preeminent *Institutes* of Research, each with a specific research agenda and independent ability to set its own funding priorities and strategies, at NIH in 2010, as part of The Patient Protection and Affordable Care Act (Public Law 111–148), or colloquially known as 'Obamacare', with the stated mission to "lead scientific research to improve minority health and eliminate health disparities."

More research, and obviously data, is needed to fully understand the factors that cause the overall racial health disparities, in general, and racial disparities in coronavirus cases and deaths, in particular. But, to do so, we must first understand 'what is race' and how is it related to health? [15] Earlier research on racial differences in health had been dominated by a genetic model that views race as primarily reflecting biological homogeneity, and Black-White differences in health as largely genetically-determined [15, 16]. More recent, rigorous, and comprehensive examinations of racial differences in health suggest, however, that race is a societally constructed taxonomy that reflects the intersection of particular historical conditions with economic, political, legal, social, and cultural factors, as well as mistrust of the medical care system and racism pertaining to biases in the quality of medical care received [15–17]. Macrosocial factors and position within social statuses also most often affect health through intermediary mechanisms and process such as health behavior, mistrust of the medical care system, stress, quality of medical care received, and a broad range of social, psychological, cultural, and religious resources [17]. Therefore, to understand the complex relationship between race and health, these factors have to be considered, which are known as 'social determinants of health' [18–21]. Thus, it is more correct to view race as a proxy variable for, or an influence of, many aspects of the health care experience that subsequently impact health outcome, rather than a direct influence on health outcome [14, 22].

'Health equity' -- the absence of health disparities in controllable or remediable aspects of health, i.e., social justice -- arises from having access to the social determinants of health, specifically those related to wealth, power and prestige [23, 24]. In the case of the coronavirus pandemic, the racial disparities in deaths reflect racial differences in the way that African Americans live, work, and exist as a result of their 'second-class citizenship' with respect to their lower socioeconomic status in comparison to other racial groups.

As noted, the health status of African Americans identifies a higher prevalence of cardiovascular diseases, cancer, hypertension, diabetes, obesity, and sexually transmitted infections, i.e., HIV infections, when compared with whites. Higher rates of coronavirus among African Americans may be due to being more likely to have comorbidities, which has been noted as a significant risk factor for coronavirus death [6, 7].

Minority racial groups are more likely to experience multidimensional poverty than their White counterparts [25]. Higher rates of coronavirus among African Americans may be due to being less likely to have basic resources or access to basic resources to provide protection against the virus, i.e., masks, gloves, sanitized wipes, etc.

The nation is largely segregated, leaving racial groups exposed to different health risks and with variable access to health services based on where they live [26]. Higher rates of coronavirus among African Americans may be due to being more likely to co-exist around others in their respective densely-populated neighborhoods and communities who are at higher risk from contracting the virus. And, there may be limited facilities to seek care in these neighborhoods and communities that have less resources.

As of 2018, most groups of color remained more likely to be uninsured compared to Whites. Moreover, despite the larger coverage increases for groups of color, the relative risk of being uninsured compared to Whites did not improve for some groups [27]. For example, Blacks remained 1.5 times more likely to be uninsured than Whites from 2010 to 2018 [27]. Higher rates of coronavirus among African Americans may be due to being more likely to be uninsured and, therefore, less likely to receive medical care after contraction of coronavirus.

U.S. Census Data from 2010 revealed that whites have the country's highest homeownership rate, while those identifying as being African American had the lowest homeownership rate, by almost half [28]. Higher rates of coronavirus among African Americans may be due to being more likely to live in densely-populated apartments and other multi-person dwellings, rather than single-family homes, which reduces the ability to self-isolate and increases the exposures for contracting the virus.

12.4 percent of African-American college graduates between the ages of 22 and 27 were unemployed in 2013, which is more than double the rate of unemployment among all college graduates in the same age range, 5.6 percent [29]. African American unemployment rates are typically double that of whites. African-American men working full-time earn only 72 percent of the average earnings of comparable white men and 85 percent of the earnings of white women [30]. Moreover, a national review of 2015 data on white-collar employment showed that white men are 61.3% of executives nationally and 81% above parity when compared with their 33.8% representation in non-management professionals [31]. African American men and women still represent a very low percentage of the professional white-collar workforce (less than 8%), given their overall representation in the population [31]. Higher rates of coronavirus among African Americans may be due to being more likely to work in customer service, technical, and support staff positions or in the 'gig economy' i.e., Uber and Lyft, which require more interaction with the public and increases the exposures for contracting the virus, rather than in more professional positions, which are more likely to allow the ability to work from home.

Researchers examined 2000 U.S. Census data to find that Black households were much less likely to own a car than were white households, identifying a growing gap between car ownership in white and black households that spanned income levels [32]. 19% of African Americans reported living in a household without access to a vehicle [31]. 4.6% of White Americans reported living in a home without access to a vehicle [32]. Higher rates of coronavirus among African Americans may be due to being more likely to use public transportation, i.e., subways and busses, to get to work, which reduces the ability to socially-distance and increases the exposures for contracting the virus.

The Pew Research Center 2014 US Religious Landscape Survey indicated that 47% of Blacks attend religious services at least once a week in comparison to 34% of whites [33]. Higher rates of coronavirus among African Americans may be due to being more likely to comingle in public spaces with many other individuals, rather than practice social distancing, particularly at the advent of the spread of the coronavirus and prior to public health messaging to stay at home and to avoid large gatherings.

Morbidity and mortality rates among African American may be influenced by the healthcare seeking behaviors of this population. Eley et al. findings confirm the importance of social relationships in influencing African American health-seeking behaviors and offer characterization of the nature of influence across different types of relationships: family, culture and upbringing, and peers [34]. For African American men, beliefs about masculinity and manhood that are deeply rooted in culture play a role in shaping the behavioral patterns of men in ways that have consequences for health [35]. Men are socialized to project strength, individuality, autonomy, dominance, stoicism and physical aggression, and to avoid demonstrations of emotion or vulnerability that could be construed as weakness [35]. These norms can translate into African American men "toughing it out" through fewer encounters with the health care system, delayed attention to symptoms, poor medication compliance, and an unwillingness to talk openly about health concerns [36]. For African American women, the literature on the reasons why individuals may miss healthcare appointments suggest that socioeconomic reasons may play a major factor [37]. African American women are more like to be single, employed, and the sole provider of her children in comparison to white women [38]. Pavik et al. indicated that full-time employment (not being able to get off work) is a reason for missing a breast examination appointment [39]. Taplin et al. noted that those attending a clinic more than 45 minutes from the breast cancer screening center was negatively associated with subsequently obtaining a breast mammogram [40]. Blankton et al. suggested that lack of transportation is the main reason for missed healthcare appointments [41]. Higher rates of coronavirus deaths among African Americans may be due to racial differences in healthcare seeking behavior as a result of sociocultural and/or socioeconomic issues.

In the United States, the more vulnerable segments of the population were also the most unwitting subjects of medical experimentation, but African Americans, including children, bore a disproportionate burden and suffered the most brutal, invasive, and perilous of the medical experiments [5]. The infamous Tuskegee Syphilis Study from 1932 to 1972 is most illustrative of this and may resonate the most with respect to African American's lack of trust in the medical care system [5]. Medical mistrust is thought to affect health care–based decisions and has been linked to poor health outcomes [42]. Previous work has demonstrated that medical mistrust is not significantly associated with failure to receive needed medical care; however, medical mistrust can serve as a barrier to optimal health [43]. Higher levels of medical mistrust have been found to be associated with failure to take medical advice, failure to keep follow-up appointments, and postponement of receiving needed care [43]. Higher rates of coronavirus deaths among African Americans may be due to mistrust in the medical care system, in general, and physicians, in particular, which may specifically impact compliance with healthcare instructions and more broadly, with public health messaging.

Unequal Treatment: Confronting Racial and Ethnic Disparities in Health Care, a 2003 book by a panel of national experts convened by the Institute of Medicine, revealed that racial and ethnic disparities in health care are known to reflect access to care and other issues that arise from differing socioeconomic conditions [6]. However, the book further reports that there is increasing evidence that even after such differences are accounted for, race and ethnicity remain significant predicators of the quality of health care received [6]. A number of studies by this author corroborate *Unequal Treatment* as pervasive and consistent racial differences and disparities in the medical treatment that African Americans have received in comparison to whites are indicated [44–49]. These differences and disparities exist for a myriad of medical conditions and procedures and in spite of controlling for insurance status and for income. For instance, studies have revealed that the occurrence of urinary symptoms by African American men does not necessarily result in the receipt of further diagnostic tests [50]. African Africans were less likely than whites to have regular digital rectal exams (DREs) by physicians. Moreover, African Americans were more likely to not received DREs at all. In contrast, whites were more likely to receive a DRE every year as recommended by the American Cancer Society guidelines. This result is consistent in the Flint Study of African American men with prostate cancer that showed that few of these men sought and received for urinary complaints [51]. In contrast, the solicitation of medical care for white men has been demonstrated to be a function of symptom severity, according to the Olmsted Study of white men with prostate cancer [52]. Higher rates of coronavirus deaths among African Americans may be due to inherent racial biases in the medical care system that impact the quality of medical care received after contraction of coronavirus.

Finally, satisfaction with medical care is increased when physicians are attentive, give patients the chance to relay information in their own way, provide more information, and share control of the termination of the medical interaction [53, 54]. In general, practitioners who use a more companionable communicative style characterized by warmth, empathy, genuineness, and a nonjudgmental attitude rather than a controlling, authoritative style received more favorable evaluations by patients. According to Auslander et al., ineffective communication can be caused by a lack of sensitivity to the cultural values, norms, and environmental contexts of patients of races or ethnicities other than those of the provider [54]. African Americans are less likely to be satisfied with the medical care that they do receive, which, again, may directly impact their use of health care services [55]. In a study of the impact that physicians trained at international medical schools (IMGs) in comparison with physicians trained at United States medical schools (USMGs) have on the satisfaction with medical care and health care-seeking behaviors of an oversampled racial cohort of urban and rural elders, Howard et al., found that for African Americans, perception of IMGs is directly related to issues of cultural competency, communication, and ageism [55]. Higher rates of coronavirus deaths among African Americans may be a result of dissatisfaction with the medical care system that dampens their pursuit of needed medical care services.

2. Conclusion

Challenges exist to reversing the current trend in coronavirus deaths among African Americans due to a myriad of historic, consistent, and pervasive societally-induced deficits within African American life. However, these are only a few of the possible factors that cause the overall racial health disparities and, in particular, influence the disproportionately high rate of coronavirus deaths among African Americans. Only a qualitative research assessment of the lives of these unfortunate individuals as well as analysis of the corresponding data will begin to provide the answers as to why these outcomes are occurring.

3. Implications

In general, the provision of widespread testing and monitoring for COVID-19 in African American communities would facilitate early detection among the symptomatic and asymptomatic infected; self-isolation and quarantine of both the symptomatic and asymptomatic infected will reduce the spread of the virus. Hospitalizations and adverse treatment outcomes could possibly be reduced by earlier treatment of the flu- and pneumonia-like symptoms before illness progression to the need for extensive medical stays and subsequent use of ventilation for lungs.

However, due to social determinants of health that convolute the relationship between race and health, substantial funding is necessary to promote health equity in the African American community during the coronavirus pandemic. For instance, due to the level of poverty, lower socio-economic status, and uninsured among African Americans, COVID-19 testing, vaccinations, as well as medical treatment for those suffering from coronavirus must be cost-free for these specific sub-groups of the African American community.

Further, not all adverse healthcare seeking behaviors can be address in the African American community as it relates to this current pandemic. But certainly, those healthcare seeking behaviors related to socio-economic factors, i.e., not being able to get off of work during traditional business hours, not having treatment facilities in proximity to poor, minority communities, and not having transportation to travel to these facilities, can be addressed. More COVID-19 testing and vaccination sites can be placed in African American communities and along or near major mass transportation routes. Hours of operation for testing and vaccination sites can be expanded to accommodate those African American workers with jobs that have less flexible schedules, i.e., customer service, technical, and support staff positions.

Finally, given the high level of mistrust of the medical system by African Americans, it is critical to build public health campaigns driven by leaders in the African American communities, and have oversight provided by community consortiums to ensure ethical, fair and safe practices in the administration of these tests and vaccines in order to enhance compliance that will facilitate the eradication of the coronavirus pandemic.

Conflict of interest

The author states that there is no conflict of interest.

Author details

Daniel L. Howard
Department of Psychological and Brain Sciences, College of Liberal Arts, Texas A&M University at College Station, College Station, TX, United States

*Address all correspondence to: dannhoward@tamu.edu

References

[1] LaVeist TA, Wallace JM, Howard DL. The Color Line and the Health of African Americans. *Humbolt Journal of Social Relations.* 1995 Vol.21:2, pp.119-137.

[2] DuBois WEB, 1899. The Philadelphia Negro. Millwood, NY: Kraus-Thomson Organization Limited. 1902. Of The Training of Black Men. Atlantic Monthly.

[3] Swados F. Negro Health on the Antebellum Plantations. *Bulletin of History of Medicine*. 1941; 10 (3): 460-472.

[4] Savitt T. The Use of Blacks for Medical Experimentation and Demonstration in the Old South. *Journal of Southern History*. 1982; 48 (3): 331-348.

[5] Washington, Harriet A. *Medical Apartheid: The Dark History of Medical Experimentation on Black Americans from Colonial Times to the Present*. New York: Doubleday, 2006.

[6] Smedley BD, Stith, AY, Nelson, AR (Eds.). Unequal treatment: Confronting racial and ethnic disparities in health care. Washington, DC: National Academies Press. 2003.

[7] Elflein, J. Leading causes of death among black U.S. residents in 2017. State of Health. Statista, Hamburg, Germany 2019.

[8] Thomas McAndrew. "COVID19-Expert Forecast-Survey5-20200316.pdf" (2020) Available at: http://works.bepress.com/mcandrew/2/

[9] Secretary's Task Force on Black and Minority Health (1985). Black and Minority Health Report the Secretary's Task Force. Washington, DC: Department of Health and Human Services. http://minorityhealth.hhs.gov/assets/ pdf/checked/1/ANDERSON.pdf

[10] Department of Health and Human Services, *Perspectives in Disease Prevention and Health Promotion Report of the Secretary's Task Force on Black and Minority Health*. Centers for Disease Control, Morbidity and Mortality Weekly Report February 28, 1986 / 35 (8):109-12.

[11] Carter-Pokras O, Baquet C. What is a "health disparity"? *Public Health Report*. 2002; 117(5), 426-434.

[12] Braveman P. What are health disparities and health equity? We need to be clear. *Public Health Rep*. 2014;129 Suppl 2(Suppl 2):5-8. doi:10.1177/00333549141291S203.

[13] Office of Minority Health (2011). HHS Action Plan to Reduce Racial and Ethnic Health Disparities. A nation free of disparities in health and health care. http://minorityhealth.hhs.gov/npa/files/Plans/HHS/HHS_Plan_complete.pdf

[14] Howard, Daniel L., Thomas A. LaVeist and William C. McCaughrin. *The Effect of Social Environment on Treatment Outcomes in Outpatient Substance Misuse Treatment Organizations: Does Race Really Matter? Substance Use and Misuse*. 1996; 31(5), pp.617-638.

[15] Howard, Daniel L. *The Meaning of Race Within Health Services Research: Biologically* Significant, Social/Political Label, or Composite Proxy? African American Research *Perspectives.* Spring/Summer 2002; Vol. 8, No.1, pp.55-59.

[16] LaVeist TA. Beyond Sample Selection and Dummy Variables: What Health Services Researchers Ought to Know about Race as a Variable. HSR: Health Services Research. 1994; 29:1 (April) 1-16.

[17] Williams DR. *The Concept of Race in Health Services Research: 1966-1990. HSR:*

Health Services Research. 1994; 29(3): 261-274.

[18] Secretary's Advisory Committee on Health Promotion and Disease Prevention Objectives for 2020. *Healthy People 2020: An Opportunity to Address the Societal Determinants of Health in the United States*. July 26, 2010. Available from: http://www.healthypeople.gov/2010/hp2020/advisory/SocietalDeterminantsHealth.htm

[19] World Health Organization, Commission on Social Determinants of Health. *Closing the Gap in a Generation: Health equity through action on the social determinants of health*. Available from: http://www.who.int/social_determinants/en

[20] National Partnership for Action: HHS Action Plan to Reduce Racial and Ethnic Health Disparities, 2011; and The National Stakeholder Strategy for Achieving Health Equity, 2011. Available from: http://minorityhealth.hhs.gov/npa

[21] The National Prevention and Health Promotion Strategy. *The National Prevention Strategy: America's Plan for Better Health and Wellness*, June 2011. Available from: https://www.surgeongeneral.gov/priorities/prevention/strategy/index.html

[22] Howard, Daniel L., Roy Penchansky, and Morton S. Brown. *Disaggregating the Effects of Race on Breast Cancer Survival*. *Family Medicine*. 1998; 30(3), pp.228-235.

[23] *Braveman, P; Gruskin (21 October 2002).* "Defining Equity in Health" (PDF). *Theory and Methods. 57 (4): 254-258.* doi:10.1136/jech.57.4.254. PMC 1732430. PMID 12646539 – *via* https://jech.bmj.com/content/jech/57/4/254.full.pdf.

[24] *Goldberg DS. "Justice, Compound Disadvantage, and Health Inequities", Public Health Ethics and the Social Determinants of Health, SpringerBriefs in Public Health, Springer International Publishing, 2017; pp. 17-32,* doi:10.1007/978-3-319-51347-8_3, ISBN 978-3-319-51345-4

[25] Reeves, Richard, Edward Rodrigue, and Elizabeth Kneebone. Five Evils: Multidimensional Poverty and Race in America. The Brookings Institution. April 2006.

[26] LaVeist T, Pollack K, Thorpe R Jr, Fesahazion R, Gaskin D. Place, not race: disparities dissipate in southwest Baltimore when blacks and whites live under similar conditions. Health Aff (Millwood). 2011;30(10):1880-1887. doi:10.1377/hlthaff.2011.0640

[27] Artiga, Samantha, Kendal Orgera, and Anthony Damico. *Changes in Health Coverage by Race and Ethnicity since the ACA, 2010-2018.* Henry J. Kaiser Family Foundation. March 5, 2020.

[28] U.S. Census Bureau, Home Ownership by Race. Retrieved 4/10/2020.

[29] Jones, Janelle and John Schmitt. A College Degree is No Guarantee. Center for Economic and Policy Research, Washington DC. May 2014.

[30] Rodgers III, Williams. *Understanding the Black-White Earnings Gap: Why Do African Americans continue to earn less despite dramatic gains in education?* The American Prospect. September 19, 2008.

[31] Gee, M. *Why Aren't Black Employees Getting More White-Collar Jobs?* Harvard Business Review. Harvard Business Publishing. February 28, 2018.

[32] Raphael, S., Berube, A., & Deakin, E. (2006). Socioeconomic Differences in Household Automobile Ownership Rates: Implications for Evacuation Policy. *UC Berkeley: University of California Transportation Center*.

Retrieved from https://escholarship.org/uc/item/7bp4n2f6

[33] The Pew Center. Religious Landscape Study. Attendance at religious services by race/ethnicity (2014). Retrieved 4/10/2020.

[34] Natalie T. Eley, Emily Namey, Kevin McKenna, Annette Carrington Johnson, Greg Guest. Beyond the Individual: Social and Cultural Influences on the Health-Seeking Behaviors of African American Men. American Journal of Men's Health, Volume: 13 issue: 1, https://doi.org/10.1177/1557988319829953 PMID: 30767594

[35] Williams, D. R. (2003). The health of men: Structured inequalities and opportunities. American Journal of Public Health, 93(5), 724-731. doi:10.2105/AJPH.93.5.724

[36] Liburd, L. C., Namageyo-Funa, A., Jack, L. (2007). Understanding "masculinity" and the challenges of managing type-2 diabetes among African-American men. Journal of the National Medical Association, 99(5), 550-552, 554-558.

[37] Howard, Daniel L., Roy Penchansky, and Morton S. Brown. Disaggregating the Effects of Race on Breast Cancer Survival. Family Medicine,30(3), pp.228-235,1998.

[38] Brundage, Vernon. Labor Market Activity Of Blacks In The United States. Division of Labor Force Statistics, U.S. Bureau of Labor Statistics. February 2020.

[39] Pavik VN, Hyman DJ, Vallbona C, et al. Response rates to randomdigit dialing for recruiting participants to an onsite health study. PublicHealth Rep 1996; Sep-Oct:444-50.29.

[40] Taplin SH, Anderman C, Grothaus L, Curry S, Montano D. Using physician correspondence and postcard reminders to promote mammography use. Am J Public Health 1994;84(4):571-4.30.

[41] Blankton ML, Goldenberg RL, Keith B. Noncompliance of high-risk pregnant women in keeping appointments at an obstetric com-plications clinic. South Med J 1994;87(6):634-8.

[42] Ballington L. Kinlock, Laurie J. Parker, Janice V. Bowie, Daniel L. Howard, Thomas A. LaVeist, Roland J. Thorpe Jr. *High Levels of Medical Mistrust is Associated with Low Quality of Life among Black and White Men with Prostate Cancer.* Cancer Control: Journal of the Moffitt Cancer Center. January 2017, Vol. 24, No. 1:72-77.

[43] LaVeist TA, Isaac LA, Williams KP. Mistrust of health care organizations is associated with underutilization of health services. Health Serv Res. 2009;44:2093-2105.

[44] Howard, Daniel L., Yhenneko J. Taylor and Louie E . Ross. *Differences in Lower Urinary Tract Symptoms, Treatment and Mortality among African-American and White Elderly Men.* Journal of the National Medical Association Vol. 100, No.10, pp. 1146-1152, October 2008.

[45] Gooden, Kyna M., Daniel L. Howard, WR Carpenter, AP Carson, YJ Taylor, S Peacock, PA Godley. The Effect of Hospital and Physician Volume on Racial Differences in Recurrence-Free Survival After Radical Prostatectomy. Medical Care 2008; 46: 1170-1176.

[46] Howard Daniel L., Nadine J. Barrett, DaJuanicia N. Holmes. *Can Cultural Competency Speak to the Race Disparities in Methadone Dosage Levels?* Review of Black Political Economy Vol. 37, No. 1, pp. 7-23, March 2010.

[47] Carpenter WR, Howard DL, Taylor YJ, Ross LE, Wobker SE, Godley PA. *Racial differences in PSA screening interval and stage at diagnosis.* Cancer Causes Control. 2010 Mar 24.

[48] Carson AP, Howard DL, Carpenter WR, Taylor YJ, Peacock S, Schenck AP, Godley PA. *Trends and Racial Differences in the Use of Androgen Deprivation Therapy for Metastatic Prostate Cancer.* Journal of Pain and Symptom Management. 2010 May; 39(5):872-881.

[49] Ballington L. Kinlock, Roland J. Thorpe Jr., Daniel L. Howard, David Fakunle, Janice V. Bowie, Louie E. Ross, Thomas A. LaVeist. *Racial Disparity in the time between being diagnosed and initial treatment of Prostate Cancer*. Cancer Control; Journal of the Moffitt Cancer Center. January 2016, Vol. 23, No. 1.

[50] Howard, Daniel L., Bennett G. Edwards, Kimberly Whitehead, M. Ahinee Amamoo, and Paul A. Godley. *Healthcare practices among blacks and whites with urinary tract symptoms.* Journal of the National Medical Association Vol.99, No.4, pp.404-411, April 2007.

[51] Wei JT, Schottenfeld D, Cooper K, Taylor JM, Faerber GJ, Velarde MA, Bree R, Montie JE, Cooney KA. The natural history of lower urinary tract symptoms in black American men: relationships with aging, prostate size, flow rate and bothersomeness. J Urol. 2001 May;165(5):1521-5. PMID: 11342910.

[52] Jacobsen SJ, Jacobson DJ, Girman CJ, Roberts RO, Rhodes T, Guess HA, Lieber MM. Treatment for benign prostatic hyperplasia among community dwelling men: the Olmsted County study of urinary symptoms and health status. J Urol. 1999 Oct;162(4):1301-6. PMID: 10492184.

[53] Anderson, B. J., W. F. Auslander, K. C. Jung, J. P. Miller, and J. V. Santiago. 1990. "Assessing Family Sharing of Diabetes Responsibilities." Journal of Pediatric Psychology 15 (4): 477-92.

[54] Auslander, W. F., S. J. Thompson, D. Dreitzer, and J. V. Santiago. 1997. "Mothers' Satisfaction with Medical Care: Perceptions of Racism, Family Stress, and Medical Outcomes in Children with Diabetes." Health and Social Work 22 (3): 190-9.

[55] Howard, Daniel L., Carol D. Bunch, Wilberforce O. Mundia, Thomas R. Konrad, Lloyd J. Edwards, M. Ahinee Amamoo, and Yhenneko Jallah. *Comparing United States Vs. International Medical School Graduate Physicians Who Serve African American and White Elderly.* HSR: Health Services Research 41:6 (December 2006).

Chapter 4

Impact of COVID-19 on Oral and Dental Health Delivery and Recommendations for Continuation of Oral and Dental Health Services

Fatih Özçelik and Dursun Ali Şirin

Abstract

COVID-19, which has caused a great panic by leaving millions of deaths in its wake worldwide, has affected the provision of oral and dental health services as in many fields. Especially dentists, who offer oral and dental health services by working in the oral region of the patients, are under a high risk of encountering the agent. This high risk has justifiably created a concern for them. Therefore, it has been quite challenging to provide oral and dental health services. In order to alleviate these concerns and to sustain oral and dental health services, many health organizations and institutions, especially the World Health Organization, have published recommendations and principles of practice, and announced financial support. In this section, we will examine the recommendations and practices regarding infection prevention and control measures by getting away from standard routine health service practices in order to be protected from COVID-19 epidemic and what areas they cover on a wide scale. By discussing the effects of these recommendations and practices on the provision of dental health services, we will try to determine the practices that will relieve concerns and are aimed at ensuring the provision of safe health services in terms of both patients' health and health professionals' health.

Keywords: SARS-CoV-2, Dental Care Delivery, Recommendations for Dental Service

1. Introduction

The novel coronavirus 2019 is a member of the Coronaviridae family. In fact, this single-stranded RNA virus, whose natural habitat is animals, was reported to be transmittable from animals to humans. The disease caused by this virus, known as SARS-CoV-2, was named Coronavirus disease-19 (COVID-19) because it was first detected in 2019 [1–4]. This virus can involve the liver and the intestinal, respiratory and nervous systems, as well as causing major damage to the lungs in severe cases, and it may also lead to acute respiratory distress syndrome (ARDS) and death [5]. The disease originated in the city of Wuhan in the Hubei province of China due to consumption of animals contaminated with the SARS-CoV-2 virus. Later, it spread around the world, causing millions of people to become ill and many of them to die. The pandemic caused by the virus changed the social life of all humanity and forced all health groups, including dental treatment providers, professionally [6–9].

All people in the world are susceptible to COVID-19. However, older people (≥55 years), those with comorbidities such as diabetes mellitus, hypertension, heart disease, chronic lung disease, malignancy and kidney disease and smokers are more susceptible to COVID-19 disease in comparison to the young and healthy population [5, 9–13]. Additionally, in a study, it was found that COVID-19 had a more severe course in those with poor oral and dental health in conjunction with immune system deficiency [14]. Healthcare professionals come first in terms of the risk of exposure to the virus. Among them, the risk of those working on the oral cavity was found to be higher [15–18]. If this risk is compared to the work done by other healthcare professionals, it is thought to be close to that of staff in laboratories where the virus is directly analyzed, or the bodily fluids of COVID-19 patients are studied. The role and risks of laboratory medicine in times of epidemics of infectious diseases are already well-known [19, 20].

Therefore, in this section, we will first discuss the possible relationships between dental and oral health and the course of COVID-19. Then, we will discuss the precautions that dental providers should take while working and the issues they should pay attention to.

2. Recommendations of international dental organizations

Many dentists have avoided making appointments except for patients in emergency cases due to the COVID-19 pandemic. The American Dental Association (ADA), American Dental Hygienist' Association (ADHA) and Centers for Disease Control and Prevention (CDC) raised a new debate by encouraging dentists and other healthcare professionals to balance the need to provide essential services while minimizing risk in caring for at-risk patients in their area [15, 21, 22]. The Interim Infection Prevention and Control Guidance for Dental Settings During the Coronavirus Disease 2019 (COVID-19) Pandemic, as the topic of discussion, chose the question "Are dentistry facilities safe?" Like these interim guides in the United States, many European and Asian countries have published guidelines based on recent information about COVID-19 or inspired by the countries where the disease was first seen. Most of the recommendations in these updated guidelines are not new. A summary of some recommendations and practices are shown in **Table 1**.

1	Recommended infection prevention and control (IPC) practices for routine dental healthcare delivery during the pandemic
2	Recommended IPC practices during dental healthcare delivery to a patient with suspected or confirmed SARS-CoV-2 infection
3	Resumption of work criteria for healthcare workers with suspected or confirmed COVID-19 (Interim Guidance)
4	Strategies to reduce the lack of health personnel and methods of working alternately
5	Risk assessment and recommendations on working restrictions for dental healthcare providers and other healthcare professionals who are likely to be exposed to the coronavirus disease 2019
6	Termination of measures and treatment due to transmission of COVID-19 during dental care delivery

Table 1.
Some recommendations and practices.

3. Measures to protect individuals from the COVID-19 outbreak

In order to be protected from the COVID-19 pandemic, CDC recommends additional infection prevention and control measures to be applied for all patients in addition to standard routine healthcare practices due to the nature of the pandemic. Some of these guidelines a applicable to all settings where healthcare services are provided, while others are not designed for environments other than health-care facilities (e.g., restaurants, cafes, shopping malls, entertainment centers). Guidelines generally include information about the ways of transmission of COVID-19, patient care and management, patient triage protocols, complications that may develop due to the disease, telehealth strategies, various transportation vehicles and medical equipment transportation, or laboratory working conditions and raising awareness. For example, while requesting a dental examination for patients with suspected or confirmed SARS-CoV-2 infection, it is recommended to use triage protocols to understand whether this appointment is necessary or whether the patient can be managed from home in quarantine conditions. COVID-19 patients who complete the 14-day isolation period at home can benefit from dental healthcare by following standard precautions. Hand disinfectants containing ≥70% alcohol, antiviral-antibacterial wipes and disposable materials are required to be kept in the entrance areas of healthcare facilities and waiting rooms, and patients are required to be informed with various warning signs. Like all citizens, all healthcare professionals, including dentists, are warned about certain safety rules. From the simplest to the most complex, publications are constantly being updated to protect people against the SARS-CoV-2 virus. Accordingly, your dentist and other healthcare professionals working with them should wash their hands before and after each procedure and sterilize the instruments. It is emphasized that especially some dental tools and needles should never be reused. Most dental procedures in dentistry produce significant amounts of droplets (>5 μm), as well as aerosols (5 μm), although not approved by the World Health Organization (WHO) as a general route of transmission. These droplets and aerosols create a potentially high risk of infection transmission [15–18, 23]. Due to this very close contact, a high viral load may be encountered when transmission through droplets occurs. However, considering that thousands of droplets or aerosols may be spread even while speaking, we need to understand well that we are facing a virus that chose the most difficult form of transmission to be protected from [24]. Transmission may occur by contact other than droplets. Direct contact with urine, tears, respiratory secretions, mouth secretions and blood is considered risky [9, 25–27].

As known, since the morbidity and mortality of COVID-19 is closely related to age, immune system deficiencies, presence of chronic diseases and especially viral load [17, 28], due to the nature of the profession (working in the oral cavity), the field of dentistry is included in the high risk category. For this reason, if procedures that can create aerosol during dental care are applied, four-handed dentistry, high evacuation suction and dental dams should be used to minimize the amounts of aerosols and droplets that are created [15, 16, 18].

In line with IPC recommendations, patients in the 14-day quarantine period based on prolonged close contact with someone with SARS-CoV-2 infection and not yet confirmed to be COVID-19-negative by a polymerase chain reaction (PCR) test should be isolated and not categorized in a cohort with patients with suspected or confirmed SARS-CoV-2 infection. Since dentists generally do not provide inpatient treatment services, while facing such a situation, they should contact their nurses or clinicians for the patient's triage [15].

Among measures to be taken in the dental clinic, the right triage is perhaps the most important. Questions about the health status of the patient calling for an

		Yes	No
1	In the last 14 days, have you had fever, cough, shortness of breath, weakness, widespread body pain, nausea-vomiting, diarrhea, or any complaint that is important to you? If your answer is yes, please state your complaint below.		
	Yes:...........		
2	Have you traveled abroad in the last 14 days?		
3	Have you been to areas where the COVID-19 pandemic is prevalent?		
4	Have you had contact with someone diagnosed with COVID-19 in the last 14 days?		
5	Have you recently attended a meeting, funeral, party or event with many people?		
If the patient's answer to the 2nd and 3rd questions is yes, the dental clinic should postpone the treatment until the incubation period (14 days) is over, unless there is an emergency.			

Table 2.
Questions about the health status of the patient who is calling for an appointment.

appointment should be asked. Dentistry personnel should also call patients and question their current health status before their scheduled appointment (**Table 2**). It is strongly recommended that questions and practices include the following information and rules [7, 11, 12, 15, 16, 25, 29–32].

3.1 Practices and rules for patient appointments

Instruct the patient to wear a facemask when entering the dental clinic and not to remove it unless the dentist instructs them to do so. Have patients have their temperature measured as a routine procedure in dental clinics during the COVID-19 pandemic. Tell patients that they should make an appointment. Make appointments so that patients do not coincidence with each other. Limit the appointments to a certain number of patients. Tell patients that they should not bring any companions except in special cases. If a patient with COVID-19 symptoms has been taken in at the dentistry clinic, isolate the patient in a pre-created area for the necessary evaluations, routine blood analysis (e.g., hemogram and routine biochemical tests) and PCR test. Postpone dental treatment until the test result comes out. In the case of a positive test result, postpone dental treatment until the incubation period (14 days) is over. Postpone treatment for patients hospitalized with COVID-19 for at least 30 days.

3.2 Recommendations for the dentist and working environment

Dentists should talk to their patients using a surgical mask. If the dentist has symptoms like those of COVID-19, they should stop performing dental treatment, take a PCR test and isolate themselves for 14 days if the disease is confirmed or suspected. Moreover, a healthy lifestyle should be maintained during isolation. To avoid cross transmission, ensure that a limited number of patients are admitted to waiting rooms and with a distance of 2 m. Remove all reading and other materials from the waiting room. Make sure that disinfection is ensured every evening after the end of working hours and that the rooms are ventilated. Post your instructions on hand hygiene (cleaning with soap and water) and respiratory hygiene (behavior while coughing or sneezing) in the waiting room and entrances with visual warnings or signs. Put a hand sanitizer in waiting rooms. Distribute information leaflets to patients. However, remind them that these brochures should not be handed over. Ensure the use of a high-volume exhaust (HVE) filter and a high efficiency particulate air (HEPA) filter to filter contaminated air in dental clinics. Have the filters disinfected every day. Prevent employees from working in the dental care room without adequate protective equipment. It should be mandatory to use protective clothing, caps, respirators, gloves, disposable shoe covers, protective glasses and/or face protective shields to protect the skin and mucous membranes of dentists and other workers from contamination with blood and secretions of patients.

Antimicrobial products are recommended for patients to rinse their mouth before dental operations (gargle with chlorhexidine and similar antiseptic solution), as it will reduce the number of germs in the oral cavity [25, 30].

Dental healthcare personnel (DHCP) should be limited to one patient each time. Contact with more than one patient at the same time will distract the staff and increase the risk of infection. The dental operator should only have clean or sterile supplies required for the dental procedure and should not use auxiliary staff unless necessary. For this reason, the setting should be kept ready so that the required tools are easily accessible. The material remaining after the process should be considered contaminated and subjected to a medical waste management procedure. During the operation, the dentist must be protected by using a shield and an N95 mask. If an aerosol- or droplet-forming procedure will not be applied, shields and surgical masks may be used. Surgical gloves and protective clothing should be changed every time. Therefore, disposable protective clothing should be preferred. Food and drinks should not be consumed during work. The environment should be sterilized with disinfectant spraying devices at the beginning and after the process. All surgical and dental instruments should be sterilized in accordance with the applicable standards, and the necessary number of materials should be available each time, because if a dental tool contaminated with SARS-CoV-2 comes into contact with the oral mucosa, the virus will enter the organism due to the highly expressed ACE-2 receptors, especially in the epithelial cells of the tongue [11, 16, 33]. Therefore, dental procedures to be performed should be designed in such a way that they do not create aerosols, and if possible, only hand tools should be used. This is because dentistry professionals work in the patient's mouth, and this carries a high risk of COVID-19 infection. While working in the mouth, droplets will be scattered with the patient's saliva and inhaled through breathing. Meanwhile, people in the immediate area will be at a high risk of infection. Therefore, all asymptomatic patients should be assumed COVID-19-positive, and action should be taken accordingly. There are recommendations to prevent SARS-Cov-2 virus transmission, such as the use of a suction cannula for rapid spray/saliva aspiration or the use of Tyvek garments and sprays designed for protection of dental care workers [15, 34–37]. Moreover, although there are no data that it reduces SARS-CoV-2 viral load, the mouth should be rinsed with preprocedural mouth rinses (PPMR) containing an antimicrobial product (chlorhexidine gluconate, essential oils, povidone-iodine or cetylpyridinium chloride) before the procedure. Two different studies showed that mouth rinsing before a routine procedure inhibits most bacterial aerosols produced by the usage of an ultrasonic unit, and chlorhexidine is more effective [38, 39]. Furthermore, Kaufman et al. [39] reported that universal barrier measures for protection from infections and effective routine infection control will prevent infections in dentistry. The virus is very sensitive to ultraviolet light and heat, and if it is kept at 56°C for 30 minutes, the virus will be inactive. Lipid solvents such as ether, 75% ethanol, chlorine-containing disinfectants, peracetic acid and chloroform can kill the virus [11, 40]. These lipid solvents are used to disinfect the environment of the dental clinic and the surfaces of objects. As a result, antiviral mouthwash application of the patient to reduce viral load, use of suction cannula for rapid spraying/saliva aspiration, use of N95 masks as well as dentist's shield, continuous environment disinfection and vaccination are known as the most effective measures. However, since it would be possible to evaluate the effectiveness of the recommendations offered through long term prospective studies, these recommendations should be considered as confidence increasing approaches towards oral and dental health for the time being. In addition, through meta-analysis studies to be conducted by using the data to be obtained from these recommendations that could be applied in different centers, the problems related to the application of these recommendations and the concerns about their effects on the efficiency of oral and dental health can be eliminated. Hence, we believe that these recommendations would be a good topic for research in various areas related to dental health.

In addition to all these precautions above that need to be followed, scientific authorities suggest that vaccination of healthcare personnel working in the frontlines is seen as the most effective method in countering the COVID-19 pandemic [41–43]. According to the results of a study conducted in the UK, vaccination, even if it provides limited protection against infection, can have a significant effect in preventing the spread of COVID-19 and reducing its outbreaks [44].

4. The importance of physical distance in the work environment

It is known that COVID-19, which has caused great concern worldwide, is asymptomatic in many people. Test positivity is quite common before the symptoms of the disease appear. Laboratory findings of these asymptomatic people are also normal. However, since COVID-19 causes hyperinflammation, significant changes such as lymphopenia, high neutrophil to leukocyte ratio, increase in CRP, ferritin, D-dimer and procalcitonin levels are found in the biochemical results of many symptomatic people [45, 46]. People who are asymptomatic are highly effective transmitters in spreading COVID-19. These are called asymptomatic carriers [47, 48]. Moreover, studies have shown that the viral load in the airway samples of asymptomatic patients is similar to that of symptomatic patients [49]. For this reason, dental health and other healthcare professionals should also continue their work in compliance with physical distancing principles (at least one meter) [50, 51] because transmission from healthcare workers to healthcare workers is a danger that should be taken seriously for healthcare institutions [52]. In cases of suspected COVID-19 cases, personnel working together are also recommended to have SARS-CoV-2 PCR tests.

If the patient who is treated in a dentistry clinic shows signs or symptoms immediately (within one to two days) after the treatment, or if they are diagnosed with COVID-19, the situation must be reported to the dental clinic [21]. Procedures for providing this feedback should be established because almost all people are susceptible to COVID-19. The incubation period is usually 3–7 days but may extend up to 14 days. Moreover, many cases showing that it takes up to 24 days have been reported. During this incubation period, patients can transmit the virus to others. It was even found that people may be infected during their recovery period. The symptoms of the disease are usually fever, dry cough and fatigue. These may be accompanied by nasal congestion, runny nose, sore throat, myalgia and diarrhea. In severe cases, acute respiratory distress, septic shocks, metabolic acidosis and multi-organ failure may develop [11, 12, 25, 30, 53, 54].

In a review conducted by Marcelo Coelho Goiato, 47 articles and 9 websites were examined, general information about SARS-CoV-2 was collected, and forms of transmission and measures in dentistry were reviewed. In the review, it was reported that the SARS-CoV-2 virus was transmitted to 213 countries as of May

2020 [8]. With 208 countries registered with the United Nations and an estimated 13 unregistered countries in the world, SARS-CoV-2 has spread almost all over the world, and millions of people have already lost their lives. There are worries that these numbers will increase even more. These figures show that the SARS-CoV-2 virus should be taken seriously. As to be understood from here, it is not possible that oral and dental health services will not be affected by this. The main question is what kind of precautions we can take to maintain these healthcare services. In clinical practice, oral and dental healthcare providers continue their profession with fear, as they come into contact with many patients every day and are exposed to many infection risks, including SARS-CoV-2 [11, 27]. The best way to overcome this fear is to have a broad knowledge of COVID-19 and follow the recommendations of the authorities working on this issue. This way, dentists will protect both their own health and the health of their patients and other people.

Another fear of all healthcare professionals, including dentistry professionals, is the possibility of transmitting this infection to their close relatives, since they work closely with infected patients [11, 16, 54]. In a study by Sabino et al., the finding that 29% of 138 patients who received hospital treatment in the city of Wuhan in the Hubei province of China for COVID-19 were healthcare workers [26] justifies this concern.

5. Oral and dental healthcare practices for the COVID-19 outbreak in Turkey

With the first cases in Turkey at the beginning of March 2020, the Turkish Ministry of Health, Coronavirus Science Board members took urgent measures in accordance with the available recommendations of international organizations, 'guidelines for working in health institutions and Infection Control Measures' were published, and individuals were instructed to comply with these guidelines and measures [55]. Accordingly, during the pandemic, it was recommended to intervene in emergency cases and avoid aerosol-producing procedures in dental practices. According to this guide, emergency and compulsory services in dental practices are defined. These are summarized below:

- Severe toothache caused by acute pulp diseases and pericoronitis,
- Osteitis or alveolitis,
- Dental abscess or bacterial infection with localized pain and swelling,
- Traumatic jaw and tooth fractures, avulsion/luxation,
- Broken brackets and dental wires causing pain and infection in patients receiving orthodontic treatment,
- Temporomandibular joint luxation,
- Acute painful ulcerations of the oral mucosa and severe uncontrolled bleeding,
- Oral infections that narrow the respiratory tract,
- Treatment of patients who are planned to receive or receiving organ transplantation, radiotherapy and chemotherapy,

- Dental consultations requested for severe medical problems,
- Taking stitches from the wound site after an intervention,
- Treatment of restoration and removable denture fractures in a way that does not create droplets and aerosols,
- Making feeding plates for newborn patients with cleft lip and palate,
- Biopsy performed for suspicion of malignancy.

In the normalization period, it was reported that planning was made by giving priority to emergency and compulsory services to manage the patient density that may occur in all institutions providing oral and dental health services.

The Turkish Ministry of Health was one of the best among the health departments of countries in the management of the COVID-19 pandemic in terms of the measures it took, the rules it set and its supply of healthcare materials. Furthermore, more positive results were obtained thanks to the cooperation with the World Health Organization (WHO). These practices encouraged all healthcare professionals, including dental healthcare professionals, to ensure the smooth continuation of healthcare services, except for minor problems. In this context, dentists were also included among healthcare professionals who directly combat COVID-19. They contributed significantly to the fight against this disease by participating in contact-tracing teams and working in the job of taking a throat and nose swab for PCR tests. The effective factors that enabled dentists to offer this contribution were provision of adequate protective equipment as well as the knowledge and skills provided by training programs. According to a study conducted by Tokuc and Coskunses [56], dentists in Turkey reporting that they have significant knowledge and skills about COVID-19 and its clinical symptoms are the proof of this. However, the opposite case was reported in a similar study conducted in Pakistan [57].

6. Importance of financial and social support

During the epidemic period, the Turkish government directly supported all healthcare professionals at high risk of contact with COVID-19, including those working in oral and dental health, as well as providing a significant quantity of medical equipment and device support to health institutions. Additionally, it took measures that would lead to improvements in the social status of healthcare personnel and encouraged them to increase the respect in the society for healthcare professionals. This attitude has had a doping effect in the fight of healthcare personnel against COVID-19. Of course, in a period when the economy and work life were unstable due to the COVID-19 pandemic, the financial support provided to fight against the pandemic had strained the Turkish economy. However, the psychological gain it created has prevented economic difficulties. Additionally, considering the humanitarian aspect and the long-term reflections of the outcomes gained from the lives that were saved, from the bodies that were freed from pain and from the brains that were restored to their normal thinking capacity, it is certain that the fight against the COVID-19 pandemic will be worth all kinds of economic difficulties. Considering the economic, psychosocial and health losses suffered by the USA, which is accepted as the most developed country in the world but caught unprepared for the pandemic due to its wrong decisions in terms of health [58], the value of the support to be given to the field of health has been understood better. Additionally, in a study on the effect of COVID-19 on healthcare workers, it was emphasized that healthcare workers should be encouraged to continue to provide high-quality and effective healthcare services [59]. In another study, it was determined that the rapid spread of COVID-19 and the lack of personal protective equipment, as well as witnessing deaths caused by the pandemic, fear of carrying the virus to family members and the deaths of colleagues, have seriously affected the mental health of healthcare professionals. For this reason, it was reported that the mental health of all healthcare professionals should be supported during and after the COVID-19 pandemic [60]. All these points show that it is important to support all healthcare professionals, including oral and dental healthcare professionals, financially and socially throughout the pandemic period.

Developments related to COVID-19 and many issues that remained in the dark initially caused anxiety in Turkey's dentistry community. However, as uncertainties and lack of information about COVID-19, which were a cause of fear, disappeared, and the necessary measures were taken, the desire to fight replaced anxiety. The measures taken, the training programs provided, and most importantly, the support of the Turkish state to healthcare professionals have enabled the people to come out of this process. The SARS-CoV-2 virus will continue to be effective for years to come. For this reason, the struggle against the pandemic should continue responsibly. As dental service providers, we exemplify our own struggle in this regard.

7. Conclusion

Scientific evidence shows that the oral cavity and its components have a very important role in the pathogenicity and morbidity of SARS-CoV-2. Since dentists work in the mouth area, they carry a high risk of COVID-19 disease. Therefore, by providing adequate personal protection equipment and administering vaccination to all staff, as well as rational practices, the concerns of dentists and other healthcare professionals about the COVID-19 pandemic may be alleviated. Additionally, financial and social support should be continued. This way, it may be ensured that dental treatment services can be maintained without any problems.

Author details

Fatih Özçelik[1] and Dursun Ali Şirin[2*]

1 Department of Medical Biochemistry, Sultan 2, Abdülhamid Han Training Hospital, University of Health Sciences Turkey, Istanbul, Turkey

2 Department of Endodontics, Hamidiye Faculty of Dentistry and Sultan 2, Abdulhamid Han Training Hospital, University of Health Sciences Turkey, Istanbul, Turkey

*Address all correspondence to: dtalisirin@gmail.com

References

[1] Drosten C, Günther S, Preiser W, et al. Identification of a Novel Coronavirus in Patients with Severe Acute Respiratory Syndrome. *N Engl J Med*. 2003;348(20):1967-1976. doi:10.1056/NEJMoa030747

[2] Gorbalenya AE, Baker SC, Baric RS, et al. The species Severe acute respiratory syndrome-related coronavirus: classifying 2019-nCoV and naming it SARS-CoV-2. *Nat Microbiol*. 2020;5(4):536-544. doi:10.1038/s41564-020-0695-z

[3] Wax RS, Christian MD. Practical recommendations for critical care and anesthesiology teams caring for novel coronavirus (2019-nCoV) patients. *Can J Anesth Can d'anesthésie*. 2020;67(5): 568-576. doi:10.1007/s12630-020-01591-x

[4] Zhou P, Yang X-L, Wang X-G, et al. A pneumonia outbreak associated with a new coronavirus of probable bat origin. *Nature*. 2020;579(7798):270-273. doi:10.1038/s41586-020-2012-7

[5] Xu L, Liu J, Lu M, Yang D, Zheng X. Liver injury during highly pathogenic human coronavirus infections. *Liver Int*. 2020;40(5):998-1004. doi:10.1111/liv.14435

[6] Zhou F, Yu T, Du R, et al. Clinical course and risk factors for mortality of adult inpatients with COVID-19 in Wuhan, China: a retrospective cohort study. *Lancet*. 2020;395(10229):1054-1062. doi:10.1016/S0140-6736(20)30566-3

[7] Adhikari SP, Meng S, Wu Y-J, et al. Epidemiology, causes, clinical manifestation and diagnosis, prevention and control of coronavirus disease (COVID-19) during the early outbreak period: a scoping review. *Infect Dis Poverty*. 2020;9(1):29. doi:10.1186/s40249-020-00646-x

[8] Melo Neto CLDM, Bannwart LC, de Melo Moreno AL, Goiato MC. SARS-CoV-2 and Dentistry–Review. *Eur J Dent*. 2020;14(S 01):S130-S139. doi:10.1055/s-0040-1716438

[9] Guo Y-R, Cao Q-D, Hong Z-S, et al. The origin, transmission and clinical therapies on coronavirus disease 2019 (COVID-19) outbreak – an update on the status. *Mil Med Res*. 2020;7(1):11. doi:10.1186/s40779-020-00240-0

[10] Lauer SA, Grantz KH, Bi Q, et al. The Incubation Period of Coronavirus Disease 2019 (COVID-19) From Publicly Reported Confirmed Cases: Estimation and Application. *Ann Intern Med*. 2020;172(9):577-582. doi:10.7326/M20-0504

[11] Peng X, Xu X, Li Y, Cheng L, Zhou X, Ren B. Transmission routes of 2019-nCoV and controls in dental practice. *Int J Oral Sci*. 2020;12(1):9. doi:10.1038/s41368-020-0075-9

[12] Yi Y, Lagniton PNP, Ye S, Li E, Xu R-H. COVID-19: what has been learned and to be learned about the novel coronavirus disease. *Int J Biol Sci*. 2020;16(10):1753-1766. doi:10.7150/ijbs.45134

[13] Vardavas CI, Nikitara K. COVID-19 and smoking: A systematic review of the evidence. *Tob Induc Dis*. 2020. doi:10.18332/tid/119324

[14] Sirin DA, Ozcelik F. The relationship between COVID-19 and the dental damage stage determined by radiological examination. *Oral Radiol*. January 2021. doi:10.1007/s11282-020-00497-0

[15] Center for Disease Control and Prevention (CDC). Guidance for Dental Settings, Interim Infection Prevention and Control Guidance for Dental Settings During the Coronavirus

Disease 2019 (COVID-19) Pandemic, 2020. https://www.cdc.gov/coronavirus/2019-ncov/hcp/dental-settings.html. Published October 4, 2020. Accessed February 6, 2021.

[16] Ge Z, Yang L, Xia J, Fu X, Zhang Y. Possible aerosol transmission of COVID-19 and special precautions in dentistry. *J Zhejiang Univ B*. 2020;21(5):361-368. doi:10.1631/jzus.B2010010

[17] Pan Y, Zhang D, Yang P, Poon LLM, Wang Q. Viral load of SARS-CoV-2 in clinical samples. *Lancet Infect Dis*. 2020;20(4):411-412. doi:10.1016/S1473-3099(20)30113-4

[18] Mazumdar P, Kaushik M, Chandrasekhar V, Mohan Kumar R, Rajawat A. Position statement of IACDE for managing dental patients during COVID-19. *J Conserv Dent*. 2020;23(2):114. doi:10.4103/JCD.JCD_361_20

[19] Lippi G, Plebani M. The critical role of laboratory medicine during coronavirus disease 2019 (COVID-19) and other viral outbreaks. *Clin Chem Lab Med*. 2020;58(7):1063-1069. doi:10.1515/cclm-2020-0240

[20] Lippi G, Plebani M. Laboratory medicine resilience during coronavirus disease 2019 (Covid-19) pandemic. *J Bras Patol e Med Lab*. 2020;56:1-2. doi:10.5935/1676-2444.20200035

[21] American Dental Association. *ADA Patient Reports COVID Post Treatment. Steps to Take If a Patient Reports COVID-19 Exposure After Treatment*.; 2020. https://success.ada.org/~/media/CPS/Files/COVID/Patient_Reports_COVID-19_Post_Treatment.pdf. Accessed February 6, 2021.

[22] *American Dental Hygienist' Association. ADHA Interim Guidance on Returning to Work*.; 2020. https://www.adha.org/resources-docs/ADHA_TaskForceReport.pdf. Accessed February 6, 2021.

[23] Zuo YY, Uspal WE, Wei T. Airborne Transmission of COVID-19: Aerosol Dispersion, Lung Deposition, and Virus-Receptor Interactions. *ACS Nano*. 2020;14(12):16502-16524. doi:10.1021/acsnano.0c08484

[24] Xie X, Li Y, Chwang ATY, Ho PL, Seto WH. How far droplets can move in indoor environments ? revisiting the Wells evaporation?falling curve. *Indoor Air*. 2007;17(3):211-225. doi:10.1111/j.1600-0668.2007.00469.x

[25] Singhal T. A Review of Coronavirus Disease-2019 (COVID-19). *Indian J Pediatr*. 2020;87(4):281-286. doi:10.1007/s12098-020-03263-6

[26] Sabino-Silva R, Jardim ACG, Siqueira WL. Coronavirus COVID-19 impacts to dentistry and potential salivary diagnosis. *Clin Oral Investig*. 2020;24(4):1619-1621. doi:10.1007/s00784-020-03248-x

[27] Ahmed MA, Jouhar R, Ahmed N, et al. Fear and Practice Modifications among Dentists to Combat Novel Coronavirus Disease (COVID-19) Outbreak. *Int J Environ Res Public Health*. 2020;17(8):2821. doi:10.3390/ijerph17082821

[28] Pujadas E, Chaudhry F, McBride R, et al. SARS-CoV-2 viral load predicts COVID-19 mortality. *Lancet Respir Med*. 2020;8(9):e70. doi:10.1016/S2213-2600(20)30354-4

[29] Samaranayake LP, Peiris M. Severe acute respiratory syndrome and dentistry: a retrospective view. *J Am Dent Assoc*. 2004;135(9):1292-1302. doi:10.14219/jada.archive.2004.0405

[30] Meng L, Hua F, Bian Z. Coronavirus Disease 2019 (COVID-19): Emerging and Future Challenges for Dental and Oral Medicine. *J Dent Res*.

2020;99(5):481-487. doi:10.1177/0022034520914246

[31] Al-Sehaibany F. Middle East respiratory syndrome in children. Dental considerations. *Saudi Med J*. 2017;38(4):339-343. doi:10.15537/smj.2017.4.15777

[32] Okba NMA, Müller MA, Li W, et al. Severe Acute Respiratory Syndrome Coronavirus 2–Specific Antibody Responses in Coronavirus Disease 2019 Patients. *Emerg Infect Dis*. 2020;26(7):10.3201/eid2607.200841. doi:10.3201/eid2607.200841

[33] Kutter JS, Spronken MI, Fraaij PL, Fouchier RA, Herfst S. Transmission routes of respiratory viruses among humans. *Curr Opin Virol*. 2018;28:142-151. doi:10.1016/j.coviro.2018.01.001

[34] Bartoszko JJ, Farooqi MAM, Alhazzani W, Loeb M. Medical masks vs N95 respirators for preventing COVID-19 in healthcare workers: A systematic review and meta-analysis of randomized trials. *Influenza Other Respi Viruses*. 2020. doi:10.1111/irv.12745

[35] Smith JD, MacDougall CC, Johnstone J, Copes RA, Schwartz B, Garber GE. Effectiveness of N95 respirators versus surgical masks in protecting health care workers from acute respiratory infection: a systematic review and meta-analysis. *Can Med Assoc J*. 2016;188(8):567-574. doi:10.1503/cmaj.150835

[36] Tan LF. Preventing the transmission of COVID-19 amongst healthcare workers. *J Hosp Infect*. 2020;105(2):364-365. doi:10.1016/j.jhin.2020.04.008

[37] Gandolfi MG, Zamparini F, Spinelli A, Sambri V, Prati C. Risks of aerosol contamination in dental procedures during the second wave of COVID-19—experience and proposals of innovative IPC in dental practice. *Int J Environ Res Public Health*. 2020. doi:10.3390/ijerph17238954

[38] Gupta G, Mitra D, Ashok KP, et al. Efficacy of Preprocedural Mouth Rinsing in Reducing Aerosol Contamination Produced by Ultrasonic Scaler: A Pilot Study. *J Periodontol*. 2014;85(4):562-568. doi:10.1902/jop.2013.120616

[39] Kaufmann M, Solderer A, Gubler A, Wegehaupt FJ, Attin T, Schmidlin PR. Quantitative measurements of aerosols from air-polishing and ultrasonic devices: (How) can we protect ourselves? Eickholz P, ed. *PLoS One*. 2020;15(12):e0244020. doi:10.1371/journal.pone.0244020

[40] Klompas M. Coronavirus Disease 2019 (COVID-19): Protecting Hospitals From the Invisible. *Ann Intern Med*. 2020;172(9):619-620. doi:10.7326/M20-0751

[41] Kaur SP, Gupta V. COVID-19 Vaccine: A comprehensive status report. *Virus Res*. 2020;288:198114. doi:10.1016/j.virusres.2020.198114

[42] Samrat SK, Tharappel AM, Li Z, Li H. Prospect of SARS-CoV-2 spike protein: Potential role in vaccine and therapeutic development. *Virus Res*. 2020;288:198141. doi:10.1016/j.virusres.2020.198141

[43] Dong Y, Dai T, Wei Y, Zhang L, Zheng M, Zhou F. A systematic review of SARS-CoV-2 vaccine candidates. *Signal Transduct Target Ther*. 2020;5(1):237. doi:10.1038/s41392-020-00352-y

[44] Moghadas SM, Vilches TN, Zhang K, et al. The impact of vaccination on COVID-19 outbreaks in the United States. *medRxiv Prepr Serv Heal Sci*. November 2020. doi:10.1101/2020.11.27.20240051

[45] Huang I, Pranata R, Lim MA, Oehadian A, Alisjahbana B. C-reactive protein, procalcitonin, D-dimer, and ferritin in severe coronavirus

disease-2019: a meta-analysis. *Ther Adv Respir Dis*. 2020;14:175346662093717. doi:10.1177/1753466620937175

[46] Mehta P, McAuley DF, Brown M, Sanchez E, Tattersall RS, Manson JJ. COVID-19: consider cytokine storm syndromes and immunosuppression. *Lancet*. 2020;395(10229):1033-1034. doi:10.1016/S0140-6736(20)30628-0

[47] Gao M, Yang L, Chen X, et al. A study on infectivity of asymptomatic SARS-CoV-2 carriers. *Respir Med*. 2020;169:106026. doi:10.1016/j.rmed.2020.106026

[48] Zhao H, Lu X, Deng Y, Tang Y, Lu J. COVID-19: asymptomatic carrier transmission is an underestimated problem. *Epidemiol Infect*. 2020;148:e116. doi:10.1017/S0950268820001235

[49] Zou L, Ruan F, Huang M, et al. SARS-CoV-2 Viral Load in Upper Respiratory Specimens of Infected Patients. *N Engl J Med*. 2020;382(12):1177-1179. doi:10.1056/NEJMc2001737

[50] Chu DK, Akl EA, Duda S, et al. Physical distancing, face masks, and eye protection to prevent person-to-person transmission of SARS-CoV-2 and COVID-19: a systematic review and meta-analysis. *Lancet*. 2020;395(10242):1973-1987. doi:10.1016/S0140-6736(20)31142-9

[51] MacIntyre CR, Wang Q. Physical distancing, face masks, and eye protection for prevention of COVID-19. *Lancet*. 2020;395(10242):1950-1951. doi:10.1016/S0140-6736(20)31183-1

[52] Schneider S, Piening B, Nouri-Pasovsky PA, Krüger AC, Gastmeier P, Aghdassi SJS. SARS-Coronavirus-2 cases in healthcare workers may not regularly originate from patient care: lessons from a university hospital on the underestimated risk of healthcare worker to healthcare worker transmission. *Antimicrob Resist Infect Control*. 2020;9(1):192. doi:10.1186/s13756-020-00848-w

[53] Radzikowska U, Ding M, Tan G, et al. Distribution of ACE2, CD147, CD26, and other SARS-CoV-2 associated molecules in tissues and immune cells in health and in asthma, COPD, obesity, hypertension, and COVID-19 risk factors. *Allergy Eur J Allergy Clin Immunol*. 2020;75(11):2829-2845. doi:10.1111/all.14429

[54] Sohrabi C, Alsafi Z, O'Neill N, et al. World Health Organization declares global emergency: A review of the 2019 novel coronavirus (COVID-19). *Int J Surg*. 2020;76:71-76. doi:10.1016/j.ijsu.2020.02.034

[55] Scientific Advisory Board Work. *Health Institutions Study Guide and Infection Control Measures in the COVID-19 Pandemic.* Ankara; 2020. https://covid19.saglik.gov.tr/TR-66532/saglik-kurumlarinda-calisma-rehberi-ve-enfeksiyon-kontrol-onlemleri.html. Accessed February 7, 2021.

[56] Tokuç B, Coşkunses FM. Knowledge, Attitude and Practice of Dentists in Coronavirus Disease 2019 Pandemic in Turkey. *Eur Oral Res*. 2020;54(2):86-91. doi:10.26650/eor.20200049

[57] Kumar J, Katto MS, Siddiqui AA, et al. Knowledge, Attitude, and Practices of Healthcare Workers Regarding the Use of Face Mask to Limit the Spread of the New Coronavirus Disease (COVID-19). *Cureus*. 2020. doi:10.7759/cureus.7737

[58] Kaye AD, Okeagu CN, Pham AD, et al. Economic impact of COVID-19 pandemic on healthcare facilities and systems: International perspectives. *Best Pract Res Clin Anaesthesiol*. November 2020. doi:10.1016/j.bpa.2020.11.009

[59] Shreffler J, Huecker M, Petrey J. The Impact of COVID-19 on Healthcare

Worker Wellness: A Scoping Review. *West J Emerg Med*. 2020;21(5):1059-1066. doi:10.5811/westjem.2020.7.48684

[60] Hall H. The effect of the COVID-19 pandemic on healthcare workers' mental health. *J Am Acad Physician Assist*. 2020;33(7):45-48. doi:10.1097/01.JAA.0000669772.78848.8c

Chapter 5

Global Impact of COVID-19 Pandemic on Public Health Supply Chains

Ukamaka Gladys Okafor, Modinat Aderonke Olaleye, Hillary Chukwuemeka Asobara and Ebuka Fidelis Umeodinka

Abstract

Health commodity supply chains are vital to a well-functioning health system and advancing national and regional health security goals. This study describes impacts of the COVID-19 pandemic on these chains, learnings from it and the challenges faced by countries. It also provides futuristic strategic recommendations for the building of the supply chain to manage the impacts and guide pandemic responsiveness. We used the PRISMA guideline for systematic review to collate relevant information from both published and unpublished literature. Out of 622 screened records, 38 were included in the review. Major impacts were innovation, collaboration, increased technology, research and development, increased prices and shortage of health products, depletion of supply chain personnel. Challenges were lack of visibility, coordination, resilience and strategy for pandemics, potential substandard medicines epidemic, travel restrictions and inadequate scientific knowledge. The studies recommended increased local production and resilience of supply chains. The pandemic disrupted national and international supply chain systems of medical devices, essential medicines and pharmaceutical products due to border closures, transportation and international trade restrictions. It however exposed hidden potentials in Sub-Saharan Africa. There is need to develop supply chain strategy for emergencies, increase local production and talent pool for supply chain management particularly in Africa.

Keywords: COVID-19, impact, health supply chain, pandemic

1. Introduction

The COVID-19 pandemic has escalated into the largest health crisis of the 21st Century. According to the COVID-19 situation dashboard of the World Health Organization (WHO), the virus has infected more than 117,132,788 people worldwide to date, and has also killed over 2,600,839 [1]. Epidemiological projections show that the outbreak overwhelmed even well-developed healthcare systems [2]. Many countries have thus imposed pandemic suppression measures such as lockdowns and community quarantines in an effort to stem the progress of the pandemic [3].

Health commodity supply chains are a critical element of a well-functioning health system and a vital input to advancing national and regional health security goals. Strong medicine and health commodity supply chains improve health outcomes and build trust in health systems. Robust supply chains provide critical vaccines, medicines, diagnostics, and other essential health supplies to support communicable disease prevention, control, and response activities [4]. A public health supply chain is a network of interconnected organizations or actors that ensures the availability of health commodities to people who need them. Essentially there are four parts to a supply chain; product manufacturers or the suppliers, distributors, service providers (hospitals, pharmacies, retail medicine sellers) and finally the customers or patients [5].

The coronavirus pandemic is having a clear impact on the supply chains of virtually all manufacturers, retailers, and wholesalers. As the world attempts to navigate through this difficult time, most companies are struggling to maintain a steady flow of required goods and services. Whether it is frozen foods and grocery items, or ventilators and masks, medicines or even the services clinic visits etc), the supply chain has been facing multiple obstacles [6]. This disruption is mainly due to COVID 19 pandemic, emanating from China being the second largest economy in the world and the major supplier of inputs for manufacturing companies around the world. Majority of the original equipment manufacturers in China have stopped production [7]. At present, most of the production capacity of these drugs and chemical precursors are in the United States, China and India. Global supply chains have been disrupted due to loss of labor and raw material inputs, creating ripple effects that cross national boundaries [3].

This chapter describes the impacts of the pandemic on public health supply chain, challenges that countries are facing, learnings from the pandemic and provides futuristic strategic recommendations for the building and rebuilding of the supply chains to manage the impact of the pandemic and guide responsiveness towards future pandemics.

2. Data collection process

This chapter is an outcome of a systematic review done by using Purdue libraries online access and e-resources centre 'All Databases" search tool. The search was conducted from June to August, 2020 using the PRISMA checklist. We screened 622 records and reviewed 31 peer reviewed publications and 7 unpublished papers from across the countries.

Literature search was done using keywords like "impact of COVID-19", "effects of COVID-19", "supply chain and COVID-19", "health impacts of COVID-19", "global and public health supply chain during pandemics", "public health and supply chain", and "impact of outbreaks" on databases like Pubmed, ProQuest, Google Scholar, Web of Science, Science Direct (Elsevier). We have excluded literatures that did not report challenges, effect or impact of COVID-19 on health supply chain and as well those not reported in English.

Figure 1 shows the flow chart of this review.

After careful review of the articles, 38 out of 622 screened publications were selected for inclusion in this study. Extracted data were analyzed and sectioned into positive impact, negative impact, challenges, learnings and recommendations.

All the 38 studies included in the review were conducted between February and August, 2020. Majority of the studies reviewed were conducted globally [8], in Africa [9], Asia [2] and United States [5]. A survey published on March 28 by the Chartered Institute of Procurement and Supply found that 86% of supply chains are impacted by the COVID-19 pandemic while another study by the Institute for Supply Management found that between early March and late March, 2020, the number of companies experiencing supply chain impact rose from 80 to 95% [9].

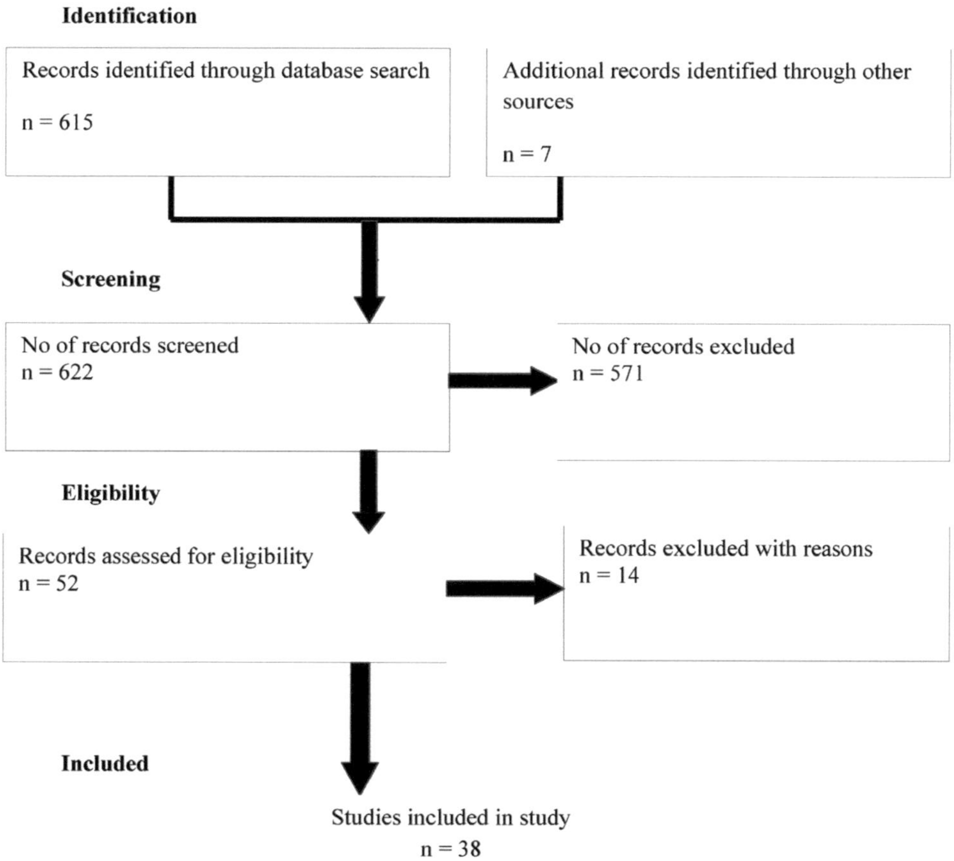

Figure 1.
Flow of information through the different phases of the review.

2.1 Outcome of systematic review

Our review revealed the following:

2.1.1 Positive impacts

While Covid-19 has been blamed for economic downturns, it has shifted organizational focus towards a sustainable supply chain [6]. Other positive impacts include:

1. Creativity and Flexibility among Companies and Countries. Due to the impact of COVID-19, many companies around the world started to re-purpose or re-adjust their production, with many brewing companies and distilleries producing hand-sanitizers, fashion companies producing masks and automotive companies looking to produce ventilators. Some governments and businesses developed a variety of innovative prevention measures such as drive-through testing kits and products that can be utilized all over the world. Countries that have never produced surgical masks, gloves, sanitizers, or ventilators turned to domestic production [7, 10–13].

2. Increased Availability and Utilization of Technology and Innovation in the Health Sector:

- Technology driven health services which was largely considered a novelty or luxury, now has the opportunity to demonstrate real value as traditional healthcare services become overwhelmed by patient load demands [7, 14].

- Some organizations were able to quickly mobilize by leveraging existing tools for source-code dissemination, accelerating innovation and targeted problem-solving. Notably, the COVID-19 emergency has highlighted the power of the Maker community to make a real and immediate impact [13].

3. Diversification of suppliers and logistics models:

    - The pandemic has thrown up opportunities for entrepreneurs to take advantage of the need for sourcing raw materials along more efficient commodity routes and methods such as railways, increase in dual sourcing of key components and a preference for larger, more financially stable suppliers with multiple manufacturing sites [14, 15].

    - Companies that operate regularly in the supply chain should expect to see the emergence of stronger, more conservatively financed, multi-site suppliers as a long-term outcome of the pandemic [14].

4. Increased Capacity in Research and Development: As the world manages to contain Covid-19 outbreak, various countries and firms are focusing on finding a vaccine, developing protocol to treat infected patients, adopting capabilities which ensure the integrity of the processes and the quality of the products and creating a safe working environment for employees [6, 7, 13].

2.1.2 Negative impacts

Unlike other disruption risks, the epidemic outbreaks start small but scale fast and disperse over many geographic regions causing simultaneous disruptions in supply, demand, and logistics infrastructure [16]. A report published on 21 February 2020, indicated that 94% of the companies listed in the Fortune 1000 list were already facing SC disruptions due to the COVID-19 [17]. Other negative impacts include:

1. Shortage in essential and non-essential medicines, raw materials, medical and pharmaceuticals products: As a result of the surge in the pandemic which led to the inevitable lock down of the economy across affected countries, there has been a noticeable decrease in production and exportation of equipment, raw materials, as well as finished products across different countries [6]. Production supply shortages, transport interruption and the virus containment measures taken by the government was limiting market access, hampering manufacturing activities and nudging the economy towards an inflationary recession which is adversely affecting the manufacturing sector, including that of health products production [7, 16, 18–20]. It has certainly surprised many to discover just how much western countries (in which shortages are particularly prevalent) rely upon global supply chains to obtain medical supplies from China and low-cost economies [21]. However, these networks have poor resilience to global disruptions, with nearly 35% of manufacturers reporting disturbances due to the global Corona virus pandemic [8, 11, 22]. Given the expected increase in COVID-19 cases and global competition for sourcing PPE, many medical facilities currently do not have enough stock and/or reliable resources to meet the anticipated demand [10].

2. Congestion of cargo terminals and delays in transportation of food and health commodities due to travel ban and movement restrictions: The severe spread of the virus into Europe and the United States has blocked the movement of the products and materials worldwide [8]. Many manufacturers and service providers experienced disruptions as more than $100 million worth of goods were stuck in China during the China lockdown [7]. For many countries and firms, the inability to respond to the Covid-19 outbreak lies in its transportation services [23]. The world's largest 1,000 companies had over 12,000 factories, warehouses and operations in quarantined regions in early March, 2020 [19]. If cargo does not flow, within days, there will be no space in the terminals to discharge other cargo and some of the cargo waiting to be discharged includes food and medicine [7].

3. Depletion of human resource for supply chain: COVID-19 has cost hundreds of thousands of human lives globally including healthcare professionals, and exposed the weaknesses of national health systems worldwide [12]. Global supply chains have been disrupted due to loss of labor and raw material inputs, creating ripple effects that cross national boundaries [3].

4. Some big multi- nationals have left themselves dangerously exposed to supply-chain risk owing to strategies designed to bring down their costs [24].

5. Reduced access to medicines due to increase in prices of medicines and movement restrictions: In Nigeria, the lockdown which was accompanied with the closure of borders and travel ban across states led to a significant drop in the quantity of essential medicines in the health facilities with a consequent increase in the prices of medicines, hand sanitizers, face masks, personal protective equipment, and other medical equipment used for providing health care, making it difficult for consumers to get the medicines they need [25].

6. Reduced patronage to small scale suppliers: An increase in dual sourcing of key components and a preference for larger, more financially stable suppliers with multiple manufacturing sites presents new challenges for smaller and more leveraged companies, regardless of their expertise [14, 15].

2.1.3 Challenges

The COVID-19 pandemic has triggered a number of challenges that have led to shortages and price hikes, and could potentially fuel an epidemic of fake and substandard medicines [26]. Findings from the reviewed literature reported the following challenges:

1. There is lack of visibility, collaboration and coordination of real demand and supply [7]. A survey with over 700 respondents conducted by Bass ware found that 60% of responding procurement managers experience a lack of transparency in their supply chain [9]. Absence of supply chain strategy for pandemics: Decision-making is executed under epistemic and stochastic uncertainty [27, 28].

2. Some supply chain disruption are not included in regular supplier performance metrics and such, unplanned for. Most supply chains are still based on reactive or transactional model, therefore, it could take several days or month to adjust supply chains during pandemics [7]. It has become extremely challenging to continue the operations of supply chains as the operations of some

parts of the supply chain in some firms has stopped with little or no alternatives during disruption [7, 29]. ISM also found that 44% of respondents to its survey did not have plans in place to cope with supply disruptions from China [9].

3. It is a great challenge to provide medical supplies (such as masks and protective clothing etc.) and equipment (for checking, testing, and monitoring the disease etc.) to meet the needs of treatment, protection, and control [7]. In a pandemic situation, the demand of the essential products increases expressively; on the other hand, the supply of the raw materials decreases considerably with a constraint of production capacity. These dual disruptions impact the production process suddenly, and the process can collapse without immediate and necessary actions [8, 16, 30]. Limitation on international trade and travel; The ban on the international travel during this pandemic may pose a serious challenge to the healthcare system in Nigeria and across Africa because of heavy reliance of Nigeria and other developing countries on importation of medicines, API and other needed resources for drug manufacturing from other countries [31]. Due to severe disruptions (e.g., manufacturers closed or partially closed, air- ports operating with harsh restrictions, shortages of medical equipment and supplies) recorded, a good number of industries including health commodity manufacturers may experience ripple effects [17, 29].

4. Cost and legal issues: Another challenging part is keeping cost under control which includes higher production costs, shipping costs and agreed costs of pending orders. A legal issue related to disagreeing the agreed cost as a Force Majeure clause or not, poses legal challenge for every company [32].

5. Wrong supply chain success function shift, which focuses on just cost savings and not revenue-assurance or sustainability [7]. A lot of the resilience challenges have arisen from a cost obsession and short-term cost focus in supply chain management [9].

6. Once effective pharmaceutical treatments are found, there will be the major engineering challenge of ramping up production at a rate that matches the pandemic [27]. Planning will be hindered by the lack of solid scientific knowledge about COVID-19 and inadequate literature on pharmaceutical supply chain (PSC) network design in the disastrous situations and other uncertainties (current literature on disruption recovery strategies and modeling during pandemics is mostly limited to humanitarian logistics) which make demand projections highly uncertain [16, 22, 27].

7. Limited supply chain talents in Africa [28].

2.1.4 Learnings

1. Social Resilience among Supply Chain Partners, Healthcare professionals and Patients: Most supply chains are transactional in nature but transactional supply chain will not be beneficial during and post Covid-19 [6] Thus;

    - It is critical to prepare health care professionals to build resilience in their interactions with patients and other stakeholders [12]

- By developing a culture of collaboration across its supply network, a firm can develop trust among supply chain partners that can help in data-sharing and joint problem-solving [6]

- Covid-19 has forced companies to lay greater emphasis on the environmental and social aspects of public health supply chain and not just the economical aspect [6, 33]

2. Inflexibility of Supply Chains: Most firms follow strict rules for their supply chain such as; specific number of days for distribution, specific production time, delivery rules, etc. These responses have proved to be inadequate during the crisis. Thus, reacting to the Covid-19 requires flexibility in the supply chain and the overall ecosystem of a firm;

    - The central learning from Covid-19 is to diversify production, sourcing, and logistics whenever and however required such that external shocks cannot disrupt the supply chain [6].

    - We also found evidence that centralized procurement and tendering can achieve direct cost savings, while supply chain management program can reduce drug stock outs and increase drug availability for populations [34].

3. The Decoupling from China's Supply Chains: COVID-19 has accelerated two powerful trends for the future, the decoupling from China's supply chains and the relocation of strategic manufacturing operations out of China [12]. A study by corporate data analytics firm, Dun & Bradstreet, reported that 51,000 companies around the world have one or more direct suppliers in Wuhan and at least 5 million companies around the world have one or more tier-two suppliers in the Wuhan region, where COVID-19 originated [18]. In US, there's been bipartisan support for legislation that would study the current medical equipment supply chain and develop an action plan to potentially address the country's dependence on foreign-made products [21].

4. Strategies to deal with Major Outbreaks

    - Designing an appropriate pharmaceutical supply chain network for pre-positioning and distributing drugs at post-disaster plays an important role in decreasing the response time and the number of casualties.

    - Pre-positioning of emergency supplies belongs to the preparedness phase of a disaster that brings about some advantages for the Humanitarian organizations [22].

5. Analysis of the Italian production network has found that sectors are both highly connected and asymmetrically connected. Hence, a local shock due to lockdown policy propagates through the whole economy and generates a sizeable global disturbance. This confirms the importance of value chain analysis in investigating how the economy adjusts to dislocation and destruction of parts of its productive capacity [35].

6. The current impact of the COVID-19 outbreak on the manufacturing firms is already very severe and medium-to-long-term impacts are predicted to be

higher than that of any other previous major outbreaks such as 2003 SARS and 2009 H1N1 [21, 36–38].

2.1.5 Recommendations

Key levers for de-risking the supply chain include the need to balance global sourcing with near shore and local sourcing, the adoption of multiple sources and a greater utilization of information technology to drive more complete and immediate information availability. Talent management in supply chain management needs to promote a focus not just on costs, but also on resilience as well as on learning from current events to improve decision-making [10, 30]. Findings from the reviewed literature reported the following recommendations:

1. Strengthen Local Manufacturing Capacity and Fortify local supply chain: The global scientific community has been galvanized into action in a frantic search for a cure for COVID-19. Greater collaboration between governments and industries will be needed to ensure minimum disruption in global supply chains Firms also need to collaborate with multiple stakeholders and be more strategic in their approach to supply chain management. Companies have to come up with alternative means of raw materials sourcing and identify other modes of cost benefit transportation. This will also involve identifying urgent research and development challenges for pharmaceutical supply chains. There should be increased R & D by local universities who should create specialized post-graduate schools that focus on research, while also recruiting and training fresh lecturers who focus on research and product/ process development to grow the domestic manufacturing sector [6, 12, 15, 16, 22, 28, 29, 32, 39].

2. Technological Augmentation and Utilization: Studies have recommended new supply chain technologies that dramatically improve collaboration, visibility, agility and optimization across the end-to-end supply chain, understand complexities and support companies' ability to resist such shocks from impact of any pandemics or rare events. Block chain systems can assist in keeping the data needed for recoveries such as information and data for production capacity, human resources requirements, information of supplier capacities, and emergency suppliers [6, 17, 30, 32, 38, 40].

3. Policymakers and program managers should examine the root causes of inefficiencies in pharmaceutical supply chain and procurement processes in order to determine how best to improve health systems performance in their specific contexts. In addition they should consider the root causes of programmatic challenges to purchasing and distributing health products in their context and identify specific interventions that can strengthen these processes. As the evolution and implications of the COVID-19 crisis are still unfolding, we posit that exploring the experiences and strategic responses of Asian countries may shed some useful light on ways to combat COVID-19 for the policymakers and suuply chain managers in the rest of the world [12, 34].

4. Development and Assessment of supply chain strategies: Optimal supply chain planning taking into account agility, resilience and sustainability are important. The negative impact of the pandemic has fostered the need for development and implementation of health supply chain strategy. The next-generation supply chain needs a significant change in outlook. Based on our analysis,

we recommend firms adopt a forward looking approach. These forward-looking strategies must comprise of multiple facets of the supply chain including people, processes, and technology.

Devoting resources for supply network mapping as a risk-mitigation strategy. A firm can design its supply network in such a way that it can balance risk and operational flexibility, manage supply chain disruptions, and keep supply chain agile. Brian Higgins, a principal Supply Chain & Operations Leader of KPMG, US has recommended some very pertinent action points for the long term:

- Build agility and speed into your supply chain by creating Micro-Supply Chains;

- Assess opportunities to diversify the supplier base and identify geographically diverse suppliers to onboard in the event of emergency. Consideration should be given to dual-sourcing for critical components.

- Move towards a Supplier-Centric approach to procurement, further integrating your supply chain with those of your direct suppliers to Original Equipment Manufacturers and direct suppliers to Tier-1 and Tier 2 suppliers

- Look to develop more collaborative relationships with critical suppliers in other to build organizational resilience as it is highly unrealistic to completely exit the Chinese market because of the supplier ecosystem in the place, however, organizations should understand their supply chain more deeply.

  A study proposed a framework for operations and supply chain management at the times of COVID-19 pandemic spanning six perspectives, i.e., adaptation, digitalization, preparedness, recovery, ripple effect, and sustainability. Assessment of COVID-19-related procurement and supply chain risks and life-cycle sustainability assessment of pharmaceutical product systems and development of drug allocation strategies under resource or supply constraints were recommended [6, 17, 41].

5. Human resource supply chain strategy that includes the selection of the critical workforce that can handle the turbulence in any environment. The supply chain initiatives will require a focused Crisis Management head whose skills and responsibility will be to communicate to all stake holders, consolidating requirements and setting priorities and work on risk mitigating methods of supply chain during non-crisis period. This will need scenario planning, resource optimization, and efficiency management. There is a greater need for a firm to look beyond profitability. Ensuring the well-being of not only a firm's employees but also those employed even with suppliers is critical if a firm wants to avoid disruptions in the supply chain [6, 32].

6. Utilize suitable resilience strategies for designing pharmaceutical relief networks, employ other types of supply contracts, consider the coordination and collaboration of multiple humanitarian organizations in a collaborative setting and address the case in which successive disasters may happen. Relief managers can ensure the high availability level of pre-positioned pharmaceutical items by paying attention to their procurement time and shelf-lives. By utilizing mobile pharmacies the distance between relief shelters and drug supply sites can be reduced, and the distribution of drugs to inaccessible areas can be

possible. Infectious disease outbreak preparedness strategies should incorporate primary healthcare services and other health system modalities to cater for non– pandemic-related conditions [18, 22].

Suppliers should manage the perception of their readiness to adapt to changing situations. Those that demonstrate competence will be rewarded as their customers look back in the coming years. Rather than ignore or complain about uncertainty, suppliers will be well-served if they can demonstrate plans that show customers they can reliably manufacture regardless of societal disruptions. Suppliers also need to be dynamic by focusing on multiple best practices explored by other suppliers, competitors and ecosystem in order to optimize cost and delivery, improve visibility across the network, and accelerate reaction times to issues in production and delivery [6, 14, 15].

2.2 Discussion and conclusions

The COVID-19 pandemic has impacted global health product supply chains, affecting key materials and ingredients, finished health products, logistics, and shipping medical devices, essential medicines and pharmaceutical products as a result of border closures, international trade restrictions and transportation problems [42]. The COVID-19 pandemic clearly shows the lack of resilience in supply chains and the impact that disruptions may have on a global network scale as individual supply chain connections and nodes fail [41].

As did HIV, the COVID-19 is likely to have profound and long-term consequences on global health care supply chains. The HIV pandemic transformed health care supply chains globally and in particular in lower and middle-income countries, (LMICs) leading to the mobilization of new financial resources for health care products, service delivery, and the creation of international bodies (including The Global Fund and PEPFAR) [43].

The short-term effects of COVID-19 on global health care supply chains have been severe; factory and border closures, transportation disruption, shifting demand, and price increases but it is more important to reflect on what the long-term consequences will be and how global changes will affect the LMICs. This is because LMICs are in their early stages of pharmaceutical development; thus they rely on importation of drugs, raw materials and equipment from countries outside the region, notably India and China.18 Researchers wonder whether the changes will be positive overall or if countries will revert to the same systems that left us unprepared for an international pandemic. This review was unable to find answer to these questions. However, crises like pandemics tend to have lasting impacts, and it is likely that the short-term disruption of health care supply chains we are seeing will result in longer-term structural changes. This highlights the need for policymakers to address challenges to large-scale and sustainable drug manufacturing, using the COVID-19 situation as a learning opportunity. It is interesting that some companies are offering strong technological solutions, which may help them survive and even prosper. While the hope is that COVID-19 will increase recognition of the importance of strong health care supply chains with commensurate investment, there will also be pressure on funders to rebuild their own shattered economies. There will be pressure to turn inward, certainly over the short term. There may also be opportunities for alternative financing mechanisms including venture capital [43]. The review has noted the fact that disruption does not necessarily mean negative outcomes and that it is incumbent on all health supply chains organizations to turn this disruptive event into positive change.

The COVID-19 pandemic is a disruption of an unprecedented magnitude, which is testing the resilience of global supply chains. The ability for a supply chain's operators to effectively plan, enabling a means for the supply chain to absorb, recover from, and adapt to disruptions of various lengths, impacts, and probabilities, is essential to ensuring the supply chain's function and success. For a supply chain, resilience measures the ability to prepare for and provide essential functions during a disruption, and then to recover from and adapt post-disruption into a form that is better suited to the new "present." Although sustainability, robustness, risk mitigation, leanness, and other supply chain management practices are important for business success, supply chain resilience is unique in its focus on recovery following a disruptive event [44].

Maintaining the supply chain of pharmaceutical products is not only paramount to cover the immediate medical response but will be fundamental to reducing disruption of the healthcare delivery system, which requires constant medicines, diagnostic tools and vaccines for smooth functioning.

In Nigeria, for example, over 70% of the prescribed medications are produced from active pharmaceutical ingredients (API) primarily sourced from firms in China and India. Uninterrupted access to medicine is an integral part of healthcare systems much needed and essential for the well-being of the population, but the COVID-19 pandemic has threatened this [31].

There is need to consider the new digital technologies that have potential to improve the ripple effect control in cases of epidemic outbreaks. Making innovations and data work for the supply chain resilience in crisis times, understanding and progressing the research of how these technologies can be used boost supply chains resilience, are important future research areas with a particular focus on data analytics, artificial intelligence, and machine learning [45].

There is minimal risk of bias in this study as articles were merely reviewed as presented and reviewers were not privy to the original data of the individual studies. Reviewers were also not interested in the outcome of the review but aimed at providing recommendations to country supply chains for the benefit of public health. None of the reviewers is a publisher of any of the articles reviewed. The review is limited to the competences of the reviewers in interpreting the results and to the fact that the coverage of included articles was flexible and neither restricted the review to articles conducted in homogenous settings nor compared their findings.

This study buttresses the need to devise and institute clear strategies on supply chain management in country and regional emergency responses, promotion of local manufacturing of medicines and other health products to reduce the extensive dependency on importation from international markets and increase the talent pool of supply chain management especially in Africa.

The review concluded that many manufacturers and service providers in some countries are already experiencing severe shortage of essential and non-essential raw materials including medical and pharmaceutical products, in addition to intermediate inputs, due to the COVID-19 pandemic and it's consequent border closures, trade restrictions among nations, and transportation problems. The COVID-19 pandemic however exposed some hidden potentials in many countries especially in Sub Saharan African. There is need for health supply chain resilience through development of a reliable supply chain strategy for pandemics and other such emergencies.

Conflict of interest

The authors declare no conflict of interest.

Author details

Ukamaka Gladys Okafor[1*], Modinat Aderonke Olaleye[2], Hillary Chukwuemeka Asobara[3] and Ebuka Fidelis Umeodinka[4]

1 Office of the Zonal Director, Pharmacists Council of Nigeria, Lagos, Nigeria

2 Department of Education and Training, Pharmacists Council of Nigeria, Lagos, Nigeria

3 Department of Registration and Licensing, Pharmacists Council of Nigeria, Lagos, Nigeria

4 Department of Pharmacy Practice, Pharmacists Council of Nigeria, Lagos, Nigeria

*Address all correspondence to: chinaemelum9291@yahoo.com; ukamaka.okafor@pcn.gov.ng

References

[1] WHO Corona virus Disease (COVID-19) Dashboard. Available from: https://covid19.who.int/

[2] Ferguson N.M, Laydon D, Nedjati-Gilani G, Imai N, Ainslie K, Baguelin M, Bhatia S, Boonyasiri A, Cucunubá Z, Cuomo-Dannenburg G, Dighe A, Dorigatti I, Fu H, Gaythorpe K, Green W, Hamlet A, Hinsley W, Okell L.C, van Elsland, S., Thompson, H., Verity, R., Volz, E., Wang, H., Wang, Y., Walker, P.G.T., Walters, C., Winskill P, Whittaker C, Donnelly C.A, Riley S, Ghani A.C (2020). Impact of Non-Pharmaceutical Interventions (NPIs) to Reduce COVID-19 Mortality and Healthcare Demand. COVID-19 Reports. Faculty of Medicine, Imperial College, London, UK. Available from: https://doi.org/10.25561/77482.

[3] Yu K.D.S., Aviso K.B (2020). Modelling the economic impact and ripple effects of disease outbreaks. Process Integration and Optimization for Sustainability. Available from: https://link-springer-com.ezproxy.lib.purdue.edu/content/pdf/10.1007/s41660-020-00113-y.pdf.

[4] Donato S., Roth S., Parry J. (2016). Strong supply chain public health. By ensuring the efficient and effective delivery of medicines and commodities, supply chains support healthy populations and regional health supply.

[5] OTL blog. Three components of an effective healthcare supply chain. Available from: https://www.google.com/amp/s/www.otlusa.biz/components-effective-healthcare-supply-chain/amp/. Accessed August, 2020.

[6] Amalesh S, Anirban A , Sourav B.B (2020). Covid-19's impact on supply chain decisions: Strategic insights from NASDAQ 100 firms using Twitter data. Journal of business research – Elsevier. Availablefrom:https://www-sciencedirect-com.ezproxy.lib.purdue.edu/science/article/pii/S0148296320303210. Accessed July, 2020.

[7] Adepoju B. [2020]. Impact of COVID-19 on Supply chain operations in Nigeria. International Journal of Business and Management Invention (IJBMI) Volume 9 Issue 4 Sr. 1; PP. 43-52. Available from: https://www.researchgate.net/publication/341055496_Impacts_of_COVID_19_on_supply_chain_operations_in_Nigeria.

[8] Lee, H.L., Zhao, X., Li, X. and Voss, C. (2020). "The effects of COVID-19 on global supply chains: responsiveness, resilience, and restoration (3Rs): special issue call for papers", Journal of Operations Management.

[9] Van Hoek R (2020). Research opportunities for a more resilient post-COVID-19 supply chain – closing the gap between research findings and industry practice. *International Journal of Operations & Production Management* Vol. 40 No. 4, 2020 pp. 341-355. DOI 10.1108/IJOPM-03-2020-0165

[10] Alborz S, Evripides G.L, Edward E, Alexandra J.G.L (2020). Exploration of alternative supply chains and distributed manufacturing in response to COVID-19; a case study of medical face shields. Available from: https://www-sciencedirect-com.ezproxy.lib.purdue.edu/science/article/pii/S0264127520
302835. Accessed July, 2020.

[11] Osseni I.A, (2020). COVID-19 Pandemic in Sub-Sahara Africa; Preparedness, Response and hidden potentials. *Tropical Medicine and Health* 48. Available from: https://tropmedhealth.biomedcentral.com/articles/10.1186/s41182-020-00240-9

[12] Yipeng L, Jong M.L, Celia. L. [2020]. The challenges and opportunities of a global health crisis: the management and business implications of COVID-19 from an Asian perspective. Available from: https://link-springer-com.ezproxy.lib.purdue.edu/content/pdf/10.1057/s41291-020-00119-x.pdf. Accessed July, 2020.

[13] Andrea M.A, Darrell E.H, Darryl H, Megan C.M and Alexis S (2020). Low-tech solutions for the COVID-19 supply chain crisis. Available from: https://www-nature-com.ezproxy.lib.purdue.edu/articles/s41578-020-0205-1.pdf. Accessed July, 2020.

[14] Freeman T.(2020)."COVID-19's Impact on the Medical Device Supply Chain." Medical Product Outsourcing 18.3(2020): 8. Business Insights: Global. Available from: http://bi.gale.com.ezproxy.lib.purdue.edu/global/article/GALE%7CA621802094/7e9204dc72c2876bbd01fd1fcfa56926?u=purdue_main. Accessed July 30, 2020.

[15] Akinyele B [2020]. COVID-19; Impact on supply chain and the implications for Business. Available from: https://www.proshareng.com/news/World-of-Business/COVID-19--Impact-On-Supply-Chains-and-Th/50529. Accessed July, 2020.

[16] Dmitry I. (2020). Predicting the impacts of epidemic outbreaks on global supply chains: A simulation-based analysis on the coronavirus outbreak (COVID-19/SARS-CoV-2) case. Available from: https://www-sciencedirect-com.ezproxy.lib.purdue.edu/science/article/pii/S1366554520304300. Accessed July, 2020.

[17] Maciel. Queiroz M.M, Ivanov D, Dolgui A, Wamba S.F (2020). Impacts of epidemic outbreaks on supply chains: mapping a research agenda amid the COVID-19 pandemic through a structured literature review. *Annals of Operations Research*. Available from: https://doi.org/10.1007/s10479-020-03685-7. Accessed July 2020.

[18] Nwoke E.A., Ofomata C. J., Amadi C.M., Jibuaku C.H., Akahome I.D. and Nwagbo E.C. Impact of the COVID-19 Pandemic on Consumers' Access to Essential Medicines in Nigeria. Available from: https://doi.org/10.4269/ajtmh.20-0838. Accessed July 2020.

[19] Linton, T. and Vakil, B. (2020). "Coronavirus is proving we need more resilient supply chains", Harvard Business Review. Available from: https://hbr.org/2020/03/coronavirus-is-proving-that-we-need-more-resilient-supply-chains. Accessed July 2020.

[20] Koonin, L.M. (2020), "Novel coronavirus disease (COVID-19) outbreak: now is the time to refresh pandemic plans", Journal of Business Continuity and Emergency Planning, Vol. 13 No. 4, pp. 1-15. Accessed July 2020.

[21] Fenske S. (2020). "COVID-19's Lasting Impact on Healthcare's Supply Chain." Medical Product Outsourcing 18.3 (2020): 8. Business Insights: Global. Available from: http://bi.gale.com.ezproxy.lib.purdue.edu/global/article/GALE%7CA621802089/843c4973e4b47d3a8008568cab2da024?u=purdue_main Accessed July 30, 2020.

[22] Akbarpour M, Tohrabi S.A and Ghavamifar A. (2020). Designing an integrated pharmaceutical relief chain network for demand uncertainty. *Transportation Research Part E. Available* from: https://doi.org/10.1016/j.tre.2020.101867

[23] Ranney, M. L., Valerie, G., & Jha, A. K. (2020). Critical supply shortages—the need for ventilators and personal protective equipment during the Covid-19 pandemic. New England

Journal of Medicine, 382, e41. Available from: https://www.nejm.org/doi/10.1056/NEJMp2006141

[24] The Economist February 15th 2020. Available from: https://shop.economist.com/products/the-economist-in-print-or-audio-february-15th-2020. Accessed May, 2020.

[25] Akasike C, Akinkuotu E, Adebayo F (2020). Coronavirus: Demands, Prices Soar for Face Masks, Hand Sanitizer. Available from: https://healthwise.punchng.com/coronavirus-demand sprices-soar-for-face-masks-hand-sanitiser. Accessed May 10, 2020.

[26] McDonnell A, Chalkidou K, Yadav P and Rosen D (2020). Understanding the impact of COVID-19 on essential medicine supply chain. Centre for Global Development. Available from: https://www.cgdev.org/blog/understanding-impact-covid-19-essential-medicine-supply-chains. Accessed July, 2020.

[27] Yua D.E.C, Razonb L. F, Tanb R.R (2020). Can global pharmaceutical supply chains scale up sustainably for the COVID-19 crisis? Chemistry Department, De La Salle University, Manila, Philippines. Available from: https://www-sciencedirect-com.ezproxy.lib.purdue.edu/science/article/pii/S0921344920301877. Accessed July, 2020.

[28] Okeke A. (2020). COVID-19 Impacts on healthcare supply chain in Africa. A webinar sponsored by: International Medical Procurement Agency (IMPA). Available from: www.iscea.org/impa. Accessed August, 2020.

[29] Breen L. and Hannibal C. (2020). "Learning from the Covid-19 pandemic: planning, controlling and driving change for greater resilience in supply chains: special issue call for papers", Supply Chain Management: An International Journal. Accessed July, 2020.

[30] Sanjoy K.P and Priyabrata C (2020). A production recovery plan in manufacturing supply chains for a high-demand item during COVID-19. International Journal of Physical Distribution & Logistics Management June 2020. DOI: 10.1108/IJPDLM-04-2020-0127

[31] Akande-Sholabi W, Adebisi Y.A (2020). The impact of COVID-19 pandemic on medicine security in Africa: Nigeria as a case study. *Pan African Medical Journal*;35(2): 73. [dio:10.11604/pamj.supp.2020.35.2.23671]. Available from: https://www.panafrican-med-journal.com/content/series/35/2/73/full

[32] Arloph J.V. [2020]. Supply Chain Disruptions & Challenges Post COVID-19 Crises in India context. Available from: https://search.proquest.com/open view/8e745a5a210c832bb4585d0c4178fca5/1?pq-origsite=gscholar&cbl=2068963. Accessed August, 2020

[33] Villena, V. H., & Gioia, D. A. (2020). A more sustainable supply chain companies tend to focus on their top-tier suppliers, but the real risks come lower down. Harvard Business Review, 98(2), 84-93. Available from: https://www.google.com/amp/s/hbr.org/amp/2020/03/a-more-sustainable-supply-chain. Accessed August, 2020.

[34] Gabriel S, Rifat A (2017). Do changes to supply chains and procurement processes yield cost savings and improve availability of pharmaceuticals, vaccines or health products? A systematic review of evidence from low-income and middle-income countries. BMJ Global Health 2017;2: e000243. doi:10.1136/bmjgh-2016-000243

[35] Raffeale G, Luca P, Désirée T, Davide T (2020) The Italian value chain in the pandemic: the input–output impact of Covid-19 lockdown. Available from: https://link-springer-com.

ezproxy.lib.purdue.edu/article/10.1007/s40812-020-00164-9. Accessed July, 2020.

[36] Mogaji, E. (2020), "Financial vulnerability during a pandemic: insights for coronavirus disease (COVID-19)", SSRN Electronic Journal, Vol. 2020 No. 5, pp. 57-63, doi: 10.2139/ssrn.3564702. Accessed August, 2020.

[37] Laing, T. (2020), "The economic impact of the Coronavirus 2019 (Covid-2019): implications for the mining industry", The Extractive Industries and Society, Elsevier, doi: 10.1016/j.exis.2020.04.003. Accessed August 2020

[38] Kilatrick J. (2020). COVID-19: Managing supply chain risk and disruption: The pandemic highlights the need to transform traditional supply chain model. Available from: https://www2.deloitte.com/us/en/pages/operations/articles/covid-19-managing-supply-chain-risk-and-disruption.html. Accessed, August 2020

[39] Lim, G. & Lee, C., (2020). Catching-up and the way forward in the electronics industry: The case of China (pp. 1-14). NCPA Case Study-2020-01. Accessed August, 2020.

[40] Laluyaux F. (2020). Covid-19 crisis shows supply chains need to embrace new technologies. Available from: https://www.weforum.org/agenda/2020/04/covid-19-crisis-shows-supply-chains-need-to-embrace-new-technologies/. Accessed August, 2020.

[41] Craighead C.W, Ketchen D.J. Jr, Darby J.L (2020). Pandemics and Supply Chain Management Research: Toward a Theoretical Toolbox. Decision Sciences Volume 51 Number 4.

[42] Covid-19 Impact on health product supply chain: Assessment and Recommendations. Available from: https://www.theglobalfund.org/media/9440/psm_covid-19impactonsupplychainlogistics_report_en.pdf?u=637330173950100000. Accessed July, 2020.

[43] Dowling P (2020). Health Care Supply Chains after the pandemic – John Snow Inc. (JSI). Available from: https://www.jsi.com/health-care-supply-chains-after-the-pandemic. Accessed July, 2020.

[44] Golan M.S, Jernegan L.H, Linkov I (2020). Trends and applications of resilience analytics in supply chain modeling: systematic literature review in the context of the COVID 19 pandemic. Available from: https://link-springer-com.ezproxy.lib.purdue.edu/content/pdf/10.1007/s10669-020-09777-w.pdf. Accessed July, 2020.

[45] Dubey R., Gunasekaran A., Childe J.S., and Wamba S.F (2020). Empirical investigation of data analytics capability and organizational flexibility as complements to supply chain resilience. *International journal of production research*. Available from: https://www.researchgate.net/deref/http%3A%2F%2Fdx.doi.org%2F10.1080%2F00207543.2019.1582820.

Chapter 6

'Silent Pandemic': Evidence-Based Environmental and Public Health Practices to Respond to the COVID-19 Crisis

Raimi Morufu Olalekan, Aziba-anyam Gift Raimi and Teddy Charles Adias

Abstract

Given the unprecedented novel nature and scale of coronavirus and the global nature of this public health crisis, which upended many public/environmental research norms almost overnight. However, with further waves of the virus expected and more pandemics anticipated. The COVID-19 pandemic of 2020 opened our eyes to the ever-changing conditions and uncertainty that exists in our world today, particularly with regards to environmental and public health practices disruption. This paper explores environmental and public health evidence-based practices toward responding to Covid-19. A literature review tried to do a deep dive through the use of various search engines such as Mendeley, Research Gate, CAB Abstract, Google Scholar, Summon, PubMed, Scopus, Hinari, Dimension, OARE Abstract, SSRN, Academia search strategy toward retrieving research publications, "gray literature" as well as reports from expert working groups. To achieve enhanced population health, it is recommended to adopt widespread evidence-based strategies, particularly in this uncertain time. As only together can evidence-informed decision-making (EIDM) can become a reality which include effective policies and practices, transparency and accountability of decisions, and equity outcomes; these are all more relevant in resource-constrained contexts, such as Nigeria. Effective and ethical EIDM though requires the production as well as use of high-quality evidence that are timely, appropriate and structured. One way to do so is through co-production. Co-production (or co-creation or co-design) of environmental/public health evidence considered as a key tool for addressing complex global crises such as the high risk of severe COVID-19 in different nations. A significant evidence-based component of environmental/public health (EBEPH) consist of decisions making based on best accessible, evidence that is peer-reviewed; using data as well as systematic information systems; community engagement in policy making; conducting sound evaluation; do a thorough program-planning frameworks; as well as disseminating what is being learned. As researchers, scientists, statisticians, journal editors, practitioners, as well as decision makers strive to improve population health, having a natural tendency toward scrutinizing the scientific literature aimed at novel research findings serving as the foundation for intervention as well as prevention programs. The main inspiration behind conducting research ought to be toward stimulating and collaborating appropriately on public/environmental health action. Hence, there is need for a "Plan B" of effective behavioral, environmental, social as well as systems interventions (BESSI) toward reducing transmission.

Keywords: Interprofessionalism, Living' reviews, Collective learning, Evidence-informed decision, COVID-19 pandemic, Environmental policy process, Team-based care, Credibility/trust, Timeliness, Systems thinking, Nigeria

1. Introduction

For each complicated challenges, there are simple, neat, as well as discreet solutions. It is therefore regularly obligatory toward making a decision on sufficient evidence for action, but then deficient toward satisfying the intellect. In this COVID-19 pandemic era where the public and the mass media attention are about serious health issues, it is important to explain why taking action should not be based on the basis of research study conducted individually, even though it remained prudently designed, effectively conducted, as well as appropriately interpreted and evaluated, which need to be highlighted. COVID-19 pandemic has been identified as a generation-defining, impacting economic shocks, families, communities and other unforeseen events in any country in the world, and has led to long-term economic financial conditions that have beset as well as create an "extinction-level event" which has cast an eerie shadow around the world long after the COVID-19 pandemic is behind us. Just over eighteen months ago, the flu-like news of a deadly virus affecting central China region started making headlines around the world. It was the start of what become a worldwide news and press conference; one that will constitute an exceptional problem for the environmental and public health practices and pose a series of lethal threats to environmental/public health. However, it is becoming increasingly "clear that the peril is not only in the form of a deadly virus". While the COVID-19 pandemic is likewise being used through maligning forces as an opportunity toward disrupting unforeseen as well as unprecedented circumstances, to sabotage and even to prevent the free flow of trusted, independent information toward the impact of the COVID-19 pandemic, which present an acute case of reliability. The highly contagious COVID-19 pandemic has been weaponised to undermine freedom of expression and has offer valid reason toward ushering in a series of reporting limitations on a descending severity scale from limiting data access, right through toward corrective legislation and even life threatening [1–3]. Additionally, the persistent disinformation onslaught as well as misinformation piercing platforms like the social media has formed a physical obstacle to COVID-19 truth-telling. Indeed, COVID-19 vaccines offer much-needed protection from disease, but there has so far been no evidence of whether they also curb transmission. Recently, around the world, concern is growing about the impact the new, fast spreading SARS-CoV-2 variants will have on the pandemic. Most countries are facing a widespread variant of SARS-CoV-2 known as B.1.351 and B.1.1.7, which appears to somewhat decrease the efficacy of some vaccines and have raised increasing apprehensions around the degree toward which their mutations are likely to aid them in evading present antibody treatments as well as extremely active vaccines. The news heightens concerns about B.1.351 and B.1.1.7, nonetheless researchers remain hopeful that the vaccine prevents severe disease and death. However, the chance of dying is around 35% higher for people who are confirmed to be infected with the new variant. Although, the data are preliminary, and it is not clear whether the variant is deadlier than previous strains or is spreading to more people who are vulnerable to severe disease. In fact, the COVID-19 vaccine might offer the necessary protection against some of these novel variants, current outcomes have recommended that the AstraZeneca vaccine might not offer much needed defense against that of South African variant, while there's still sufficient defense in most other existing vaccines toward preventing hospitalization, serious illness, as well as death. At the moment, the public health emergence of this novel variants ought to inspire us all toward taking steps to reduce SARS-CoV-2 spread. Meaning the three W's must be strictly followed: Wash your hands, watch your distance, wear a mask regularly. This likewise means we have to wrap up our sleeves toward getting vaccinated once the opportunity arises. Hence, the global health, economic, and social events that rattled series of activities around the world in 2020 have kicked off a new, uncertain era of environmental/public health practices, and it may take a long time for such uncertainty to ease. As many environmental/public health experts are predicting that it could even outlast the pandemic itself. While the world remains alarmed to panic at the grip of the demonic novel COVID-19 infection, there is still plenty of bearish perception as 2020 will certainly and no doubt be etched in the minds of health-care professionals, including environmental health officers all over the globe for several years to come which is unprecedented in the modern health care setting [4–6]. While, the national response toward COVID-19 varies, from the swift and most proactive to haphazard and negligent to the worst. That nations have already managed the spread of the pandemic in a different way is expected, nonetheless COVID-19 pushes all health systems toward their limits, thereby revealing serious gaps in environmental/public health structure, even in countries that are acclaimed as the popular centers for readiness. Thus, the response toward COVID-19 shows a glaring lack of social health determinants as well as meaningful collective learning, community participation and engagement on important issues in a health emergency. The outbreak of COVID-19 triggered severe acute respiratory syndrome of coronavirus 2 (SARSCoV-2) and has adversely affected social, economic events that rattled businesses as well as environmental health determinants and has challenged health professionals such as doctors, nurses, health workers, researchers, decision-makers and many others working in the health sector in many ways, while suspending the usual daily businesses [7].

2. How SARS-CoV-2 infects cells

To better understand SARS-life CoV-2's cycle and how it evades detection, as well as what makes the Delta variant so hazardous, scientists are working to unravel the virus's life cycle (**Figure 1**). Researchers have identified crucial modifications that enable viruses infect and hide inside of human cells with remarkable force. SARS-CoV-2 then performs a key processing phase as it exits the cells, preparing its particles to infect even more human cells.

Accordingly, COVID-19 pandemic has presented an acute case and also tested and assesses the national capacity of health systems toward withstanding health shocks while maintaining routine functions in many ways [9–11]. Hence routine reopening of service/activities toward approaching normalcy could continue for months or else years, but some positive results have been emerged and achieved in its wake. At the same time, global effort is being made to develop relevant international technologies, resources as well as available information that would create and accelerate data-driven results for all facets of this coronavirus pandemic. The coronavirus crisis is a global changing phenomenon and has become a top priority for our healthcare system, halting patient care processes which ranges from disrupting childhood vaccination as well as campaigns on polio eradication [12], maternal and child mortality are projected toward rising sharply, and health of young people

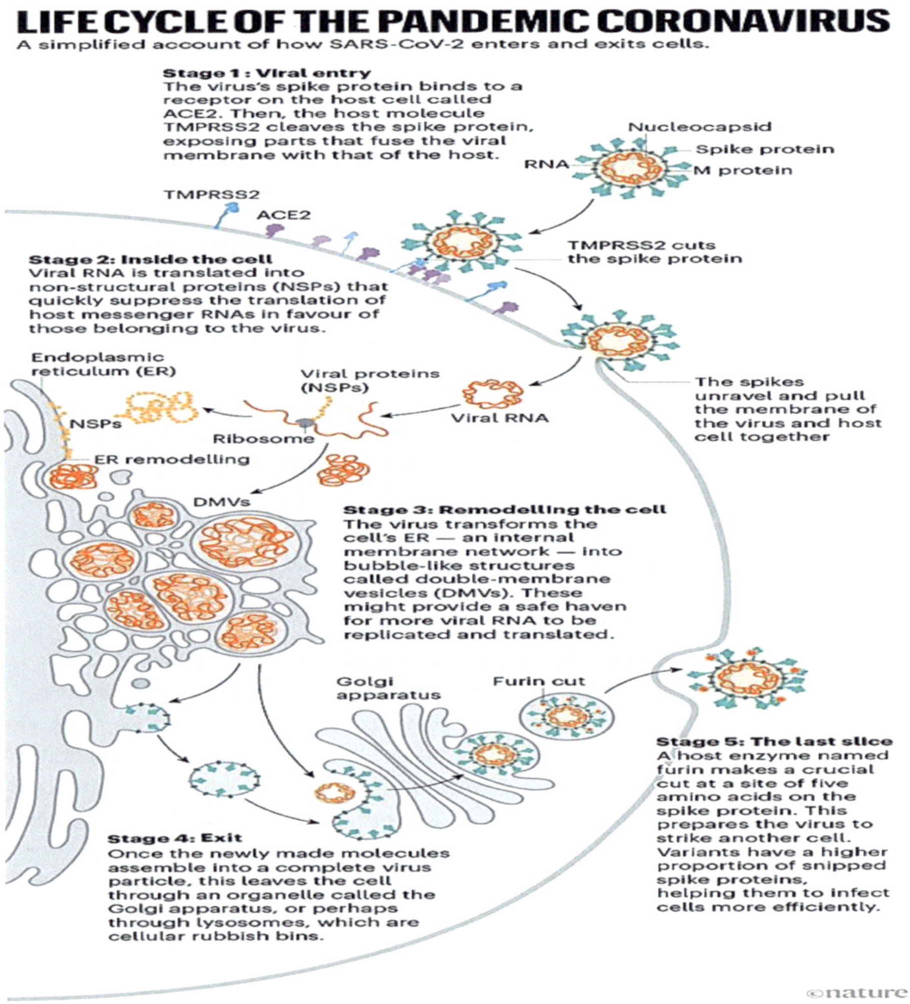

Figure 1.
Life cycle of the pandemic coronavirus: a simplified account of how SARS-CoV-2 enters and exists cells. Source: Adapted from [8].

to injuries, non-communicable diseases, as well as universal health coverage, despite unleashing enormous social, economic and health crises that threaten the world with antimicrobial resistance which threatens our ability to treat common infections, disrupting many research activities as well as overwhelmingly impacting medical education in various research activities. The coronavirus pandemic is not the first and foremost serious health challenge facing the world, nevertheless its long-term achievement will largely depend on rapid data synthesizing and information, appropriately AND responsibly into comprehensive public and environmental health policies both national and international. In the face of great uncertainty around Covid-19 pandemic future, epidemiologic models become an important planning tools for decision makers, clinicians as well as public health practitioners [1–3]. COVID-19 has made visible major global weaknesses, vulnerabilities and highlighted the necessity for health reforms toward promoting global access toward affordable care. At the same time, countries are examining their different policies toward protecting people at increased severe risk of disease. It may be the policies intended at preventing transmission in the general population, immunization (as the Oxford AstraZeneca vaccine and Pfizer BioNTech COVID vaccine has turn out to be available) because the world has received the Oxford AstraZeneca vaccine and Pfizer BioNTech COVID vaccine and has been roll-out to millions of people in the United States of America (USA), India, United Kingdom (UK), Ghana, Cote d'ivoire and Nigeria, also its distribution and immunization has commenced without political, religious or ethnic affiliation. Up until now, the seemingly bulletproof important priority is to rebuild and reenergize the country toward acting rather than reacting. As uncertainty around the peril of COVID-19 calamity grows continuously and geometrically, long-term protection policies need to be developed such as specific public safety measures toward protecting vulnerable populations at increased risk through reducing contacts between individuals in danger, etc. Recognizing that promoting sustainable development is risky, difficult and exhausting, particularly as the spread of SARS-CoV-2 pandemic increased geometrically, as those living in poverty which is leading to growing anger and frustration are currently at increased peril of setbacks with more than thirteen (13) million children out of school [1, 3, 9, 10, 13]. This stresses the importance of linking the results of environmental research with human health has mentioned. This necessitates understanding of the significance of interventions toward addressing system inequalities, universal health care as well as coverage issues, and wide-ranging public protection schemes as being part of response.

Now is the time toward realizing that we are not at equal peril of severe COVID-19 consequences and that there is need to work with stakeholders and development partners toward developing and improving effective response as well as solutions [3, 14–19]. This paper offers research evidence to inform decision makers about people that could remain at increased peril or severe high risk of COVID-19 pandemic in diverse countries. Hence, scientific research evidence is required to investigate the environmental as well as public health practices in the coronavirus diseases era, which ought to place emphasis on diverse policies guidelines toward preventing those that are vulnerable and at increased risk. It is imperative toward comparing those individuals at high peril of severe COVID-19 pandemic toward helping nations to design as well as develop improved interventions measures toward protecting vulnerable populations as well as reducing straining on health complications as well as health systems [1–3, 10, 19]. These evidences can offer as well as advise a wide-ranging health assessment, social, as well as economic significances of protecting diverse groups [9, 16–18, 20–22], highlighting the prerequisite toward developing and providing a long-term Covid-19 management policy as well as given the unprecedented scale of policy-makers', scientific evidence require large-scale partnership as well as collective learning in the scientific evidence synthesis community. Henceforth, outcomes improvement across countries can be attained through successful high-quality evidence certification that is properly implemented. To accomplish this, national systems, policies as well as political milieus require to be hospitable toward evidence informed methods, besides there is prerequisite toward fostering partnership, facilitate negotiation, promote as well as advance scientific evidence-informed decision-making (SEIDM) in Sub-Saharan Africa as well as the world at large toward achieving effective greater performance and worldwide sustainable implementation.

Since the 2019 coronavirus disease (COVID-19) has triggered seismic economic and societal changes which grapple with an uncertain future, that has consumed and changed our lives, the COVID-19 global crisis also revealed that the country is deteriorating in terms of environmental/public health readiness. As COVID-19 has become an imminent emerging, rapidly evolving situation of environmental/public health concern with 'threat multiplier to health in the 21st century [11, 23, 24]. As confusion, disorientation, agitation and even psychosis have been associated with symptoms of COVID-19. The body of research is making the link among infection as a result of virus and neurological symptoms. The number of publicly reported deaths rate of the population due to the 2019 coronavirus disease (COVID-19) might underrate the death toll from the pandemics. These estimates are based on provisional data that are frequently incomplete as well as might rule out unreported COVID-19 deaths. In addition, the pandemic restrictions imposed (for example, stay-at-home orders, school closures, quarantine measures, personal hygiene, physical distancing measures used to contain the spread of the virus) may possibly and indirectly claim lives through delayed care for acute emergencies, exacerbations of chronic diseases, as well as psychological distress (for instance, drug overdoses). As a result, the severe burden of acute respiratory syndrome coronavirus 2 (SARS-CoV-2) pandemic remains to rise, both due to morbidity as well as pandemic mortality along with the impact of mitigation strategies [2, 3, 9, 10, 25]. Tailoring policies based on emerging evidence on the conditions associated with the severity of COVID-19 is essential toward actions informing of both decision-makers as well as individuals. Meaning moving from generalized population-based mitigation strategies toward focusing on people exposed to the risk of severe COVID-19 outcomes [16–18, 20–22].

Too often, Jenicek [26] has repeatedly described evidence-based environmental/public health (EBEPH) as "the conscientious, explicit, as well as judicious usage of available evidence in decisions making process towards communities care as well as populations in the realm of health maintenance and protection, disease prevention and development (health promotion)." Similarly, a succinct definition arisen from Kohatsu [27]: "Evidence-based public health is the process of integrating science-based interventions with community preferences to improve populations health". While, public health has succeeded in solving numerous problems, but almost all successes have a double-edged sword. Programs as well as policies have remained enacted as well as, in most cases, results that are positive which shows an increase in the improvement number of population health. However, some people suffer from health disparities as well as social inequalities. This raises such questions like, is there a way to approach the lessons learned directly from successful interventions as well as applies them toward other topics and situations? Are we using evidence that is based on scientific research/evidence? How can we greatly foster political will toward supporting evidence-based policy making? How do we promote and influence inducements so that practitioners can make effective evidence usage? Just as evidence-based environmental/public health has turn out to be a topic of conversation for both practitioners and policymakers, it is so fundamental toward people concept of justice, it is likewise important for environmental/public health. Therefore, it ought to notify our decisions on how the intervention will be implemented, and in what populations, when as well as how to assess both the negative and occasionally positive impact of such interventions. Justice commitment also bears the obligation of finding effective approaches toward reducing disparities in health between groups existing in practically entirely geopolitical units. For environmental and public health professionals, evidence is a type of data that includes (quantitative) epidemiologic data, program policy evaluations or outcomes, as well as the qualitative data to be used in establishing decisions or judgments [2, 3, 28, 29] (see **Figure 2**). Indeed, Brownson and colleagues identify a (6) six-stage procedure through which environmental and public health practitioners remain able toward taken an approach that is evidence-based toward policy making, with the community members perspectives, fostering an added population-centered method, which seems toward a combination of consensus that are of scientific evidence, along with resources, values, as well as contexts, ought to cross the threshold of policy making. Hence, "Evidence-based public/environmental health is the process of integrating science-based interventions with community preferences

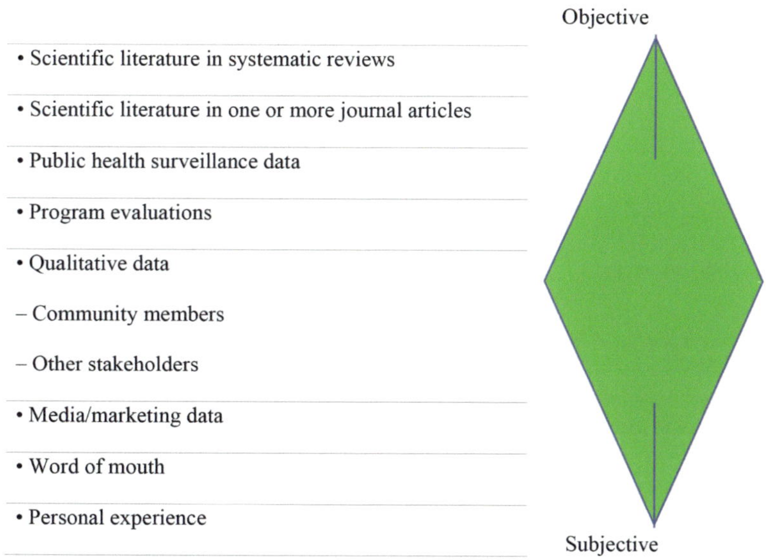

Figure 2.
Different forms of evidence. Source: Adapted from chambers and Kerner [28] and Raimi et al., [2].

toward improving populations health" or it involves "the available body of facts or information indicating whether a belief or proposition is true or valid." [2, 30].

Evidence in public and environmental health is often the outcome of a complicated concepts of theory, observation, as well as experiment [3, 31]. The evidence value, on the other hand, remains in the beholder eyes (for example, the value of evidence might differ from a stakeholder type) [2, 3, 32]. Research not only encompasses medical evidence, then also patient characteristics, readiness of patients toward undergoing a therapy, as well as society's values [33]. Decision-makers pursue distributional penalties (i.e., who pays, how much as well as who profits) [34, 35], and practically, settings anecdotes and occasionally provide detailed experimental data [2, 3, 36]. The evidence is typically imperfect, as Gray Muir note [37], "The absence of excellent evidence does not make evidence-based decision making impossible; what is needed is the best available evidence, not the best evidence possible." Some authors describe diverse types of scientific evidence for public health practice [38, 39] (see **Table 1**). Evidence from Type 1 identifies the diseases causes as well as the degree, severity, as well as risk factors preventability associated with the diseases. They suggest that a specific disease or risk factor needs to be done. Evidence from Type 2 establishes the absolute effects of a particular actions that cause or do not advance health, with the caveat that, "In particular, this must be done" [39]. The situation has remained observed that strict adherence toward regulatory study designs guidelines can strengthen an "inverse (see **Figure 2**) evidence law" through which most probable toward influencing the public interventions (e.g., change in policy) remain least appreciated from an evidence matrix highlighting randomized designs [29, 40–45]. In comparison to descriptive/epidemiologic research (Type 1), a recent study showed a paucity of research intervention (Type 2). In a randomized controlled trial of cigarette use, alcohol consumption [46–48], as well as insufficient physical activity, the team discovered that in 2005–2006, 14.9 percent of subjects reported an intervention, while, 78.5 percent of research articles reported remained descriptive or epidemiologic. Less research is probable published on Type 3 evidence showing in what way as well as beneath what circumstantial interventions conditions remained implemented, as well as by what method they remained received, indicating "how it

S/N	Characteristic	Type 1	Type 2	Type 3
1	Typical data/ relationship	Size and strength of preventable risk - disease relationship (measures of burden, etiologic research)	Relative effectiveness of public health intervention	Information on the adaptation and translation of an effective intervention
2.	Common setting	Clinic or controlled community setting	Socially intact groups or community-wide	Socially intact groups or community-wide
3.	Example	Smoking results in lung cancer.	Price upsurges from a targeted media campaign decrease the rates of smoking.	Comprehending the political problems of increase in price or aiming at media messages toward specific audience segments
4.	Quantity	More	Less	Less
5.	Action	Something must be done.	These specific priorities must be implemented.	How can this intervention be implemented

Source: Adapted from Brownson et al., [39] and Raimi et al., [2].

Table 1.
Comparison of the types of scientific evidence.

should be done" [38]. So far, research has focused on internal validity (for examples, well-controlled trials efficacy) with external validity while receiving sparse consideration (e.g., adaptation of scientific knowledge to a different context) [2, 3, 49, 50].

3. Comprehending the framework for evidence

Evidence of type 3 from an intervention context [38]. While many scholars have written around the context role it plays in providing information on the subject of evidence-based practice [32, 38, 51], there is not much consensus on its meaning. Context turn into more unknown as well as unpredictable, variable, and multifaceted as we move from scientific interventions toward population-level as well as policy interventions. Relevant definitions to the context highlight's evidence required toward modifying as well as implementing an information-based intervention in a specific population or context [38]. There are five overlapping domains in the conditions for Type 3 evidence (see **Table 2**). First, there are features of the intervention targeting demographic, for instance educational attainment as well as medical history. This is the reason why interpersonal variables provide the most important context. People with cancer history, for example, may be more susceptible toward getting cancer screening. Finally, organizational variables must be taken into account. For instance, if an organization succeeds in implementing an evidence - based program in which it is influenced through capacity (for example, agency leadership, a trained personnel) [51, 52]. Fourth, it is known that social norms and cultural traits are closely linked toward shaping several health behaviors. Ultimately, the greatest political as well as economic forces will influence the context. For example, large-scale measures of certain disease can impact a state's political will toward addressing the problems in a logical as well as methodical way. There is an urgent evidence need for contextual determinants as well as approaches

Category	Examples
Individual	Personal/Individual health history Education level Basic human needs[a]
Interpersonal	History of family health Social capital Peers support
Organizational	Organizational culture Staff expertise Staff configuration Physical infrastructure
Sociocultural	Values Social norms History Cultural traditions
Economic and political	Political ideology Political will Lobbying as well as special interests costs and benefits

[a]Basic human needs include food, shelter, warmth, and safety.
Source: Adapted from Brownson et al., [39] and Raimi et al., [2].

Table 2.
Contextual variables for intervention design, implementation, and adaptation.

toward adapting programs as well as policies across contexts as well as demographic subgroups. Predominantly aimed at high-risk as well as understudied populations. Circumstantial COVID-19 pandemic questions remain being addressed in novel "realist review," which remains a systematic review procedure that not only examines if the recent intervention is working effectively but then again, in what manner interventions actually work in real-world contexts [53].

4. Related challenges toward public/environmental health evidence

Evidence on public and environmental health has been described as underpopulated, dispersed, as well as varied. The situation remains underpopulated since there are comparatively limited well-done appraisals of how public/environmental health impacts interventions (Type 2 evidence) while applying across varied cultural groups (Type 3 evidence). The criteria for making public/environmental health decision are much more varied than the clinical interventions evidence. Health impact evidence on built milieu, for instance, could be discovered in transportation planning. Lastly, evidence in public and environmental health is varied, in part since much of the interventions base science remains obtained from "natural experiments" or nonrandomized designs.

5. Triangulating evidence

Triangulation is the process of combining multiple evidence from various sources toward gaining understanding into a specific topic as well as typically includes both qualitative as well as quantitative data [39]. It often entails the application of several ways of data collection as well as analysis toward determining disagreement or commonality points. Due to the corresponding nature of evidence from varied sources, triangulation is generally useful. Even though quantitative data offer an outstanding opportunity toward determining by what method, variables are made in the lives of many individuals, these data does not provide much insight into why such associations exist. Qualitative data, on the other hand, can aid in providing information toward explaining quantitative results, or what is known as "illuminating meaning". Many instances of the application of qualitative as well as quantitative data triangulation toward evaluating health programs as well as policies, together with AIDS & HIV prevention programs [54], policies as well as programs on occupational health [35], and programs in community settings toward chronic disease prevention [2, 55].

6. Geographic and cultural differences

The concept of EBPEH was developed largely by a context of Western, European American [56]. The epistemologic grounds of logical positivism, which discovers meaning by a rigorous observation as well as measurement, are revealed in the reality through the conceptual method. This is apparent in a professional preference aimed at randomized controlled trial between clinicians designed for research designs. Additionally, most research in the EBPEH literature are academic research, typically through well-established investigators receiving external financial support. In dissimilarity, even if the problem scope might be huge, the information base aimed at how best toward addressing mutual public/environmental health glitches is generally limited in emerging countries as well as some impoverished areas of affluent countries, Cavill and colleagues [57] likened interventions that are evidence-based across European countries, demonstrating that considerable evidence base is restricted toward experimental observations in various domains. Even in nations that remain developed (such as United States), much of peer-reviewed published information in journals or data made available by websites as well as government agencies might not sufficiently epitomize entirely interested populations. There are (4) four prime user evidence groups in environment and public health, namely: practitioners of environmental and public health as well as their partners, who are likely to recognize the scope as well as quality of evidence in certain strategies (for example, policies, programs)? In actual fact, nevertheless, practitioners of environmental and public health often possess a comparatively narrow selection process option. Funds resulting from local, state and federal sources are usually earmarked for definite purpose [for example, sexually transmitted diseases as well as surveillance treatment [54], establishments of retail food inspection [58–60]. However, there is an opportunity for environmental and public health professionals, including the responsibility, toward cautiously examining the evidence to find alternative methods toward achieving required health goals [3, 15, 35, 61, 62]. Decision-makers at regional, state, local, national, as well as international levels (deciding at the macro level in what way toward allocating public resources aimed at which they have remained nominated stewards [2, 16–18, 20–22, 63] make up the next generation user group. This group is also in charge of extra responsibility for formulating policies for complex and controversial public issues), Stakeholders (This group consist of many development partners i.e., NGOs whose missions' emphasis on or incorporate health improvement, either directly or by improving the social as well as physical milieus that remain significant demographic health determinants for example whether the community water supply should be fluoridated, dumpsite should be sited in a community cemetery or burial ground) and researchers on population health issues (They create as well as apply exploring research hypotheses using evidence. Some remain principally interested in used methodologies toward determining the quality as well as research implications on population-based interventions studies). Both enhance and use the evidence to answer research questions. However, the additional increased benefits of evidence-based environmental/public health (EBE/PH) have many indirect as well as direct benefits, including access toward a more as well as better quality evidence toward improving public's/environmental health, an effective and efficient probability of successful policies as well as programs implemented, better workforce productivity, as well as greater efficient usage of private as well as public resources [10, 64]. Therefore, in most areas of environmental, public health as well as clinical practice, decisions about when to intercede as well as what policy or program to execute remain not simple as well as straightforward. These choices are generally based on (3) three essential questions: (1) Should public and environmental health intervention remain taken toward addressing a specific environmental/public health concern (Type 1, etiologic information or evidence of behavioral knowledge)? (2) What measures or action must be taken (Type 2, intervention evidence or proof of intervention)? (3) In what manner can a specific policy or program remain implemented most effectively at the local setting (Type 3, contextual evidence)? **Table 1** presents a range of systematic evidence aimed at public and environmental health practice [2, 38, 64]. Evidence from Type 1 assesses the diseases causes as well as its severity, magnitude, and risk factors preventability as well as diseases. Also, evidence from Type 2 describes the comparative effects of specific interventions that may or may not advance health and evidence from Type 3 comes from the context of the intervention and specifies the five (5) overlapping domains (**Table 2**).

Firstly, there are features of the number of populations for intervention like, for instance education level as well as health history. In addition, interpersonal variables make available an important context. For instance, an individual with cancer family history might be more probable toward undergoing screening of cancer. Thirdly, institutional variables ought to remain considered. For instance, whether an organization is successfully implementing an evidence-based program that may remain influenced through the aforementioned capacity (example, professional workforce, organizational leadership) [1, 2, 7, 64].

Fourth, it is argued that social norms and cultural norms cause and shape a lot of health behaviors. Lastly, more economic as well as political forces tend to affect context. For instance, the occurrence of high rate aimed at certain disease like the recent COVID-19 pandemic, has claimed far too many lives worldwide. Fortunately, as environmental health officers and doctors continue to gained more experience at monitoring, contact tracing, communicating and treating COVID-19 patients, and many people hospitalized eventually recover, this might impact a state's political will toward addressing the problem meaningfully, logically as well as in a systematic method [1–3, 9, 10, 19]. Particularly because of the understudied populations at high-risk, there is a great requirement for more evidence between contextual variables as well as process toward adapting program change as well as policies in context as well as population subgroups. Problem-solving questions are addressed in novel detail known as "realist review," which remains a systematic assessment procedure that explores not only how intervention works, but then again by what method, interventions measures work in a real-world situation [1–3, 53, 65, 66]. Numerous ideas are important in achieving a greater evidence-based method toward the practice of public and environmental health. Essentially, scientific knowledge is required on programs as well as policies that can be effective toward promoting and improving health (i.e., conducting evaluation research toward generating sound evidence) [2, 3, 64, 67]. Second, in order to transform science into scientifically sound practice, there is a necessity toward marrying evidence-based interventions information from peer-reviewed literature through the realities of a definite real-world milieu [2, 3, 64]. To achieve this, there is prerequisite to properly define decision making procedures that must be evidence-based. Lastly, widespread dissemination of proven effectiveness interventions must arise more constantly at levels of state as well as local [3, 35, 68, 69]. Therefore, the main characteristics of evidence-based features of public and environmental health decision making comprise:

i. Making Decision founded on the most up-to-date peer-reviewed evidence (both research on qualitative and quantitative): The scientific literature as well as guidelines issued through expert panels serve as a starting point of advice. Additionally, researchers as well as practitioners are frequently presenting preliminary findings in national, regional, as well as international professional conferences.

ii. Using data and information systems systematically: Data remain being created more for issues at local level and a few initial efforts to improve the public and environmental health policy surveillance systems are under way. For instance, policy surveillance systems for alcohol, tobacco, and more recently, school-based nutrition as well as physical education have currently developed by a consortium of federal as well as voluntary agencies [46–48].

iii. Developing and application of robust program planning frameworks (which is often rooted in behavioral science theory): For instance, ecological models or systems are progressively used where "appropriate cultural changes take place in the social milieu brings about individual's changes, and support population considered critical to the implementation of changes in the environment" [11, 61–63, 65, 66, 70–73]. These models emphasize the need toward solving remarkable multiple levels problems as well as emphasize the interaction as well as integration of elements within and between interpersonal, individual, organizational, community and governmental levels. The aim is toward creating a healthy positive community milieu that offers information that enhances health-promotion as well as social support toward helping the population live healthier and better lifestyles. Interventions that are effective are most frequently grounded on the principles of health-behavior theory [31].

iv. Community assessment involvement and decision-making: Community-based methods include research community members as well as projects intervention and demonstrates progress made toward improving public health as well as addressing disparities in health. Academicians, practitioners, as well as members of the community who collaboratively highlight key concern issues, develop intervention strategies, as well as evaluate outcomes. This method integrates knowledge as well as action that seek toward leading a fair distribution of the benefits of an intervention for all partners, builds on data from "stakeholder" input [2, 3, 74], while also, building on existing resources and facilitates collaboration between all partners.

v. Conducting sound and appropriate evaluation: In most cases in population health, programs as well as policies are implemented without fully focusing on methodical evaluation. Additionally, even if the programs are not effective, sometimes, they are sustained due to political or historical reasons. Evaluation criteria should be based on the development of early program as well as had better consist of both formative as well as result evaluation.

For instance, the injury management program remained properly discontinued after evaluating its effectiveness. This program evaluation demonstrates the usage of both multiple critical quantitative as well as qualitative data toward framing the evaluation model.

vi. Disseminating what is being taught to key stakeholders in decision-makers: If a policy or program is implemented, or if final outcomes is recognized, other public and environmental health such as community medicine, social medicine, community health and preventive medicine (environmental health) can draw on their research findings toward enhancing their own evidence use, while making decision. It can be disseminated or communicated to health practitioners through scientific literature, toward overall public through the media, toward decision-makers through individual meetings, as well as toward training public/environmental health professionals. In many settings, effective interventions remain required, comprising worksites, health care settings, schools, as well as wide-ranging community environments etc. Hence, accomplishing these activities in EBE/PH is likely to require a synthesis of scientific skills, enhanced communication, common sense, and political acumen.

7. Systematic techniques and methods to enhance environmental/public health evidence-based uptake

Several tools as well as planning methods can help practitioners in environmental/public health in responding to questions like: What are the magnitude of the environmental/human health challenges relating to COVID-19 pandemic; If there is an effective priorities aimed at resolving the challenges; What about the local environmental information as well as specific intervention that is useful in determining its possible use in relation to the current state of affairs at hand (Covid-19 pandemic); Is it that a specific program is policy worth having or worth doing (i.e., is it better than having substitutes), as well as will it yield suitable investment return, measured in terms of monetary or health consequences? These tools include:

8. Public/environmental health surveillance

According to the public/environmental health adage, which state that "what gets measured, gets done." This measurement often begins with public/environmental health monitoring, the continuing systematic collection, analysis, interpretation, as well as distribution of COVID-19 pandemic health data with the aim of preventing as well as managing illness, injury, along with other health snags. Public/environmental health monitoring is an important instrument for those using EBEPH. It includes building a systematic analysis, collection as well as routinely interpreting detailed health information/data, and combining the strengths and weaknesses of disseminating data over time toward those accountable for prevention as well as disease control or injury [3]. Public/Environmental health monitoring systems must have the ability toward collecting as well as data analyzing, disseminating data toward human health programs, as well as frequently appraise the efficiency of the usage of disseminated data [2, 3, 75]. For instance, the ongoing prevalence of COVID-19 pandemic documentation as a justification for eliminating COVID-19 spread along with documenting the impacts of such actions [2, 3, 10, 19]. In substance use control in the core Niger Delta region of Nigeria, a common agreement metric for substance use across Bayelsa states was recognized [46–48]. While, systems of surveillance are supported at local, state as well as federal levels and could be used toward determining the diseases frequency as well as other conditions of health in a defined population. At minimum, five main objectives of the surveillance systems could be stated: (1) health assessment and monitoring status as well as general health risks; (2) to provide a disease-specific understanding of events as well as trends; (3) planning, implementation, monitoring, as well as appraising health policies and programs; (4) put in place financial management as well as information monitoring; and (5) conduct research in environmental/public health [1–3]. Some systems of surveillance presently existing can now offer deaths, births, birth defects, cancers, infectious diseases as well as health behaviors information. Individual system frequently has enough information toward assessing the prevalence or incidence rates as well as toward describing diseases frequency or condition of health through a person, place, as well as time. Even the surveillance systems data could be used toward obtaining a baseline as well as follow-up measurements aimed at specific populations.

9. Systematic reviews and evidence-based processes

Systematic reviews involve comprehensive syntheses of collections of databases on specific topic. Good review reading may remain one of the utmost resourceful ways toward getting acquainted with advanced research as well as practice on several precise environmental/public health topics [76, 77]. The usage of explicit and consistent systematic methods (i.e., decision-making rules) in reviews decrease bias as well as decrease's chance impacts, hence providing a more trustworthy outcomes on which decisions are made [78]. One utmost important critique for public/environmental interventions in health is the "Guide toward Community Preventive Practices" (the Community Guide), providing a synopsis of contemporary scientific literature using a well-defined and rigorous approach where existing important research are units of analytical analysis [79, 80]. The Public Guide offers to addressed (1) What interventions statements are been considered or evaluated as well as what are their implications? (2) What interventions aspects could support clients in choosing between proven interventions set that are effective? (3) How much does this intervention cost, as well as how much does it costs in relation to probable impacts on health? A respectable systematic critique should enable professionals to comprehend local contextual situations required for fruitful implementation [81].

10. Economic evaluation

The costs-benefits comparison to establish the most effective allocation of scarce resources is known as economic evaluation. We always carry out economic evaluations, albeit we rarely openly think about the process. It is a key component of evidence-based practice [82]. It could make available evidence toward evaluating the absolute alternative value of expenditures provided to the public/environmental health programs as well as policies. In cost–benefit analysis, all decision options based on costs as well as consequences remain valued in economic terms. Most frequently, placement on financial investment is related to an intervention likened to its effects on health, for instance, cases of disease prevented or saved life years. The absolute worth of some alternative interventions (for instance, health return on euro/dollars invested) may show this method of cost-effectiveness analysis (CEA), [82].

Cost-effectiveness analysis (CEA) has turn out to be an increasingly essential instrument for academics, practitioners, as well as policy makers. Nevertheless, appropriate data toward supporting this analysis type are not permanently accessible, particularly in the context of potential public policies considered in health improvement [3, 36, 83, 84]. While, four (4) related kinds of economic assessment namely: cost utility analysis (CUA), cost-effectiveness analysis (CEA), cost–benefit analysis (CBA), as well as cost-minimization analysis (CMA). The four techniques vary chiefly in the mode of how benefits are measured. The cost–benefit analysis (CBA) measures the benefit in economic units (e.g., euros, dollars), while the cost-effectiveness analysis (CEA) measures the benefits in the relevant health unit (e.g., saved lives). Cost utility analysis (CUA) is a form of cost-effectiveness analysis (CEA) in which the benefits (such as life expectancy) are adjusted for life quality as well as quantified through a measure of health utility (typically quality-adjusted life years [QALYs]). Cost-minimization analysis (CMA) remain used once the two benefits interventions are the same, so the benefits measurement remains not a problem. Since cost–benefit analysis (CBA) uses the utmost "generic" outcome measure (several factors could remain measured through currency, together with the value of public health projects as well as educational interventions), it enables for a comparison of multiple programs. Its outcomes (see **Figure 3**) illustrate the possible results of the economic evaluation [2]. In view of the four (4) squares of the graph. Programs toward improving health as well as saving money (Quadrant IV) are certainly valuable as well as ought to be implemented. Likewise, programs that undermine health as well as costs affordability (Quadrant II) are unwelcome as well as must not remain continued or initiated. The two quadrants remaining (I and III) are in critical condition as well as where monetary appraisal can be more informative. In history, systems of environmental/public health as well as nations develop, interventions as well as programs began in Quadrant IV, through these programs that remain cost saving as well as improve and maintain health. Several initial public/environmental health interventions, like systems of sanitation, drop in Quadrant IV. When interventions are used as well as implemented, attention turns to programs in Quadrant I that improve and maintain health at an affordable cost. After all, as pressures in budgetary activities rise, programs in quadrant III are bear in mind: programs that lessen costs, nevertheless add loss toward health status. Aiming at the four (4) quadrants, the key question is, what is investment return

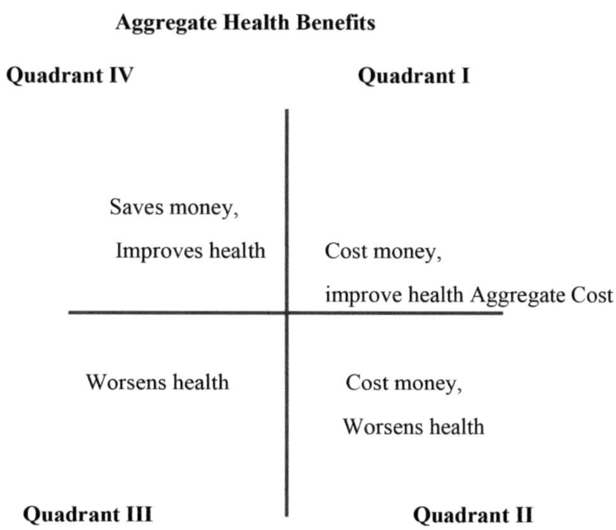

Figure 3.
Possible outcomes of an economic evaluation. Adapted from Raimi et al., [2].

(or disinvestment) toward public's funds? Economic evaluation offers a means toward answering this pertinent question, so programs can be selected for the highest investment return.

Using the above conceptual framework (**Figure 3**) for the case of COVID-19 pandemic, numerous important conceptual economic evaluation elements can remain recognized. Before bearing in mind the procedure of conducting economic evaluation, it can be helpful toward determining the overall elements as well as all economic evaluations approach. The primary step is toward choosing the economic evaluation opinion. Each intervention could be thought of in several ways, often categorized as going from narrow toward broad. Health agencies or organization opinion should directly take part in delivering projected intervention. The next step which may be the insurers opinion, or payers, particularly in the health care industry, where consumers as well as payers remain two (2) distinct groups. The widest opinion is that of the whole society. Recommendations has been based on this wide-ranging economic evaluation opinion for all, as well as it is obligatory in quite a few countries having an established national health system. The viewpoint of the society is importantly suitable in public/environmental health as it seeks interventions designed toward benefiting taxpayers as well as the public funding the costs.

11. Health impact assessment

Health impact assessment (HIA) is an evidence-based forward-looking instrument used toward informing stakeholders as well as policymakers around the possible health impacts of projects as well as policies being anticipated, while identifying opportunities aimed at maximizing possible health benefits as well as limiting potential damage. Similarly, Health Impact Assessment (HIA) is a blend of several methodologies in the assessment of the possible health impact on a population and its distribution, arising from policies, programmes, or projects is instrumental in linking with other sectors to deal with the root cause of health challenges and thereby fostering the successful actualization of the sustainable development goals, having sprung into prominence in the last few decades [16–18, 20–22, 63]. Health impact assessment (HIA) is a somewhat recent way of assessing the likely impact of policy or intervention in non-health sectors, for instance economic development, transportation, as well as agriculture, on population health [2, 6, 22, 29, 42–45, 63, 85–87]. Other HIAs is aimed to ensure the participation of the actors involved in a particular project development. This latter method, which forms the foundation of the environmental impact assessment that several massive place-based projects is obligatory through law, which is comparable toward the nonregulatory method that has remained accepted for other HIAs. In general, HIA, in all its procedures, has remained acceptable by way of a tool due to the growing evidence that the social as well as physical milieus remain a significant health determinant as well as health inequalities in populations (see **Figure 4**). Hence, social determinant of health (SDoH) could be influenced through policies as well as programs, and are related through improved health outcomes. Social Determinant of Health (SDoH) is strongly influenced through policies, systems, as well as the environments (PSE). Diagram in **Figure 4** shows County Based Health Rankings as well as Roadmaps recognize the interplay amongst health outcomes, the Social Determinant of Health (SDoH), are policies as well as programs. For instance, tobacco being a foremost health outcomes determinant (e.g., quality of life, mortality), as well as the reduction in the use of tobacco and is strongly influenced through cigarettes prices as well

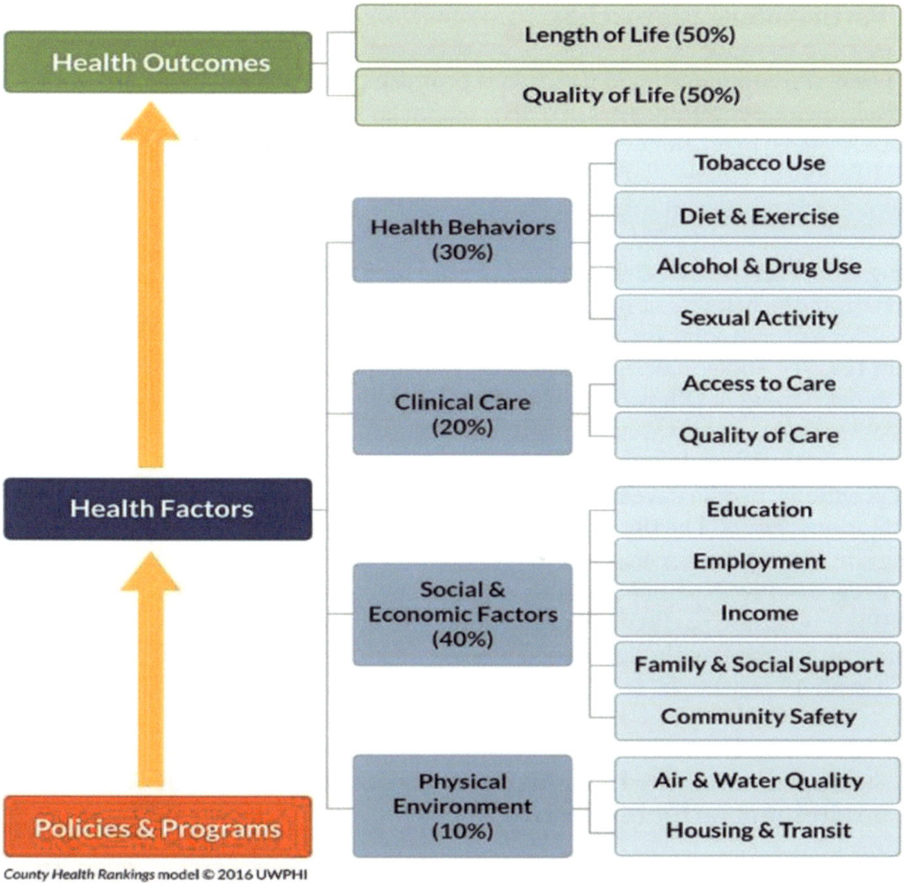

Figure 4.
County Health Rankings & Roadmaps. Source: Reprinted with permission from County Health Rankings & Roadmaps, [88].

as environmental determinism in the community that are smoke-free using cessation clinics availability.

It is currently utilized toward helping in assessing the prospective health consequences and outcomes of several policies as well as health status programs [16–18, 20, 21]. HIA is a systematic procedure aimed at recognizing as well as communicating the possible health-associated impacts of anticipated projects along with policies and formulating recommendations toward reducing probable health benefits as well as lessening possible harm [16, 18]. It combines several multidisciplinary approaches in the assessment of health-related consequences that may arise from a project, policy, and programme that does not clearly define health as is major focus, based of evidences of health effects from a well-structured framework. HIAs application spans over its use in a wide range of situations, such as the appraisal of national policies, infrastructural development, transportation and national/regional agricultural projects. Public participation and interagency synergy are two key positive outcomes; however, the setback is that there are no globally accepted methods in the evidence-based health impacts. Despite being a promising emerging practice, it has proven to be a great tool in the understanding of possible human health consequences, thereby informing decision-making and public policies [16, 17, 21].

12. Participatory approaches

Involving communities in EBE/PH is promising in participating techniques that actively include community people in research and intervention programs [2, 27, 89]. Academicians, practitioners, as well as members of the community collaboratively identify concern issues, devise intervention strategies, as well as evaluate results. This method relies on the input of "stakeholder" [3, 74], builds on current resources, enhances collaborative synergy between all parties, as well as integrates knowledge along with activities which it is hoped, would lead toward a fair distribution for all partners to the benefits of project intervention [14, 90]. Stakeholders, or important development partners, are persons or agencies with an interest in the problem at hand [14, 91]. Policymakers for instance, remain particularly significant stakeholders in developing health policies [92]. Stakeholders must include people who might possibly receive, use, as well as profit from the policy or program being considered. The three (3) stakeholders' groups remain pertinent viz.: people affected through interventions, people developing programs as well as those who used the program evaluations results. The three groups of people involved include: the creators of the program, those who participated in the program and those who used the results of the program. Participatory methods can also be an existing challenge in following EBEPH guidelines, particularly in attainment of appropriate agreement through which appropriate methods are used aimed at addressing a specific health problem i.e., Covid-19 pandemic [1–3, 9, 10, 19, 93].

13. An approach toward increasing evidence use in the practice of environmental/public health

Education as well as training backgrounds are needed to improve and strengthen EBEPH proficiencies workforce. The prominence on EBEPH principles is not taught in the same way in all the subjects epitomized by public/environmental health professionals. For instance, a public/environmental health professional may not be sufficiently trained to pinpoint the most recent evidence as well as interpret other possibility than what an epidemiologist can do. A newly health educator graduate having a master's degree in public/environmental health is expected to have an expanded understanding of the significance of EBEPH better than a specialist in environmental health with a bachelor's degree. Perhaps less than half of environmental/public health practitioners have little prescribed training or education in the discipline of environmental/public health like health education, environmental health ethics and epidemiology [4, 5, 94]. Most of these specialists receive formal regular graduate education or training in a college of health sciences or other programs in public health. Presently, it seems that limited public/environmental health departments need more ongoing education and training around mandatory EBEPH. Although the recognized EBEPH concept is relatively novel, but not fundamental skills. For instance, evaluating a program intervention through reviewing scientific literature aimed at evidence are skills frequently taught in postgraduate programs in environmental/public health or other areas of academic disciplines, as well as they are the basis for the practice of public/environmental health. While, the most frequently EBEPH applied outline is perhaps that identified by Brownson and his colleagues (**Figure 5**), which tends to use a seven-steps procedure [52, 64, 95]. The framework procedure used for applying is not linear as well as involves several iterations [2, 52, 96]. Competencies are becoming increasingly evident in terms of more effective public/ environmental health practice [1–3, 97, 98]. For instance,

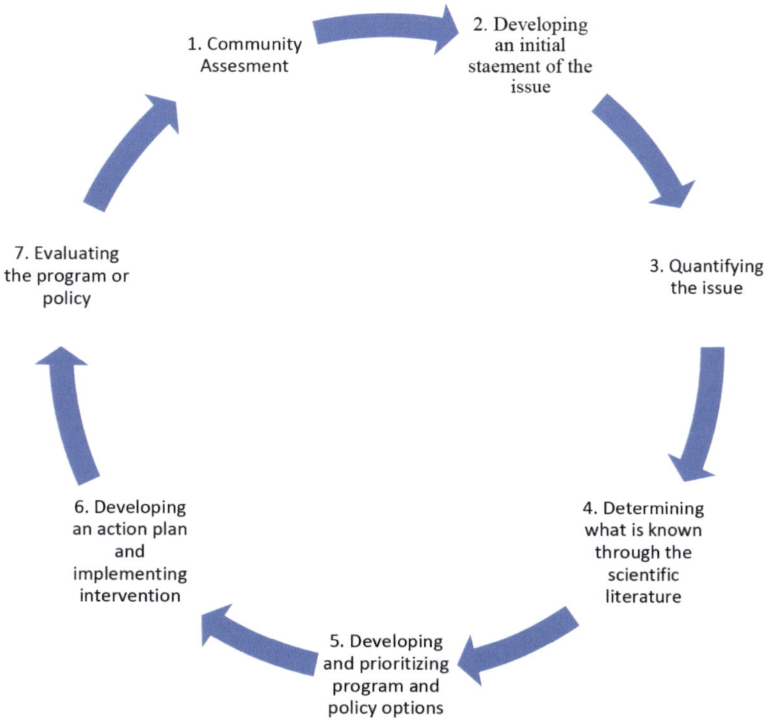
1. Community Assesment
2. Developing an initial staement of the issue
3. Quantifying the issue
4. Determining what is known through the scientific literature
5. Developing and prioritizing program and policy options
6. Developing an action plan and implementing intervention
7. Evaluating the program or policy

Figure 5.
Training approach for evidence-based environmental/public health. Adapted from Brownson et al., [64]; Hallfors et al., [93].

S/N	Characteristic	Description
1.	Holistic and comprehensive	Collaborate to resolve problems deemed important; A good example is the Ottawa Charter for promoting health.
2.	Flexible and responsive	Coalitions to answer emerging problems as well as adapt its strategies to meet the new needs of the community.
3.	Build a sense of community	Members regularly express and report that they value as well as obtain professional and personal support for their participation in collaborative relationships.
4.	Build as well as improve resident engagement in community life	Make available a structure for renewed civic engagement; Collaborate as a forum where multiple sectors can engage together.
5.	Offer a vehicle for empowering community	When community coalitions address indigenous issues, it often develops social capital, permitting residents toward having an impact on multiple problems.
6.	Permit diversity to be valued as well as celebrated	When communities become more diverse, integration offers a vehicle to bring together diverse group toward solving common challenges.
7.	Incubators for innovative solutions toward large challenges	Solving problem happens not only at local levels, but also at regional as well as national levels; local leaders may become national/global leaders.

Source: Adapted from Wolff, [109].

Table 3.
Characteristics of effective community coalitions.

S/N	Title	Domain[b]	Level[c]	Competency
1.	Community input	C	B	Understand the importance of soliciting public opinion before planning as well as implementing interventions that is evidence-based.
2.	Etiologic knowledge	E	B	Understand the relationship amongst risk factors as well as diseases.
3.	Community assessment	C	B	Understand how health issue is defined based on the needs as well as assets of the population/community of interest.
4.	Partnerships at multiple levels	P/C	B	Understand the importance of recognizing as well as developing partnerships to meet the need for routine evidence-based strategies at various levels.
5.	Developing a concise statement of the issue	EBP	B	Understand the important of developing a concise statement of the challenges in order to build support for it.
6.	Grant writing need	T/T	B	Identify the importance of skills in grant writing which comprise the phases used in the application process.
7.	Literature searching	EBP	B	Understand how scientific literature is searched as well as summarize the results of health issue.
8.	Leadership and evidence	L	B	Identify the need for a strong leadership from environmental/public health professionals regarding the need and importance of evidence-based environmental/public health interventions.
9.	Role of behavioral science theory	T/T	B	Comprehend the role of behavioral science theory in implementing, designing, as well as evaluating strategies.
10.	Leadership at all levels	L	B	Comprehend the importance of commitment from all stages of environmental/public health leadership while improving the use of evidence-based strategies.
11.	Evaluation in "plain English"	EV	I	Identify the importance of translating the programs impacts or policies in language that can be understood by practice sectors, communities as well as policy makers.
12.	Leadership and change	L	I	Identify the importance of effective leadership from professionals environmental/public health when making decisions in the middle of ever-changing milieus.
13.	Translating evidence-based interventions	EBP	I	Identify the importance of translating evidence-based strategies to unique "real-world" settings.
14.	Quantifying the issue	T/T	I	Comprehend the importance of descriptive epidemiology (concepts of person, place, time) in quantifying the environmental/public health problems.
15	Developing an action plan for program or policy	EBP	I	Comprehend the importance of developing an action plan that will shows how goals and objectives are to be achieved, what resources are needed, and how to share responsibility for achieving assigned objectives.

S/N	Title	Domain[b]	Level[c]	Competency
16.	Prioritizing health issues	EBP	I	Comprehend the selection process and implement relevant criteria as well as processes for prioritizing program and policy options.
17.	Qualitative evaluation	EV	I	Make sure that the value of qualitative evaluation approaches together with the steps involved in conducting qualitative evaluations.
18.	Collaborative partnerships	P/C	I	Comprehend the importance of collaborative partnerships amongst researchers as well as practitioners when implementing, designing and evaluating evidence-based policies and programs.
19.	Nontraditional partnerships	P/C	I	Comprehend the importance of traditional partnerships and those that have been considered nontraditional for instance those with planners, transportation department, and others.
20.	Systematic reviews	T/T	I	Comprehend the rationale, uses, as well as systematic reviews usefulness that document effective strategies.
21	Quantitative evaluation	EV	I	Comprehend the importance of quantitative evaluation methods together with the concepts of measurement validity as well as reliability.
22	Grant writing skills	T/T	I	Demonstrate the ability toward creating a grant together with an outline of the steps involved in the application procedure.
23	Role of economic evaluation	T/T	A	Identifying the importance of using economic data as well as strategies toward evaluating costs and consequences when making public/environmental health decisions.
24	Creating policy briefs	P	A	Comprehend the importance of writing concisepolicy briefs toward considering the problem using evidence-based strategies.
25	Evaluation designs	EV	A	Understand the different designs that is useful in program evaluation with a specific focus on quasi-experimental (nonrandomized) designs.
26	Transmitting evidence-based research to policy makers	P	A	Comprehend the importance of coming up with creative as well as novel ways of transmitting what we know works (evidence-based interventions) toward policy makers in order to gain interest, political support, and funding.

[a] *Adapted from Gebbie et al., [97]; Brownson et al., [99].*
[b] *C, community-level planning; E, etiology; P/C, partnerships and collaboration; EBP, evidence-based process; T/T, theory and analytic tools; L, leadership; EV, evaluation; P, policy.*
[c] *B, beginner; I, intermediate; A, advanced.*

Table 4.
Competencies in evidence-based environmental/public Health.[a]

the EBEPH procedure, requires a certain set of competences to be capable of making evidence-based decisions [99] (see **Table 4**). EBEPH training programs in the developed countries aimed at public and environmental health professionals in their various state health agencies were created toward addressing these as well as other related competencies, [2, 3, 52, 100], community-based organizations as well as local health departments [2, 3, 101, 102], along with related programs have remained established in many countries [96, 99]. Some programs demonstrate evidence of efficacy [52, 102]. In the most frequent format, the faculty team with competence in EBEPH employs didactic lectures, computer workshops, as well as scenario-based exercises. The training programs scope could remain increased through stressing a train-the-trainer method [96, 99]. Other formats were employed, together with Internet-based self-study [101, 103], CD-ROMs, [99] distance as well as distributed networks learning, along with technical support that are targeted. Educational training programs can be very effective in delivering "change agents" who are seen as professionals, but also share general goals as well as characteristics through the trainees [104]. A leadership and staff commitment aimed at life-long learning are also key ingredient toward training successes [105]. Training implementation toward addressing EBEPH competencies must be in accordance with the principles of adult education and learning. These occurred problems remained recently articulated with Bryan along with his collaborators [106], who have stressed the need toward (1) recognize the reason why the audience is learning; (2) use a fundamental motivation toward learning the necessity of problems solving; (3) build as well as respect preceding experience; (4) developing learning methods that are aligned with the development background as well as recipient's diversity; and (5) actively participating with the participants in the education/learning process. Below are a sequential framework seven-stage steps, toward promoting better evidence use in everyday policy making (see **Figure 5**). It is remarkable to remember that this procedure is rarely a stringently linear or prescriptive one, nonetheless it must include several feedback "loops" as well as common processes that exist in multiple models' program-planning.

14. Community assessment

Community (or needs) assessment is "a systematic set of procedures undertaken for the purpose of setting priorities and making decisions about program or organizational improvement and allocation of resources. The priorities are based on identified needs" [107]. Diverse forms of data, together with epidemiologic (quantitative) data, qualitative information, health inequalities on data, as well as health resource utilization patterns, might include a variation of community assessment. The first part of community or need assessment is very important in identifying a problem or an issue. A community assessment typically could begin through looking at baseline sources or background information about health issues in a community. These may comprise data from primary as well as secondary sources. Primary data encompass novel information collection on specific programs or study through using techniques like a community examination, focus groups and interviews, etc. Although, the community might mean people who reside inside a specified geographic area or as people sharing a communal experience or share a specific cultural or social identity sense [100]. When doing the assessment, it is likewise necessary in order to appropriately portray the spectrum of community members, toward recognizing any subgroups around the community of interest (for instance, adolescence, adults on lower-income). Hence, community assessments might thus involve an attempt to recognize mortality as well as morbidity, environmental and organizational circumstances, current policies, along with significant associations between stakeholders. Community assessments examine the community health concerns, the variables influencing the health in a community (for instance, health determinants), and the resources, assets, as well as difficulties influencing these factors [107]. Assessment, ideally is a community process by which stakeholders together with members of the community and a wide range of community-based as well as government organizations turn out to be partners in community assessment as well as a shift from assessment toward action planning. While, community assessments remain critical toward ensuring appropriate priorities are been carried out. This is for the reason that they can make available an understanding of the importance of the community setting so that priorities stay planned, designed as well as implementing ways to leverage as well as maximizing the community benefit. Additionally, the assessments can be recognized (as well as in some cases improve) support aimed at specific priorities' methods. This significant support is garnering resources as well as safeguarding an intervention that is successful. Assessments can likewise be an important baseline measure for a series of circumstances. Hence, assessing community characteristically arises before program development or policy as well as seeks toward comprehending the public/environmental health challenges as well as interventions in a specified community. It likewise begins toward recognizing recent resources previously in place toward addressing this apprehension. Data is occasionally obtained from national as well as local data sets in addition to surveillance systems. Another useful information at this level is a written contextual documentation, or setting, within which the problem of health is happening, together with social assessment, economic, as well as physical conditions. Data for assessing community may be collected with qualitative (e.g., individual or group interviews) or quantitative (e.g., questionnaires) methods. The decision concerning what to look for need to remain guided through the assessment goal. For example, a youth-focused assessment may include factors other than age assessment. For example, an adolescence focused assessment may comprise diverse elements other than focusing on adult's assessment who are older. Bearing in mind, there remain likewise some useful general guiding principle to consider when engaged in assessment planning. It is remarkable toward assessing factors in particular along the full ecologic series of factors influencing the health of population as well as well-being, in doing so, including the community assets, besides not just the challenges. Ecologic frameworks indicate the influence on the behavior modification as well as social health of the individual and contextual factors [101]. Numerous changes have been proposed to the ecologic framework [55]. Based on work conducted, it is useful to consider assessment of factors at five levels:

1. Individual factors: individual characteristics include knowledge, skills, attitudes, and developmental history of a persons.

2. Interpersonal factors: social networks of formal as well as informal, including social support systems such as friends and family.

3. Organizational factors: organizational features, social institutions, as well as operational rules or regulations. Organizational factors assessments might not only include the institutional existence nevertheless change readiness as well as organizational capacity (e.g., organizational support, communication within and amongst policy making structures, organizations, leadership as well as availability of resources [100].

4. Community factors: associations amongst economic forces, organizations, the physical milieu, as well as cultural changes that could shape people behavior

5. Government and policy issues: national, state and local laws, rules, as well as regulations

The use of the ecologic framework makes it possible to assess indigenous community people (their health as well as wellness and people's behaviors), the agencies as well as the organizations serving the community, and the milieu within which members of the community reside [35, 69, 108]. In detail, the greatest effective priorities act at multiple levels because societies are people who communicate with each other on different social networks within a specific context; thus, need assessment should help to understand this extensive variety of factors in general. Hence, **Table 3** shows a number of probable ecologic framework indicators aimed at each of these stages.

15. Developing an initial statement of the issue

Professionals must start with developing a brief description of the problem or issue being considered. In order to receive support on any issue (by the organization, a funding agency or decision makers), the issue should remain evidently articulated. This part of the problem definition corresponds to the initial stages of the strategic program planning process, which typically includes a description of the internal strengths as well as weaknesses, mission, threats and external opportunities as well as future vision. This typically helps define the gaps amongst the program current status or organization as well as the goals desired. The main mechanisms in statement issue comprise the condition of health or perceived risk factor, number of affected population(s), the size and the problem scope, potential stakeholders as well as prevention opportunities.

16. Quantifying the issue

Once important information about a public health problem has been established, it is often helpful to identify the root sources of the prevailing data. Just as such data might depend on recent vital statistical data (records of death/birth), special surveys, surveillance systems or other national studies. In public/environmental health, qualitative studies could take many forms. The utmost popular descriptive type of study consists of scientifically effective sample survey of the people of interest (a representative cross section). This type of cross-sectional studies was not designed toward changing health status (like an intervention) but then to help determine the prevalence of quantifying behaviors, exposures, characteristics as well as diseases at a period (or point) of time, especially in a population that is defined. This information can help to understand the magnitude toward public/environmental health challenge at hand. Qualitative studies usually offer information about the designs of occurrence according to such individual attributes place (e.g., county of residence), (e.g., gender, age, ethnicity), as well as time (e.g., seasonal changes in the patterns of disease). In addition, cross-sectional data may in certain circumstances, offer used information in the design of analytic studies (e.g., baseline information/data toward evaluating the advantages of public/environmental health intervention).

17. Determining what is known from scientific literature

When problem to be addressed are clearly defined, professionals should be knowledgeable of prior or continuing efforts toward resolving the issue. This ought to comprise a systematic method for identifying, retrieving, as well as evaluating appropriate scientific reports based on research, panels, as well as conferences associated toward the issue of interest. The best way to start this investigation is through a formal study of the official literature review. Much databases information is available toward facilitating such a review; the best known of these public/environmental health purposes remain Scirus (Elsevier), MEDLINE Ovid, PubMed, ProQuest Dissertations and theses, CINHAL EBSCO Host, Web of Knowledge, Research Gate, Scopus/Elsevier, Mendeley, Geobase/Elsevier, Environment Complete/Ebsco, Campbell Collaboration databases, Google Scholar, Google Web, SSRN, Academia etc. These subscribed databases through an institution, can selectively remain accessible in the Internet, or occasionally the public can access it from institutions (like the National Library of Medicine [110], Hinari, Universities, Research4life as well as public libraries). There are also a number of organizations that sustain Internet sites that help identify appropriate information, together with several government health departments, the World Health Organization, Centers for Disease Control and Prevention, as well as the National Institutes of Health etc. It is remarkable to note that the published literature does not cover all (Type 2) intervention studies (see **Table 1**).

18. Developing and prioritizing program options

The first three phases examine a number of policy options or health program. The options list can remain expanded from various sources. Preliminary review from scientific literature may occasionally shed light on different priorities options. In most cases, a group of expert panels can provide advice on policy recommendations or program on various issues. A summary of the available evidence is usually provided in systematic reviews and practice guidelines. There are numerous assumptions or circumstances that underlie every development options. Five key focus areas are covered through these considerations: demographic, economic, political/regulatory, social values, as well as technological [2, 3, 111]. Specifically, it is remarkable toward assessing as well as monitoring the policy process once developing a crucial option in health policy. Doing so, stakeholder contribution can be suitable. The policy stakeholder may be health policy makers, while community intervention through coalition stakeholder may be a member of the community. With regard to health policies, supportive decision makers may often offer guidance on policy initiatives timing, problem-solving strategies, identifying sponsorship strategies, as well as techniques toward improving general public support. On the topic of community priorities, additional planning information can consist of significant informant interviews, coalition member surveys or focus groups [112].

19. Developing an action plan together with implementing priorities

This reform procedure has a profound impact on strategic planning snags. As soon as the option has remained carefully chosen, a set of goals as well as objectives must remain developed. The goal is a lasting desired variable in the intervention's status of related health need, as well as short-term objective, measurable, definite action leading in the direction of goal attainment. The action course describes how to achieve the goals together with objectives, what required resources are needed, as well as how accountability aimed at achieving assigned objectives.

20. Evaluating the policy or program

Simply put, evaluation is a work experiment that has achieved policy goals as well as program objectives. After established research design, many public/ environmental health policies as well as programs are frequently examined using a "quasiexperimental" designs (i.e., people lacking haphazard assignment toward intervention as well as comparison groups). Generally, the strongest appraisal designs recognize the roles of both parametric as well as non-parametric evaluation. In addition, evaluation designs tool must be flexible as well as sensitive enough toward measuring average variability, even individuals falling short of behavioral changes. Genuine variables take incremental place over time, in many ways frequently not known toward those individuals closest to the intervention.

21. Barriers to more extensive use of evidence in decision making

Several obstacles are present in the decision-making process to better employ data and analytical processes [51, 64, 113] (**Table 5**). Others have explored possible

S/N	Barrier	Potential solution
1.	Inadequate resources	Commitment to increase funding for prevention and rectifying staff shortages
2.	Leadership lacks and uncertainty in setting a clear and focused agenda for evidence-based approaches	Commitment from all levels of environmental/ public health leaders to increase the understanding of the value of EBEPH approaches
3.	Inadequate incentives for using evidence-based approaches	Identification of new ways of shaping organizational culture toward supporting EBEPH
4.	Inadequate view of the long-term "horizon" for program implementation and evaluation	Adoption and adherence to causal frameworks and formative evaluation plans
5.	External (including political) pressures drive the process away from an evidence-based approach	Systematic communication and dissemination strategies
6.	Inadequate training in key public health disciplines	Wider dissemination of new and established training programs, including use of distance learning technologies
7.	Inadequate time to gather information, analyze data, and review the literature for evidence	Enhanced skills for efficient analysis and review of the literature, computer searching abilities, use of systematic reviews
8.	Inadequate evidence on the effectiveness of certain environmental/public health interventions for special populations	Increased funding for applied environmental/public health research; better dissemination of findings
9.	Inadequate information on implementation of interventions	A greater emphasis on building the evidence base for external validity

Source: Adapted from Brownson et al., [39].

Table 5.
Potential barriers and solutions for use of evidence-based decision making in environmental/public health.

Category	Influential Factor
Information	• Sound scientific basis, including knowledge of causality • Source (e.g., professional organization, government, mass media, friends)
Clarity of contents	• Formatting and framing • Perceived validity • Perceived relevance • Cost of intervention • Strength of the message (i.e., vividness)
Perceived values, preferences, beliefs	• Role of the decision maker • Economic background • Previous education • Personal experience or involvement • Political affiliation • Willingness to adopt innovations • Willingness to accept uncertainty • Willingness to accept risk • Ethical aspect of the decision
Context	• Culture • Politics • Timing • Media attention • Financial or political constraints

Source: Adapted from Anderson et al. [115]; Brownson et al., [39] and Raimi et al., [2].

Table 6.
Factors influencing decision making amongst environmental/public health administrators, decision makers, and the general public.

methods to overcome these obstacles [2, 3, 100]. The necessity for and relevance of evidence-based decision-making is the leadership that environmental and public health professionals need. Such leadership is apparent in training programs, for instance the regional environmental and public health leadership network [107] and continuous efforts to establish and distribute documented evidence-based recommendations for intervention [79].

However, numerous factors affect environmental/public health decision-making [114, 115] (see **Table 6**). Some of these variables are under the control of environmental/public health practitioners, while others are very difficult to change.

Also, there are quite at least four techniques in which environmental/public health policy or program cannot achieve a specific success goal:

i. Choose an intervention forms whose effectiveness in scientific literature has not yet been confirmed.

ii. Choosing a policy or program that may be effective but only attaining frail, partial implementation or "reach," thus worsening to accomplish the objectives (few call this Type III error)

iii. Assessing insufficient or improper evaluation that led to public ignorance of the impacts of a policy or program

iv. Paying insufficient consideration toward acclimatizing an intervention between population as well as background interest.

However, part of the reason that environmental/public health-policy officials have struggled in the face of the COVID-19, is that it's very difficult to identify appropriate interventions that might inspire people to change their behaviors given reasons. For instance, do people who will not wear masks think the virus is not risky, since they do not think masks work, or just as their leaders including others aren't wearing them? To make matters worse, surveys or studies often represent only a portion of the population leaving those most at risk underrepresented. "Data can be instructive, but it does not speak for itself, as data access remains one of the primary hurdles to advancing science". "Behind every data point is a person. And with something like the coronavirus, where people are so deeply affected, there is need to think about the ethics of intervening in people's lives."

22. Addressing the issue

While, the 2020 COVID-19 pandemic unlocked our eyes toward the ever-changing situations as well as uncertainty that prevail in today world, particularly with regards to environmental and public health practices disruption. Due to the unprecedented novel nature and scale of coronavirus as well as the worldwide public/environmental health crisis nature, which upended several public/environmental research norms almost overnight. Though, the virus is expected with further waves as well as more pandemics increase is anticipated. COVID-19 had demonstrated a global catastrophe that touched everybody, including the scientific community. As we respond and recover rapidly from this pandemic, there is an opportunity to guarantee that the fabric of our society includes sustainability, fairness, and care. However, approaches to environmental health attempt to decrease the populations burden of COVID-19, toward saving patients from becoming ill along with preserving the allocation of clinical resources and public safety standards.

Even though the coronavirus continues to surge globally, the COVID-19 pandemic continues to put the health as well as economic security of millions of Nigerians and the world at large at risk, evidence is building and has accumulated over the course of the COVID-19 pandemic, scientific understanding about the virus has changed. Overall, to improve evidence-based or proven practices, every option must attempt to give practical recommendations on how programs and policies based on evidence in environmental and public health settings may be selected, implemented and evaluated. It also addresses the need for a highly trained environmental/public health workforce and expands available technologies, hence study into the origins of infectious diseases and the creation of vaccinations and medicines that have triggered formerly deadly diseases such as polio, smallpox and now COVID-19. Thus, the successful EBE/PH implementation in the practice of public/environmental health is both scientific as well as art. Science is based on behavioral, epidemiologic, as well as policy research that reflects the size with the magnitude of the public/environmental health issues and which interventions probable are to be of advantage to problem solving. The policy-making art experience usually comprises understanding of what information that is significant toward a specific stakeholder at the appropriate time. Remarkable environmental/public health decisions should balance science as well as art, because rational, scientific-based policy making that frequently comprises selecting an option amongst set of choices that are rational in nature.

By using the outlined concepts in EBE/PH above, decision making are ultimately improving environmental/public health practice; this is particularly important in a times when environmental/public health practitioners should be incentivized, not disincentivized, toward providing remote and long-term care and if implemented as well as maintained successfully in the post COVID era, this could benefit from our efforts as well as welcome efficiency consequence and cost savings [3–5, 15, 16]. These efforts can assist toward adapting effective interventions strategies to improve the pandemic response to COVID-19. However, suppression of the COVID-19 pandemic, cannot depend solely on the hope that effective vaccines as well as medical treatment, especially having the new, fast spreading SARS-CoV-2 variants: thus, an effective behavioral, environmental, social and systems interventions (BESSI) known as "Plan B" is needed to cut transmission. Given the pandemic, Covid-19 is probable to remain around to at least first quarter of 2022 (hypothetically followed via seasonal outbreaks), even if an effective treatments or vaccine is established, it is essential to deal with Behavioral, Environmental, Social and Systems Interventions (BESSI) now and establish long-term research priorities and processes for improving evidence on BESSI Interventions toward preventing as well as managing outbreaks of futuristic infectious diseases through fostering research synthesis, systems thinking, incorporating interprofessionalism and team-based care, piloting, prioritization, as well as field trials in partnership with health organizations, communities, policy makers, as well as an array of relevant researchers to BESSI research strategy (see **Figure 6**).

Furthermore, there is need to fund evidence-based projects that will focus on recognizing condition of a health or disease, aimed at which there is need for community support intervention as well as engagement toward addressing the issues, articulate a cultural appropriateness process must be established and recognizing community strengths as well as resiliencies, advancing knowledge must be promoted to address the condition of health or disease by etiologic research, prevention research, building robust frameworks for governance, oversight, and accountability, treatment or research recovery, or dissemination as well as implementation research and accounting for sustainability in test communities

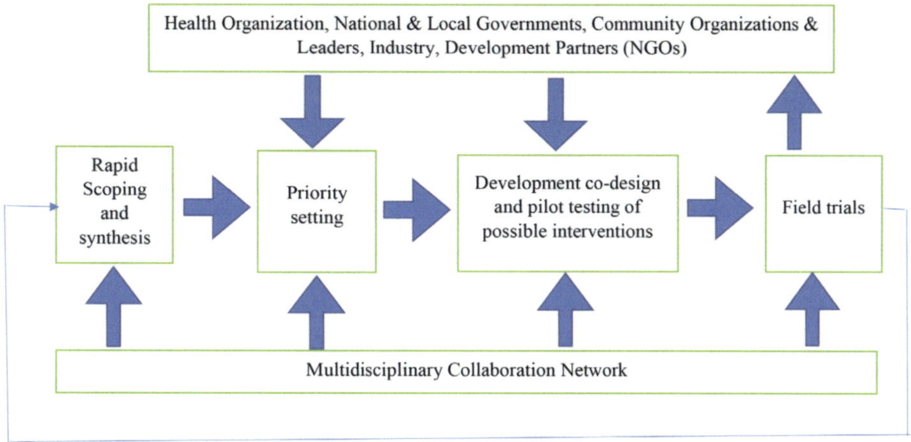

Figure 6.
Behavioral environmental social and system intervention (BESSI) (for pandemic preparedness) research strategy. Adapted from [116].

and for dissemination and scale up to other communities as indicated. Hence, real-world evidence could significantly improve public health (community medicine, preventive medicine, social medicine, as well as community health) decisions throughout the health system, eventually improving environmental health. However, expanding its usage, will need multi-stakeholder engagement on numerous priorities, along with country-specific initiatives. Therefore, the broader public/environmental health community is best positioned toward making progress in addressing individual behaviors, social circumstances, or environmental factors associated with a disorder or disease. Making improvement on such goals will thereby help contribute to the creation of a culture where evidence-based innovation may thrive, while also ensuring that the required, complementary proficiencies occur toward supporting traditional research and development (R&D) operations activities. Likewise, governments at all levels must act expeditiously and aggressively in providing robust support for crucial national public/environmental health as well as health care programs, the development of medical countermeasures, global readiness and response mechanism programs as well as international collaborations. So as to reduce the virus effects. National as well as international response prompt action are now needed to respond and prevent worst case health as well as economic repercussions. Based on the identified realities of the present COVID-19 pandemic, it seems that government must urgently take additional steps now to prepare domestically and to invest globally and to help make the shift from containment of the virus to mitigation of its effects. This shift will be difficult, and the response will be exceptionally resource intensive. Response as well as readiness toward threats to health security like COVID-19 is as critical to the safety as well as well-being of humanity. Preparedness for emergency situations have been essential for increasing national resilience and capacities to combat health risk emergencies. There is need to build systems to strengthen evidence-based research and expertise must remain sustained as well as boistered. With the intention of reducing death as well as diseases in the current dark times and time to come. The COVID-19 pandemic provides a unique opportunity to discuss critical issues related to defining living reviews and how often they should be conducted. It has significantly accelerated the production of living reviews as a useful tactic toward informing decision makers in a context where evidence is constantly evolving on a regular (sometimes even on a daily basis). Since 'living' reviews are most useful in a context where information is changing relatively frequently on a topic, so hopefully an update is expected to be happening at pace with evolving literature. From this perspective, part of the requirements of a living review should be that there is a positive plan to monitor for new relevant data or evidence, and a plan for managing this evidence when it emerges. Hence, there is needs to be a plan for incorporating new information as it emerges, with the aim that decisions that are made on the basis of the reviews can be relied on or trusted to be informed by the best current evidence. Thus, the framework above provides an important Living Evidence Network criterion from a positive sense (i.e., the question must be an important priority, there is uncertainty in the outcomes, and that new forthcoming evidence can likely improve this certainty). It is important to assess whether or not the review should no longer be updated on a living basis if at least one of these characteristics are no longer true. As we have seen with COVID-19, the frequency of updating may vary depending on the rate at which new research is coming through and its likely impact on the evidence base, but whatever frequency is adopted this needs to be communicated clearly together with the intent to keep the review under active surveillance. While, communicating with users and readers about the currency and comprehensiveness of the evidence.

23. Conclusion

Conclusively, as the Chinese proverb used to say "Problems give opportunity and changes, and the gods cannot help those who do not take advantage of this opportunity". Out of a disaster provide opportunities toward building a safer, healthier, as well as a more just world. In all these domains, addressing health toughest triage will be crucial and will help strengthen and maintain the scientific integrity as well as political neutrality of action on human and environmental health in the times of concurrent international crises. Of course, this is not only a response toward COVID-19, but also for the full gamut of health challenges. Time has come toward revitalizing and rethinking governance, policies, as well as investments in scientific research for better health, which precede a more sustainable future for global as well as national health leadership in preparedness, response, and health recovery for emergencies, which will necessitate a range of research methods and analytic decisions. Increased focused attention toward these approaches and analytic decisions has the potential toward increasing the importance of policies and its uses toward health systems strengthening, hence potentially assisting policy makers toward improving mitigation efficiency while concurrently improving global and national health, with an attempt toward drawing remarkable lessons for strengthening pandemic preparedness as well as response. While the response to COVID-19 is constantly evolving and the situation is constantly changing, how a country respond to an outbreak depends on the resilient of its health systems, effective response is needed to fight the immediate outbreak and reduce its downstream impact on health. In general, environmental and public health research analyses as well as comprehensive health systems in all countries which may include integrated core capacities for environmental/public health at all governance levels, will be the best protection/defense against other major great pandemic outbreak. Therefore, sound national planning/preparedness necessitates visibly a comprehensive states situation' of the capabilities toward predicting, managing as well as balancing public/environmental requirements at all pandemic stages. This requires leveraging data for rapid, accurate as well as reliably impacting on effective public/environmental policies on health, hence converting this intelligence into actionable solutions will thereby ensure shared accountability. The boundary amongst action as well as inaction is rarely separate. Scientific evidence along with values assessment, costs, preferences, as well as several benefits options must be carefully considered. Hence, this discovery as well as its plausible explanation therefore point to the necessity for far greater proof of evidence. There is therefore evidence requirement around the risks as well as discrete benefits of biologically tailored COVID-19 interventions as well as how these risks along with benefits differ across various population subgroups. Other recommendations include:

1. Investment in Behavioral Environmental Social and System Intervention (BESSI): Whilst the limited investment in BESSIs to date is a missed opportunity, we should learn from this pandemic to prepare for rapid, effective response to future pandemics. As BESSI collaboration should help develop rigorous "research in action", with researchers and those tasked with implementing programmes working together. Thus, there is need to consider how to efficiently set research priorities and how to work more closely with WHO which potentially has the infrastructure to collate BESSI protocols that might be developed and then adapted for future pandemics. While a few examples of this have occurred, many public/environmental health and clinical services have felt too overwhelmed to engage with researchers, but clearly it is possible and we can learn from those that did engage.

2. Collective Collaboration/Partnership: Geographical hubs for BESSI collaborators will enable meaningful research interactions and activities between the global north and south. There is need to avoid designing research in the global north and then contextualizing it for the south. This interaction needs to be bidirectional and co-designed. As BESSI need to focused on funders, researchers, and major international organizations, while there is need to start to engage with some health professional organizations such as WFPHA, EHORCON, PAHO, etc.

3. Emphasis on Practice-Based Research: Research in environmental health is incremental, through a body of scientifically compiled evidence over a period of several years or decades. Hence, environmental health information for decision making should be founded on science, and science is based on the collection, analysis, and interpretation of data. Data in environmental/public health are generally derived from two overlapping sources: research studies and environmental/public health surveillance systems. Indeed, there is the need for a more practice-based research in which environmental/public health practitioners routinely collect as well as record data on the COVID-19 treatment and outcomes of their patients in order to better care for those in the future? Hence, there is pressing need for evidence development. More and better evidence including comparative as well as longitudinal data is required to determine the effectiveness and usefulness of novel medical interventions, drugs, treatments, devices, and genetic information.

4. Clear Uncertainty: The exposed uncertainty through the information environment. An irony of the information-rich environment is that information imperative for decision making is frequently not available, or is provided in ways that are not relevant to the broad spectrum of patients with differing levels of health, socioeconomic circumstances, and preferences, as well as the issues encountered in practice. This is due to too little research effectiveness, to poor evidence dissemination that is available, and to too few incentives as well as decision supports for evidence-based care. Hence, there is need for a rapid review on public/environmental health topics driving by: 1) emergence of new evidence (sometimes even on a daily basis 2–3 months into the pandemic; 2) research designs of available evidence, and likelihood that more rigorous designs may provide greater certainty in the findings; and 3) emergence of evidence that 'add's something new'. Also, it is found that the frequency of updating a living review has changed from earlier in the pandemic to now.

5. Credible and Capable Leadership: Broad leadership that stems from any part of the world will be needed to adapt to taking advantage from changes in the healthcare milieu. Involvement of the private sectors, public, policy makers, patients, providers, insurers, as well as other development partners working together in the steps toward transformation will require a planned focus on evidence development as well as required application. Else, there is need for a shift toward a culture of collective learning. Investment in infrastructure is essential to produce best proof of evidence for environmental/public health delivery which meets the requirements of individual patients (see **Table 2**), and aimed at collecting along with analyzing healthcare data as well as information, along with standards and protocols toward ensuring their reliability and accuracy. This evolving role will necessitate a culture which promotes the application of evidence along with its generation in patients and healthcare providers.

Acknowledgements

I thank all anonymous reviewers, for feedback and discussions that helped to substantially improve this manuscript.

Authors' contributions

All authors included in the manuscript provided substantial contribution to (i) conception and design, (ii) drafting the article or revising it critically for important intellectual content and (iii) final approval of the completed manuscript.

Declaration of competing interests

We affirm that we have no conflict of interest that may be alleged as prejudicing the impartiality of the study reported. This researcher did not receive special assistance from government, not-for-profit sectors or commercial institutions.

Abbreviations

HIA	Health Impact Assessment
WFPHA	World Federation of Public Health Associations
PAHO	Pan American Health Organization
SDoH	Social Determinant of Health
BESSI	Behavioral Environmental Social and System Intervention
EHORCON	Environmental Health Officers Registration Council of Nigeria

Author details

Raimi Morufu Olalekan[1*], Aziba-anyam Gift Raimi[2] and Teddy Charles Adias[2]

1 Department of Community Medicine, Environmental Health Unit, Faculty of Clinical Sciences, Niger Delta University, Wilberforce Island, Bayelsa State, Nigeria

2 Office of the Vice-Chancellor, Federal University Otuoke, Bayelsa State, Nigeria

*Address all correspondence to: ola07038053786@gmail.com

References

[1] Morufu Olalekan Raimi, Ebikapaye Okoyen, Tuebi Moses, Aziba-anyam Gifty Raimi, Adedoyin Oluwatoyin Omidiji, Aishat Funmilayo Abdulraheem, Mariam Oluwakemi Raimi, Beatrice Oka Joseph (2021) Do Weak Institutions Prolong Crises? [#ENDSARs] in the Light of the Challenges and opportunities beyond COVID-19 Pandemic and the Next Normal in Nigeria. *Communication, Society and Media.* ISSN 2576-5388 (Print) ISSN 2576-5396 (Online) Vol. 4, No. 2, DOI: https://doi.org/10.22158/csm.v4n2p1. http://www.scholink.org/ojs/index.php/csm/article/view/3790.

[2] Raimi Morufu Olalekan, Moses Tuebi, Okoyen Ebikapaye, Sawyerr Henry Olawale, Joseph Beatrice Oka, Oyinlola Bilewu Olaolu (2020) "A Beacon for Dark Times: Rethinking Scientific Evidence for Environmental and Public Health Action in the Coronavirus Diseases 2019 Era" *Medical and Research Microbiology,* Vol. 1, Issues 3.

[3] Raimi Morufu Olalekan & Raimi Aziba-anyam Gift (2020). The Toughest Triage in Decision Impacts: Rethinking Scientific Evidence for Environmental and Human Health Action in the Times of Concomitant Global Crises. *CPQ Medicine,* 11(1), 01-05.

[4] Olalekan RM, Olawale SH, Christian A, Simeon AO (2020). Practitioners Perspective of Ethical Cases and Policy Responses by Professional Regulator: The Case of Environmental Health Officers Registration Council of Nigeria (EHORECON). *American Journal of Epidemiology & Public Health*. 2020;4(1): 016-023. https://www.scireslit.com/PublicHealth/AJEPH-ID23.pdf. https://www.scireslit.com/PublicHealth/articles.php?volume=4&issue=1.

[5] Olalekan RM (2020). "What we learn today is how we behave tomorrow": a study on satisfaction level and implementation of environmental health ethics in Nigeria institutions. *Open Access Journal of Science*; 4(3):82-92. DOI: 10.15406/oajs.2020.04.00156.

[6] Olalekan RM, Muhammad IH, Okoronkwo UL, Akopjubaro EH (2020). Assessment of safety practices and farmer's behaviors adopted when handling pesticides in rural Kano state, Nigeria. *Arts & Humanities Open Access Journal.* 2020;4(5):191-201. DOI: 10.15406/ahoaj.2020.04.00170.

[7] Gift R.A, Obindah F (2020). Examining the influence of motivation on organizational productivity in Bayelsa state private hospitals. Open *Access Journal of Science.* 2020;4(3):94-108. DOI: 10.15406/oajs.2020.04.00157.

[8] https://www.nature.com/articles/d41586-021-02039-y.

[9] Gift RA, Olalekan RM, Owobi OE, Oluwakemi RM, Anu B, Funmilayo AA (2020). Nigerians crying for availability of electricity and water: a key driver to life coping measures for deepening stay at home inclusion to slow covid-19 spread. *Open Access Journal of Science*. 2020;4(3):69-80. DOI: 10.15406/oajs.2020.04.00155.

[10] Gift R A, Olalekan RM (2020). Access to electricity and water in Nigeria: a panacea to slow the spread of Covid-19. *Open Access Journal of Science* 2020;4(2):34. DOI: 10.15406/oajs.2020.04.00148. https://medcrave.com/index.php?/articles/det/21409/

[11] Morufu Olalekan Raimi, Tonye Vivien Odubo & Adedoyin Oluwatoyin Omidiji (2021) Creating the Healthiest Nation: Climate Change and Environmental Health Impacts in Nigeria: A Narrative Review. *Scholink*

Sustainability in Environment. ISSN 2470-637X (Print) ISSN 2470-6388 (Online) Vol. 6, No. 1, 2021 www.scholink.org/ojs/index.php/se. URL: http://dx.doi.org/10.22158/se.v6n1p61. http://www.scholink.org/ojs/index.php/se/article/view/3684.

[12] Raimi Morufu Olalekan, Omidiji Adedoyin O, Ebikapaye Okoyen, Moses Tuebi, Adeolu Timothy Adedotun, Makanjuola Bosede Christianah (2019), Situational Analysis of National Immunization Programme in Nigeria, *Journal of Immunology and Inflammation Diseases Therapy.* Doi: http://dx.doi.org/10.31579/2637-8876.2019/008.

[13] Olalekan R. M, Dodeye E. O, Efegbere H. A, Odipe O. E. Deinkuro N. S, Babatunde A and Ochayi E. O (2020) Leaving No One Behind? Drinking-Water Challenge on the Rise in Niger Delta Region of Nigeria: A Review. *Merit Research Journal of Environmental Science and Toxicology* (ISSN: 2350-2266) Vol. 6(1): 031-049 DOI: 10.5281/zenodo.3779288

[14] Olalekan RM, Omidiji AO, Williams EA, Christianah MB, Modupe O (2019). The roles of all tiers of government and development partners in environmental conservation of natural resource: a case study in Nigeria. *MOJ Ecology & Environmental Sciences* 2019;4(3):114-121. DOI: 10.15406/mojes.2019.04.00142.

[15] Raimi MO, Ochayi EO, Babatunde A, Okolosi-Patani IE, Oluwaseun EO, Adio ZO and Bilewu OO (2019) "Environmental Ethics Relevance to Public Health: Current Narratives and Implications for Policy". *EC Emergency Medicine and Critical Care* 3.12:01-09.

[16] Raimi MO, Ihuoma BA, Esther OU, Abdulraheem AF, Opufou T, Deinkuro NS, Adebayo PA and Adeniji AO (2020) "Health Impact Assessment: Expanding Public Policy Tools for Promoting Sustainable Development Goals (SDGs) in Nigeria". *EC Emergency Medicine and Critical Care* 4.9 (2020).

[17] Olalekan RM, Oluwatoyin OA, Olawale SH, Emmanuel OO, Olalekan AZ (2020) A Critical Review of Health Impact Assessment: Towards Strengthening the Knowledge of Decision Makers Understand Sustainable Development Goals in the Twenty-First Century: Necessity Today; Essentiality Tomorrow. *Research and Advances: Environmental Sciences*. 2020(1): 72-84. DOI: 10.33513/RAES/2001-13. https://ospopac.com/journal/environmental-sciences/early-online.

[18] Olalekan R. M, Oluwatoyin O and Olalekan A (2020) Health Impact Assessment: A tool to Advance the Knowledge of Policy Makers Understand Sustainable Development Goals: A Review. *ES Journal of Public Health*; 1(1); 1002. https://escientificlibrary.com/public-health/in-press.php.

[19] Samson T.K., Ogunlaran O.M., Raimi O.M. (2020); A Predictive Model for Confirmed Cases of COVID-19 in Nigeria. *European Journal of Applied Sciences*, Volume 8, No 4, Aug 2020; pp:1-10. DOI: 10.14738/aivp.84.8705. URL: http://dx.doi.org/10.14738/aivp.84.8705.

[20] Omidiji A. O and Raimi M. O (2019) Practitioners Perspective of Environmental, Social and Health Impact Assessment (ESHIA) Practice in Nigeria: A Vital Instrument for Sustainable Development. Paper Presented at the Association for Environmental Impact Assessment of Nigeria (AEIAN) On Impact Assessment: A Tool for Achieving the Sustainable Development Goals in Nigeria, 7th and 8th November, 2019 In University of Port Harcourt. https://aeian.org/wp-content/uploads/2019/08/EIA-Presentations-Portharcourt.pdf.

[21] Raimi M. O, Omidiji A. O, Adio Z. O (2019) Health Impact Assessment: A Tool to Advance the Knowledge of Policy Makers Understand Sustainable Development Goals. Conference paper presented at the: Association for Environmental Impact Assessment of Nigeria (AEIAN) On Impact Assessment: A Tool for Achieving the Sustainable Development Goals in Nigeria, 7th and 8th November, 2019 in University of Port Harcourt. DOI: 10.13140/RG.2.2.35999.51366 https://www.researchgate.net/publication/337146101.

[22] Adedoyin OO, Olalekan RM, Olawale SH, *et al* (2020). A review of environmental, social and health impact assessment (Eshia) practice in Nigeria: a panacea for sustainable development and decision making. *MOJ Public Health*. 2020;9(3):81-87. DOI: 10.15406/mojph.2020.09.00328. https://medcraveonline.com/MOJPH/MOJPH-09-00328.pdf.

[23] Raimi Morufu Olalekan (2019) 21st Century Emerging Issues in Pollution Control. 6th Global Summit and Expo on Pollution Control May 06-07, 2019 Amsterdam, Netherlands.

[24] Raimi Morufu Olalekan, Tonye V. Odubo, Omidiji Adedoyin O, Oluwaseun E. Odipe (2018) Environmental Health and Climate Change in Nigeria. World Congress on Global Warming. Valencia, Spain. December 06-07, 2018.

[25] Nicola M, Alsafi Z, Sohrabi C, Kerwan A, *et al.* (2020) The socio-economic implications of the coronavirus pandemic (COVID-19): a review. *Int J Surg;* 78: 185-93.

[26] Jenicek M. (1997) Epidemiology, evidence-based medicine, and evidence-based public health. *J Epidemiol Commun Health*; 7: 187 – 197.

[27] Kohatsu ND, Robinson JG, Torner JC (2004). Evidence-based public health: an evolving concept. *Am J Prev Med*. 27 (5): 417 – 421.

[28] Chambers D, Kerner J. (2007) Closing the gap between discovery and delivery. Dissemination and Implementation Research Workshop: Harnessing Science to Maximize Health, Rockville, MD.

[29] Morufu Olalekan Raimi, Tonye Vivien Odubo, Ogah Alima, Henry Akpojubaro Efegbere, Abinotami Williams Ebuete (2021) Articulating the effect of Pesticides Use and Sustainable Development Goals (SDGs): The Science of Improving Lives through Decision Impacts. *Research on World Agricultural Economy.* Vol 2, No. 1. DOI: http://dx.doi.org/10.36956/rwae.v2i1.347.

[30] McKean E. (2005). The New Oxford American Dictionary. 2nd ed. New York, NY: Oxford University Press.

[31] Rimer BK, Glanz DK, Rasband G. (2001) Searching for evidence about health education and health behavior interventions. *Health Educ Behav*; 28 (2): 231 – 248.

[32] Kerner JF. (2008) Integrating research, practice, and policy: what we see depends on where we stand. *J Public Health Manag Pract;* 14 (2): 193 – 198.

[33] Mulrow CD, Lohr KN. (2001) Proof and policy from medical research evidence. *J Health Polit Policy Law*; 26 (2): 249 – 266.

[34] Sturm R. (2002) Evidence-based health policy versus evidence-based medicine. *Psychiatr Serv*; 53 (12): 1499.

[35] Suleiman Romoke Monsurat, Raimi Morufu Olalekan and Sawyerr Henry Olawale (2019) A Deep Dive into the Review of National Environmental Standards and Regulations Enforcement

Agency (NESREA) Act. *International Research Journal of Applied Sciences.* pISSN: 2663-5577, eISSN: 2663-5585. DOI No. Irjas.2019.123.123. www.scirange.com. https://scirange.com/abstract/irjas.2019.108.125.

[36] Brownson RC, Royer C, Ewing R, *et al.* (2006) Researchers and policymakers: travelers in parallel universes. *Am J Prev Med*; 30 (2): 164 – 172.

[37] Muir Gray JA. (1997) Evidence-Based Healthcare: How to Make Health Policy and Management Decisions. New York and Edinburgh: Churchill Livingstone.

[38] Rychetnik L, Hawe P, Waters E, *et al.* (2004) A glossary for evidence based public health. *J Epidemiol Commun Health*; 58 (7): 538 – 545.

[39] Brownson RC, Elizabeth AB, Terry LL, Kathleen NG, William RT (2011). Evidence-Based Public Health. Second Edition. Oxford University Press, Inc. ISBN 978-0-19-539789-51.

[40] Nutbeam D (2003). How does evidence influence public health policy? Tackling health inequalities in England. *Health Promot J* Aust. 2003; 14: 154 – 158.

[41] Ogilvie D, Egan M, Hamilton V, Petticrew M (2005). Systematic reviews of health effects of social interventions: 2. Best available evidence: how low should you go? *J Epidemiol Community Health;* 59 (10): 886 – 892.

[42] Hussain Muhammad Isah, Morufu Olalekan Raimi, Henry Olawale Sawyerr (2021) Patterns of Chemical Pesticide Use and Determinants of Self-Reported Symptoms on Farmers Health: A Case Study in Kano State for Kura Local Government Area of Nigeria. *Research on World Agricultural Economy.* Vol 2, No. 1. DOI: http://dx.doi.org/10.36956/rwae.v2i1.342.

[43] Isah, H. M., Sawyerr, H. O., Raimi, M. O., Bashir, B. G., Haladu, S. & Odipe, O. E. (2020). Assessment of Commonly Used Pesticides and Frequency of Self-Reported Symptoms on Farmers Health in Kura, Kano State, Nigeria. *Journal of Education and Learning Management (JELM),* HolyKnight, vol. 1, 31-54. doi.org/10.46410/jelm.2020.1.1.05. https://holyknight.co.uk/journals/jelm-articles/.

[44] Isah Hussain Muhammad, Raimi Morufu Olalekan, Sawyerr Henry Olawale, Odipe Oluwaseun Emmanuel, Bashir Bala Getso, Suleiman Haladu (2020) Qualitative Adverse Health Experience Associated with Pesticides Usage among Farmers from Kura, Kano State, Nigeria. *Merit Research Journal of Medicine and Medical Sciences* (ISSN: 2354-323X) Vol. 8(8) pp. 432-447, August, 2020. DOI: 10.5281/zenodo.4008682. https://meritresearchjournals.org/mms/content/2020/August/Isah%20et%20al.htm.

[45] Morufu Olalekan Raimi (2021). "Self-reported Symptoms on Farmers Health and Commonly Used Pesticides Related to Exposure in Kura, Kano State, Nigeria". *Annals of Community Medicine & Public Health.* 1(1): 1002. http://www.remedypublications.com/open-access/self-reported-symptoms-on-farmers-health-and-commonly-used-pesticides-related-6595.pdf. http://www.remedypublications.com/annals-of-community-medicine-public-health-home.php.

[46] Abdulraheem A. FO, Olalekan R. M, Abasiekong E. M (2018) Mother and father adolescent relationships and substance use in the Niger delta: a case study of twenty-five (25) communities in Yenagoa local government of Bayelsa state, Nigeria. *Sociol Int J.* 2018;2(6):541-548. DOI: 10.15406/sij.2018.02.00097.

[47] Funmilayo A. A, Robert O. T, Olalekan R. M, Okoyen E, Tuebi M

(2019). A study of the context of adolescent substance use and patterns of use in yenagoa local government, Bayelsa State, Nigeria. *MOJ Addiction Medicine and Therapy.* 2019;6(1):25-32. DOI: 10.15406/mojamt.2019.06.00142.

[48] Raimi MO, Abdulraheem AF, Major I, Ebikapaye O, Bilewu OO (2019). Public Health Impact of Substance Use on Adolescent: A Snapshot of Yenagoa in Bayelsa State, Nigeria. *American Journal of Biomedical Science & Research. 4(3).* AJBSR. MS.ID.000796. DOI: 10.34297/AJBSR.2019.04.000796. https://biomedgrid.com/current-issue.php.

[49] Glasgow RE, Green LW, Klesges LM, *et al* (2006). External validity: we need to do more. Ann Behav Med; 31 (2): 105 – 108.

[50] Green LW, Glasgow RE (2006). Evaluating the relevance, generalization, and applicability of research: issues in external validation and translation methodology. Eval Health Prof; 29 (1): 126 – 153.

[51] Kahn EB, Ramsey LT, Brownson RC, *et al.* (2002) The effectiveness of interventions to increase physical activity. A systematic review (1,2). *Am J Prev Med.* 22 (4 Suppl 1): 73 – 107.

[52] Dreisinger M, Leet TL, Baker EA, *et al.* (2008) Improving the public health workforce: evaluation of a training course to enhance evidence-based decision making. *J Public Health Manag Pract.* 14 (2): 138 – 143.

[53] Pawson R, Greenhalgh T, Harvey G, *et al* (2005). Realist review - a new method of systematic review designed for complex policy interventions. *J Health Serv Res Policy*; 10(Suppl 1): 21 – 34.

[54] Raimi MO, and Ochayi EO. (2017) Assessment of the Rate of Sexually Transmitted Diseases in Kubwa F.C.T. Abuja, Nigeria, *Science Journal of Public Health*. Vol. 5, No. 5, 2017, Pp. 365-376. DOI: 10.11648/J.Sjph.20170505.12.

[55] Goodman RM, Wheeler FC, Lee PR (1995). Evaluation of the Heart-to-Heart Project: lessons from a community-based chronic disease prevention project. *Am J Health Promot*; 9: 443 – 455.

[56] McQueen DV (2002). The evidence debates. *J Epidemiol Commun Health*; 56 (2): 83 – 84.

[57] Cavill N, Foster C, Oja P, *et al* (2006). An evidence-based approach to physical activity promotion and policy development in Europe: contrasting case studies. Promot Educ; 13 (2): 104 – 111.

[58] Sawyerr O. H, Odipe O. E, Olalekan R. M, *et al.* (2018) Assessment of cyanide and some heavy metals concentration in consumable cassava flour "*lafun*" across Osogbo metropolis, Nigeria. *MOJ Eco Environ Sci.* 2018;3(6):369-372. DOI: 10.15406/mojes.2018.03.00115.

[59] Raimi MO., Oluwaseun EO, Nimisingha DS, Abdulraheem AF, Okolosi-Patainnocent E, Habeeb ML and Mary F (2019) Assessment of Environmental Sanitation, Food Safety Knowledge, Handling Practice among Food Handlers of Bukateria Complexes in Iju Town, Akure North of Ondo-State, Nigeria. *Acta Scientific Nutritional Health* 3.6 (2019): 186-200. DOI: 10.31080/ASNH.2019.03.0308.

[60] Omotoso Ayodele Jacob, Omotoso Elizabeth Anuoluwa, Morufu Olalekan Raimi (2021) Potential Toxic levels of Cyanide and Heavy Metals in Cassava Flour Sold in Selected Markets in Oke Ogun Community, Oyo State, Nigeria, 01 July 2021, PREPRINT (Version 1) available at Research Square [https://doi.org/10.21203/rs.3.rs-658748/v1].

[61] Raimi Morufu Olalekan, Bilewu Olaolu Oyinlola, Adio Zulkarnaini Olalekan, Abdulrahman Halimat (2019) Women Contributions to Sustainable Environments in Nigeria. *Journal of Scientific Research in Allied Sciences*. 5(4), 35-51. ISSN NO. 2455-5800. DOI No. 10.26838/JUSRES.2019.5.4.104.

[62] Raimi M O, Suleiman R M, Odipe O E, Salami J T, Oshatunberu M, *et al* (2019). Women Role in Environmental Conservation and Development in Nigeria. *Ecology & Conservation Science*; 1(2): DOI: 10.19080/ECOA.2019.01.555558. Volume 1 Issue 2 - July 2019. https://juniperpublishers.com/ecoa/pdf/ECOA.MS.ID.555558.pdf

[63] Ajayi Folajimi Ajibola, Raimi Morufu Olalekan, Steve-Awogbami Oluseyi Catherine, Adeniji Anthony Olusola, Adebayo Patrick Adekunle (2020) Policy Responses to Addressing the Issues of Environmental Health Impacts of Charcoal Factory in Nigeria: Necessity Today; Essentiality Tomorrow. *Communication, Society and Media*. Vol 3, No 3. DOI: https://doi.org/10.22158/csm.v3n3p1. http://www.scholink.org/ojs/index.php/csm/article/view/2940.

[64] Brownson RC, Baker EA, Leet TL, *et al* (2003). Evidence-Based Public Health. New York: Oxford University Press.

[65] Raimi, O. M., Samson, T. K., Sunday, A. B., Olalekan, A. Z., Emmanuel, O. O., & Jide, O. T. (2021). Air of Uncertainty from Pollution Profiteers: Status of Ambient Air Quality of Sawmill Industry in Ilorin Metropolis, Kwara State, Nigeria. *Research Journal of Ecology and Environmental Sciences*, *1*(1), 17-38. Retrieved from https://www.scipublications.com/journal/index.php/rjees/article/view/60.

[66] Raimi Morufu Olalekan, Adio Zulkarnaini Olalekan, Odipe Oluwaseun Emmanuel, Timothy Kayode Samson, Ajayi Bankole Sunday & Ogunleye Temitope Jide (2020) Impact of Sawmill Industry on Ambient Air Quality: A Case Study of Ilorin Metropolis, Kwara State, Nigeria. *Energy and Earth Science* Vol. 3, No. 1, 2020. URL: http://dx.doi.org/10.22158/ees.v3n1p1. www.scholink.org/ojs/index.php/ees ISSN 2578-1359 (Print) ISSN 2578-1367 (Online)

[67] Black BL, Cowens-Alvarado R, Gershman S, *et al.* (2005) Using data to motivate action: the need for high quality, an effective presentation, and an action context for decision-making. Cancer Causes Control; (16 Suppl 1): 15 – 25.

[68] Kerner J, Rimer B, Emmons K (2005). Introduction to the special section on dissemination: dissemination research and research dissemination: how can we close the gap? *Health Psychol;* 24 (5): 443 – 446.

[69] Raimi Morufu Olalekan, Ayinla Lateefat Olajumoke, Ogah Alima (2021) First to Respond, Last to Leave: The Role of Para-Military Agencies in Disaster Management: Evidence from Nigeria. *Sumerianz Journal of Medical and Healthcare*, 2021, Vol. 4, No. 2, pp. 96-100 ISSN(e): 2663-421X, ISSN(p): 2706-8404 Website: https://www.sumerianz.com DOI: https://doi.org/10.47752/sjmh.42.96.100. https://www.sumerianz.com/?ic=journal-home&journal=31&info=archive-detail&month=06-2021&issue=2&volume=4.

[70] Raimi Morufu Olalekan, Adio Zulkarnaini Olalekan, Odipe Oluwaseun Emmanuel, Timothy Kayode Samson, Ajayi Bankole Sunday & Ogunleye Temitope Jide (2020) Impact of Sawmill Industry on Ambient Air Quality: A Case Study of Ilorin Metropolis, Kwara State, Nigeria. *Energy and Earth Science* Vol. 3, No. 1, 2020. URL: http://dx.doi.org/10.22158/ees.v3n1p1. www.scholink.org/ojs/index.php/ees ISSN 2578-1359 (Print) ISSN 2578-1367 (Online)

[71] Olalekan RM, Adedoyin OO, Ayibaṭonbira A, *et al* (2019). "Digging deeper" evidence on water crisis and its solution in Nigeria for Bayelsa state: a study of current scenario. *International Journal of Hydrology.* 2019;3(4):244-257. DOI: 10.15406/ijh.2019.03.00187.

[72] Raimi Morufu Olalekan, Omidiji Adedoyin O, Adeolu Timothy Adedotun, Odipe Oluwaseun Emmanuel and Babatunde Anu (2019) An Analysis of Bayelsa State Water Challenges on the Rise and Its Possible Solutions. *Acta Scientific Agriculture* 3.8 (2019): 110-125. DOI: 10.31080/ASAG.2019.03.0572.

[73] Afolabi Abiodun Segun, Morufu Olalekan Raimi (2021) Investigating Source Identification and Quality of Drinking Water in Piwoyi Community of Federal Capital Territory, Abuja Nigeria., 20 July 2021, PREPRINT (Version 1) available at Research Square [https://doi.org/10.21203/rs.3.rs-736140/v1].

[74] Green LW, Mercer SL. (2001) Can public health researchers and agencies reconcile the push from funding bodies and the pull from communities? *Am J Public Health*; 91 (12): 1926 – 1929.

[75] Thacker SB, Stroup DF (2006). Public health surveillance. In: Brownson RC, Petitti DB, eds. Applied Epidemiology: Theory to Practice. 2nd ed. New York, NY: Oxford University Press; 30 – 67.

[76] Hutchison BG (1993). Critical appraisal of review articles. Can Fam Physician. 1993; 39: 1097 – 1102.

[77] Milne R, Chambers L (1993). Assessing the scientific quality of review articles. *J Epidemiol Commun Health.* 47 (3): 169 – 170.

[78] Oxman AD, Guyatt GH (1993). The science of reviewing research. *Ann N Y Acad Sci*. 703: 125 – 133; discussion 133-124.

[79] Zaza S, Briss PA, Harris KW (2005) The Guide to Community Preventive Services: What Works to Promote Health? New York: Oxford University Press.

[80] Mullen PD, Ramirez G (2006). The promise and pitfalls of systematic reviews. *Annu Rev Public Health*. 27: 81 – 102.

[81] Waters E, Doyle J (2002). Evidence-based public health practice: improving the quality and quantity of the evidence. *J Public Health Med.* 24 (3): 227 – 229.

[82] Gold MR, Siegel JE, Russell LB, *et al.* (1996) Cost-Effectiveness in Health and Medicine. New York: Oxford University Press.

[83] Carande-Kulis VG, Maciosek MV, Briss PA, *et al.* (2000) Methods for systematic reviews of economic evaluations for the Guide to Community Preventive Services. Task Force on Community Preventive Services. *Am J Prev Med*. 18 (1 Suppl): 75 – 91.

[84] Raimi Morufu Olalekan, Emeka Chisom Lucky, Ebikapaye Okoyen, Angalabiri Clement, Christopher Ogbointuwe, Atoyebi Babatunde (2021) COVID-19 Decision Impacts: Vaccine Hesitancy, its Barriers and Impact Studies: Taking Bayelsa State as an Example., 27 May 2021, PREPRINT (Version 1) available at Research Square [https://doi.org/10.21203/rs.3.rs-566532/v1].

[85] Okoyen E, Raimi M O, Omidiji A O, Ebuete A W (2020). Governing the Environmental Impact of Dredging: Consequences for Marine Biodiversity in the Niger Delta Region of Nigeria. *Insights Mining Science and technology* 2020; 2(3): 555586. DOI: 10.19080/IMST.2020.02.555586. https://juniperpublishers.com/imst/pdf/IMST.MS.ID.555586.pdf.

[86] Deinkuro Nimisngha Sanchez, Charles W. Knapp, Raimi Morufu Olalekan, Nimlang Henry Nanalok (2021) Oil Spills in the Niger Delta Region, Nigeria: Environmental Fate of Toxic Volatile Organics. 28 June 2021, PREPRINT (Version 1) available at Research Square. DOI: https://doi.org/10.21203/rs.3.rs-654453/v1.

[87] Raimi Morufu Olalekan, Abiola Ilesanmi, Ogah Alima, Dodeye E. Omini and Aziba-anyam Gift Raimi (2021) Exploring How Human Activities Disturb the Balance of Biogeochemical Cycles: Evidence from the Carbon, Nitrogen and Hydrologic Cycles. *IntechOpen*. DOI: http://dx.doi.org/10.5772/intechopen.98533. https://www.intechopen.com/online-first/77696.

[88] http://www.countyhealthrankings.org/our-approach (accessed July 18, 2017).

[89] Cargo M, Mercer SL (2008). The value and challenges of participatory research: Strengthening its practice. *Annu Rev Public Health*. 29: 325 – 350.

[90] Leung MW, Yen IH, Minkler M (2004). Community based participatory research: a promising approach for increasing epidemiology's relevance in the 21st century. *Int J Epidemiol.* 33 (3): 499 – 506.

[91] Soriano FI (1995). Conducting Needs Assessments. A Multidisciplinary Approach. Thousand Oaks, CA: Sage Publications.

[92] Sederburg WA (1992). Perspectives of the legislator: allocating resources. MMWR Morb Mortal Wkly Rep. 41 (Suppl): 37 – 48.

[93] Hallfors D, Cho H, Livert D, *et al.* (2002) Fighting back against substance abuse: are community coalitions winning? *Am J Prev Med.* 23 (4): 237 – 245.

[94] Turnock BJ (2004). Public Health: What It Is and How It Works. 3rd ed. Gaithersburg, MD: Aspen Publishers.

[95] Brownson RC, Ballew P, Brown KL, *et al.* (2007) The effect of disseminating evidence-based interventions that promote physical activity to health departments. Am J Public Health. 97 (10): 1900 – 1907.

[96] Brownson RC, Diem G, Grabauskas V, *et al.* (2007) Training practitioners in evidence-based chronic disease prevention for global health. *Promot Educ*. 14 (3): 159 – 163.

[97] Gebbie K, Merrill J, Hwang I, *et al.* (2002) Identifying individual competency in emerging areas of practice: an applied approach. *Qual Health Res.* 12 (7): 990 – 999.

[98] Birkhead GS, Davies J, Miner K, *et al.* (2008) Developing competencies for applied epidemiology: from process to product. *Public Health Rep*. 2008; 123 (Suppl 1): 67 – 118.

[99] Brownson R, Ballew P, Kittur N, *et al.* (2009) Developing competencies for training practitioners in evidence-based cancer control. *J Cancer Educ.* 24 (3): 186 – 193.

[100] Baker EA, Brownson RC, Dreisinger M, *et al.* (2009) Examining the role of training in evidence-based public health: a qualitative study. *Health Promot Pract*. 10 (3): 342 – 348.

[101] Maxwell ML, Adily A, Ward JE. (2007) Promoting evidence-based practice in population health at the local level: a case study in workforce capacity development. *Aust Health Rev.* 31 (3): 422 – 429.

[102] Maylahn C, Bohn C, Hammer M, *et al.* (2008) Strengthening epidemiologic competencies among local health professionals in New York: teaching evidence-based public health. *Public Health Rep*. 123 (Suppl 1): 35 – 43.

[103] Linkov F, LaPorte R, Lovalekar M, *et al.* (2005) Web quality control for lectures: Super course and Amazon.com. *Croat Med J.* 46 (6): 875 – 878.

[104] Proctor EK. (2004) Leverage points for the implementation of evidence-based practice. Brief Treatment Crisis Intervent. 4 (3): 227 – 242.

[105] Chambers LW (1992). The new public health: do local public health agencies need a booster (or organizational "fix") to combat the diseases of disarray? *Can J Public Health*. 83 (5): 326 – 328.

[106] Bryan RL, Kreuter MW, Brownson RC. (2008) Integrating Adult Learning Principles into Training for Public Health Practice. *Health Promot Pract.* Apr 2.

[107] Wright K, Rowitz L, Merkle A, *et al.* (2000) Competency development in public health leadership. *Am J Public Health*. 90 (8): 1202 – 1207.

[108] Odubo Tonbra Robert and Raimi Morufu Olalekan (2019) Resettlement and Readjustment Patterns of Rural Dwellers During and After Flood Disasters in Bayelsa State Nigeria. *British Journal of Environmental Sciences* Vol .7, No .3, Pp. 45-52, July 2019. www.eajournals.org.

[109] Wolff, T. J. (2001). Special section: Contemporary issues series I community coalition building-Contemporary practice and research. *American Journal of Community Psychology*, 29.

[110] http://www.nlm.nih.gov.

[111] Ginter PM, Duncan WJ, Capper SA. (1992) Keeping strategic thinking in strategic planning: macro-environmental analysis in a state health department of public health. Public Health. 106: 253 – 269.

[112] Florin P, Stevenson J. (1993) Identifying training and technical assistance needs in community coalitions: a developmental approach. *Health Educ Res.* 8: 417 – 432.

[113] Jacobs J, Dodson E, Baker E, *et al.* (2010) Barriers to evidence-based decision making in public health: a national survey of chronic disease practitioners. Public Health Rep.

[114] Savitz DA. (2003) *Interpreting Epidemiologic Evidence. Strategies for Study Design and Analysis.* New York, NY: Oxford University Press.

[115] Anderson LM, Brownson RC, Fullilove MT, *et al.* (2005) Evidence-based public health policy and practice: promises and limits. *Am J Prev Med*; 28 (5 Suppl): 226 – 230.

[116] https://www.bessi-collab.net/.

Chapter 7

A Report of the Survey on Shelter Management under COVID-19 in Japanese Local Governments

Arisa Yasui and Muneyoshi Numada

Abstract

Japan is a disaster-prone country and natural disasters could happen under COVID-19. Shelter management is especially important because many people evacuate there and there's high risk of spreading infection. In order to establish feasible countermeasures in shelters, we conducted a survey about the current situation of preparation and experience of shelter management in Japanese local governments under COVID-19. From the answer of 346 municipalities, we found that some municipalities took measures against COVID-19 such as adding new shelters and conducting the training, and these proactive measures were very useful. However, due to the addition of infectious disease control work, it became clear that it would take time and difficulty at reception, and that it would be even more difficult to identify evacuees with the recommended distributed evacuation. These results can be useful in proceeding consideration of better shelter management under COVID-19.

Keywords: COVID-19, shelter management, infectious disease measures, Japan, local governments

1. Introduction

Currently, the infection of COVID-19 is spreading all over the world. As of April 21, 2021, the number of infected people worldwide has exceeded 140 million and the death toll has exceeded 3 million [1]. The infection has spread by an order of magnitude compared to the SARS infections of 8,096 and deaths of 794 [2] that prevailed in 2003, and the MARS infections of 971 and deaths of 356 [3] that prevailed in 2012. The development of therapeutic drugs and vaccines is progressing all over the world, and inoculation is progressing [4], but it has not yet ended in some countries such as Japan and India.

In Japan, which is a disaster-prone country, there are concerns about the occurrence of natural disasters such as earthquakes, tsunamis, and typhoons during the period when COVID-19 is spreading. Especially in recent years, disasters such as the 2011 off the Pacific coast of Tohoku Earthquake, the 2016 Kumamoto Earthquake, and the heavy rains in western Japan in 2018, have become more severe and frequent. When such disasters occur, schools and public halls become shelters and many residents evacuate [5, 6]. In these past disasters, the spread of infection in shelters has become a problem. Although the Basic Act on Disaster Countermeasures requires improvement of the living environment in shelters, such as distribution of food, clothing, medicines, and provision of health care services (Article 86–6), specific measures against infectious diseases have not been mentioned. In addition, outbreaks in shelters can be larger under COVID-19 than infectious diseases after previous natural disaster because some people have not taken COVID-19 vaccine yet. It is also possible that people are more likely to suffer damage at home if they do not evacuate to a shelter for fear of getting infected. 90% of those who died in the heavy rains in western Japan were found at home [7], and it is said that they could not evacuate to a safe place.

Based on this situation, the problem is that human damage caused by both COVID-19 and natural disasters will increase, and it is necessary to consider measures against the occurrence of natural disasters and the shelter management system under COVID-19.

Therefore, our research question is, "What is the current situation regarding the shelter management in Japanese local governments under COVID-19?" This research will contribute to realize effective disaster countermeasures under COVID-19.

2. Literature review

Infectious diseases are often prevalent after a natural disaster [8]. In particular, there are many cases of infectious diseases occurring in shelters [9–11].

The spread of infectious diseases involves multiple factors. First, stress due to major changes in the living environment [12], food shortages, and unsanitary environments increase the risk of infection [8]. Next, although an unspecified number of people live together in shelters, it has been clarified that infection is spreading in shelters where the usable area per person is small and dense [13]. In addition, disasters can paralyze medical institutions and damage healthcare workers, so inadequate provision of medical care compared to normal times contributes to the spread of infection [12].

In the Great East Japan Earthquake, there were many acute respiratory and gastrointestinal symptoms [9]. During the Kumamoto earthquake, norovirus-induced infectious gastroenteritis was prevalent [10].

The epidemic of infectious diseases after the occurrence of a natural disaster is not limited to Japan.

For example, the 2004 Sumatra earthquake and tsunami caused aspiration pneumonia, skin and wound infections [14], the 2005 hurricane Katrina spread norovirus infections in shelters [11], and the 2010 Haiti earthquake caused a cholera outbreak [15].

It is necessary to take appropriate measures against the epidemic of such infectious diseases. During the Great East Japan Earthquake, an infectious disease control team [12] and Japan Medical Association Team (JMAT) from a nearby university hospital were dispatched to shelters [16]. At the time of the Kumamoto earthquake, Kagoshima Prefecture JMAT was also dispatched, and public health activities including infectious disease control were carried out along with medical care for the victims [17]. Activities from the early stage of 5 days after the disaster are attributed to the good relationship between the medical association and the local government before the disaster and the communication function using the Web [17]. Thanks to these activities, the effects of the infection are said to have been relatively small [18].

The main activities of these organizations are the provision of medical care and surveillance of infectious diseases. As medical needs change over time, the content and scale of medical care provided by various organizations changes [19]. Early after the disaster, disaster medicine is provided, but gradually shifts to support for daily medical care in the disaster area, and the proportion of nurses decreases and the proportion of doctors increases [20]. Since conventional surveillance systems may not function or limited resources may be available in the early stages after the disaster, it is necessary to consider a system that efficiently collects infectious disease information from the early stages of the disaster [9]. In addition to relying on people with specialized knowledge, shelter operators, mainly local governments, also need basic knowledge [21] and understanding of pathogens [22] to improve the environment of shelters.

However, according to a survey conducted by Kudo et al., about 60% of local governments have prepared infection control manuals, and it cannot be said that a sufficient system is in place to prevent the spread of infectious diseases. In addition, 75% said they had insufficient knowledge about infectious diseases, and only 3% said they had sufficient knowledge [23].

As described above, infectious diseases have become prevalent in shelters after the occurrence of natural disasters, and many studies have analyzed individual cases and are considering countermeasures. However, they do not consider COVID-19 that is currently prevalent. In addition, this is a study on cases of infectious diseases that occur after natural disasters and their countermeasures, which is different from the case where natural disasters occur while infectious diseases are spreading as they are now. In order to implement effective countermeasures against COVID-19, it is necessary to understand disaster countermeasures that incorporate infectious disease countermeasures by local governments.

Therefore, the purposes of this study are i) to clarify the current status of proactive measures for shelter operation under COVID-19, and ii) to clarify the actual state and issues of shelter operation in COVID-19. These results are useful in considering countermeasures against the occurrence of natural disasters and shelter management under COVID-19.

3. Methods

3.1 Outline of the survey

As the method of this research, we used the implementation of questionnaire surveys for Japanese local governments nationwide and their statistical analysis.

In this study, the authors created a questionnaire in Excel and sent it by e-mail to the departments in charge of disaster prevention in local governments. **Table 1** shows the outline of the survey, and the number of valid answers is 346.

Table 2 shows the composition of the questionnaire. Most of them are multiple-choice, but some questions are descriptive. The contents of the survey can be roughly divided into four. The first is the proactive measures for the shelter management under COVID-19. In order to clarify what kind of measures are being taken by each local government in Japan, we have set up questions asking about the creation of shelter management manuals that incorporate infectious disease countermeasures, the implementation of training, and the addition of shelters. The second is the actual shelter management under COVID-19 in entire municipality. For local governments that have experience in opening shelters under COVID-19, we set up questions asking about the provision of evacuation information and the acceptance of support staff. The third is the actual shelter management under COVID-19 at each shelter. In order to clarify the infection countermeasures taken at the shelters and their issues, we set up questions asking about the specific contents of infectious disease countermeasures, how to grasp evacuees at home, and difficult tasks. The fourth is the attributes of the respondents. Questions were set up asking the name of the municipality, population size, name of the department in charge, title of the person in charge, and experience of opening shelters.

Item	Contents
Survey name	Survey on shelter management under COVID-19
Survey target	Municipalities nationwide
Investigation	• Preparation for shelter management under COVID-19
	• Actual shelter management under COVID-19 etc.
Survey period	From December 14th, 2020 to December 31st, 2020
Collection method	Send mail
Number of valid answers	346

Table 1.
Outline of the survey.

Proactive measures for shelter management under COVID-19
• **Addition of shelter**: Asked the question, "Did you add a new shelter as a measure against COVID-19? Please tell me all that apply." Respondents who selected "Other" are requested to provide a descriptive response.
• **Creation of a shelter management manual fur COVID-19**: In response to the question "Are you creating an evacuation shelter management manual based on COVID-19 measures?" Request a single selective answer from the three.
• **Implementation of shelter management training under COVID-19**: In response to the question "Did you conduct shelter management training based on COVID-19 measures?", You can choose from three options: "We did it for the entire municipality," "We did it independently at each shelter," and "We did not." Request a single selective answer.
Actual shelter management under COVID-19 (for the entire municipality)
• **Experience of opening a shelter under COVID-19**: "Did you open a shelter under COVID-19? Please tell us about the target disaster. If not, please enter None". We requested a descriptive answer to the question and asked the respondents who filled in the target disaster to answer the following questions.
1. **Provision or evacuation information**: In response to the question, "What kind of information did you provide in addition to the evacuation information when the above disaster occurred? Please tell me all that apply." Request multiple selective answers from "Prompted for evacuation at home", "Prompted for evacuation to house of acquaintances or relatives", "Prompted for distributed evacuation", "Request for wearing mask", and "Other", and requested respondents who selected "Other" to answer with a description of the contents.
2. **Acceptance of support staff**: In response to the question "Did you accept the support staff?", Request a single selective answer from "Yes" and "No". For respondents who selected "Yes", in response to the question "Which area did you accept support staff from? Please tell me all that apply." Request on answer and request the respondents who selected "Other to further describe the content.
3. **Acceptance of volunteers**: In response to the question "Did you accept volunteers?", Request a single selective answer from "Ye" and "No". For respondents who selected "Yes", in response to the question "Which area did you accept volunteers from? Please tell me all that apply.", request multiple selective answers from "City / town" "Prefecture" "Kyushu region" "Others", and request the respondents who selected "Other" to further describe the contents.
Actual shelter management under COVID-19 (for each shelter)
Following the above, we asked the following questions for each shelter opened.
4. **Shelter name**: Request a descriptive answer to the question "Please tell me the name of the shelter."
5. **Opening period**: In response to the question "Please tell me the opening: period of the shelter", request a single selective answer from "within 24 hours", "1–3 days", "3 days-1 week", "1 week-3 weeks", and "3 weeks or more".
6. **Maximum capacity**: In response to the question "What is the maximum number of evacuees accommodated?", request a single selective answer from "10 or less," "10–50," "50–100," "100–300," and "more", and request the respondents who selected "more" to answer with a description of the content.
7. **Utilization of shelter management manuals incorporating infectious disease countermeasures**: In response to the question "Have you been able to utilize shelter management manuals based on COVID-19 measures?", we requested a single selective answer from "Yes", "No" and a descriptive answer for each.

8. **Utilization of shelter management training incorporating infectious disease countermeasures**: In response to the question "Did the evacuation shelter management training based on COVID-19 measures help in actual management?", we requested a single selective answer from "Yes" and "No" and requested a descriptive answer for each.
9. **Grasping home evacuation and staying in the car (distributed evacuation)**: Requested a descriptive answer to the question "How did you grasp evacuation at home and staying in the car?"
10. **Acceptance of pets**: Requested a descriptive answer to the question "How did you accept evacuees' pets?"
11. **Infectious disease control items**: In response to the question "Did you have enough items for infectious disease control?", We requested a single selective answer from "Yes" and "No", and the respondents who selected "No" were asked" In response to the question "Please tell me all that apply to the missing items", request multiple selective answers from "Mask", "Disinfectant", "Gloves", "Protective clothing", "Face shield", and "Other" and select "Other". The selected respondents are requested to further describe the contents.
12. **Measures taken against infections diseases**: In response to the question "Did you take Ihe following measures against infectious diseases? Please tell me all that apply", we requested multiple selective answers from "Limited number of people" "Temperature measurement at reception" "Zoning of evacuation space" "Not crossing the flow lines of each space" "Separate toilets and water supply between healthy people and people with poor physical condition" "Social distancing in each space" "Installing disinfectant solution in various places such as reception desks" "Regular ventilation" "Disinfection of handrails and doorknobs" "Operator's sanitary equipment" and "Others", and request respondents who selected "Others" to provide a descriptive response.
13. **Shelter operator**: In response to the question "Please tell me everything that applies to the shelter operator", request multiple selective answers from "local government officials", "facility manager", "residents", and "others", and request respondents who selected "others" to provide a descriptive response to the content. In addition, we requested a descriptive answer to the question "Please tell us about the reaction of the residents who participated in the shelter management."
14. **Transportation to medical institutions**: In response to the question "Did you transport the person with poor physical condition or fever to a medical institution?", We requested a single selective answer from "Yes" and "No" and request respondents who selected "Yes" to provide descriptive answers to the question "Please tell us about the specific situation when transporting to a medical institution. (Procedures, persons in charge, issues, etc.)".
15. **Difficult work, problems**: "Which work was difficult or time consuming in the entire shelter management?" "Please tell us if there is a problem in the whole shelter management." In response, each requested a descriptive answer.
16. **Changes in evacuees' characteristics before and after COVID-19**: In response to the question "Did the evacuees change before and after COVID-19? (The number of elderly people has decreased, the number of children has decreased, the number of nights in the car has increased, etc.), request a single selective answer from "changed" and "not changed", and ask the respondents who selected "changed" to give a descriptive answer.
17. **Changes in evacuation shelter operators before and after COVID-19**: In response to the question "Did the shelter management entity change before and alter COVID-19? (For example, the residents refrained from operating it, the elderly people refrained from operating it, etc.)", we requested a single selective answer from "changed" and "not changed" and asked the respondents who selected "changed" to give descriptive answer to the content.
Attributes
• **City name**: Request a written response with the name of the prefecture and the name of the city.
• **Population size**: In response to the question "Please tell me the population size of the municipality", "10,000 or less", "10,000-30,000", "30,000-50,000", "50,000-100,000", "10", request a single selective answer from "10,000–300,000" and "300,000 or more".
• **Name of department in charge**: In response to the question "Please tell me the name of the respondent's department in charge.", requested a descriptive response.
• **Experience of opening a shelter**: Asked "Have you ever opened a shelter in a municipality before COVID-19 disaster?" and requested a single selective answer from "Yes" and "No".

Table 2.
Composition of the questionnaire.

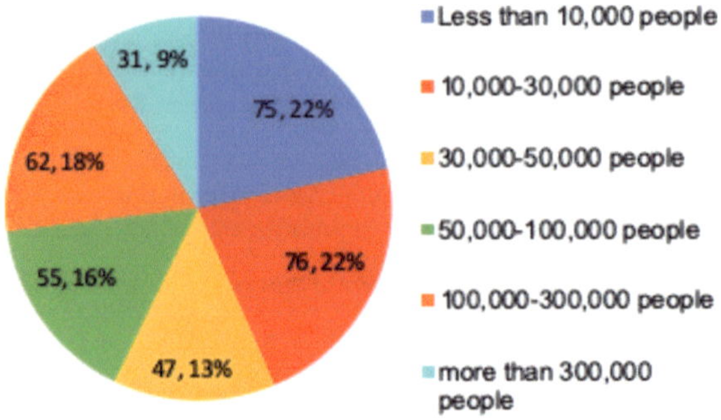

Figure 1.
Distribution of the population size.

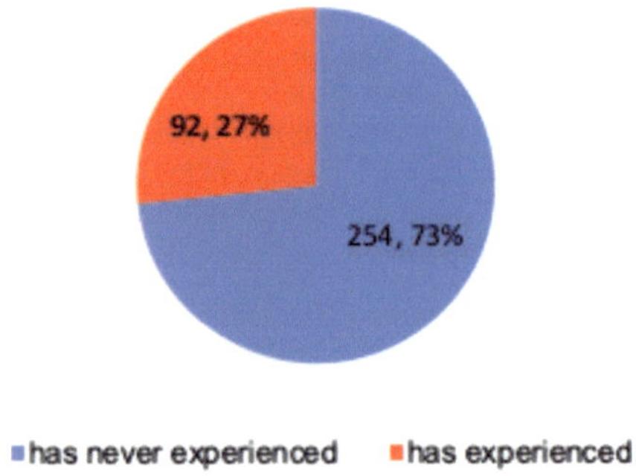

Figure 2.
Experience of opening a shelter under COVID-19.

The structure of this paper is as follows. Chapter 4 shows the proactive measures for the shelter management under COVID-19, and the following Chapter 5 shows the actual shelter management under COVID-19. Based on the above, Chapter 6 considers how shelters should be operated under COVID-19. Finally, Chapter 7 describes the limitations and prospects of this research.

3.2 Survey target

The characteristics of the local governments that responded to this survey are shown in **Figures 1** and **2**. **Figure 1** shows the distribution of the population size of the responding municipalities. About half of the municipalities have less than 30,000 people.

Figure 2 shows the experience of opening a shelter under COVID-19. About 1/4 of the local governments have opened shelters due to some natural disaster under COVID-19. In this survey, the target disaster was not specified, and each local government was requested to answer the description of the target disaster. According to their answer, heavy rains in July 2020, typhoon No. 8, typhoon No. 9, typhoon No. 10, typhoon No. 12, and typhoon No. 14 were mentioned. There are no cases of opening shelters after the earthquake, and all shelters were opened after the storm and flood damage.

4. Proactive measures for shelter management under COVID-19

4.1 Creating a manual

Figure 3 shows the status of preparation of a manual on the shelter management under COVID-19. Approximately 3/4 of the municipalities created the manuals in

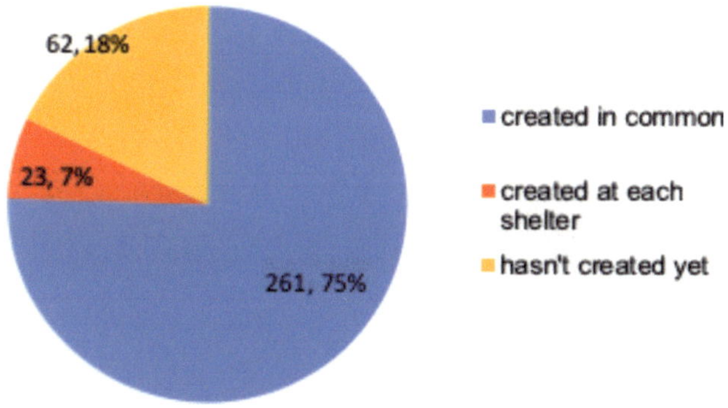

Figure 3.
Status of preparation of a manual on the shelter management under COVID-19.

common, and when combined with the municipalities created individually at the shelters, about 80% of the municipalities answered that they created the manual. The Cabinet Office [24] and NPOs [25, 26] have issued guidelines for shelter management under COVID-19, and it is probable that they were created with reference to them. It can be utilized for countermeasures by showing the overall guideline at an early stage.

4.2 Implementation of training

Figure 4 shows the implementation status of shelter management training under COVID-19. Approximately half of the local governments conducted training for the entire municipality, and when combined with the local governments that conducted individual training at shelters, about 3/4 of the local governments conducted shelter management training under COVID-19. Compared to the preparation of manuals, many local governments conducted their own training at shelters. It is thought to be because training at the shelter can be conducted in a state closer to the actual situation.

4.3 Addition of shelter

Figure 5 shows the presence or absence of shelters newly added as a countermeasure against COVID-19.

Under the Disaster Countermeasures Basic Law, as a rule, basic municipalities are obliged to designate shelters (Article 49–7), and local elementary schools and public halls are shelters.

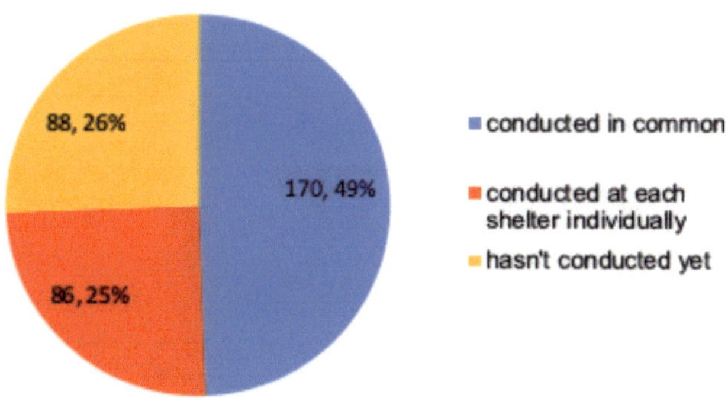

Figure 4.
Implementation status of shelter management training under COVID-19.

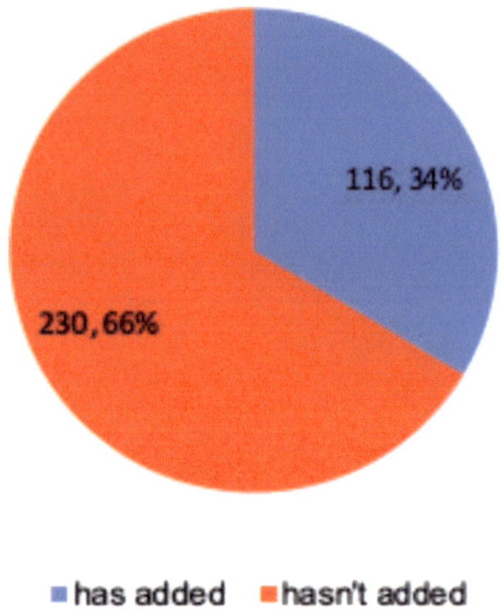

Figure 5.
Presence or absence of shelters newly added.

In addition, as a measure against infectious diseases, securing social distance will result in a shortage of conventional shelters. Therefore, it is recommended by the government to add new shelters and carry out distributed evacuation.

About 30% of local governments have added new shelters. In addition, the municipalities that answered "not added" include those that are in the process of adjustment.

Figure 6 shows the details of the newly added shelter. We asked the local governments that answered that they had "added" shelters to answer with multiple answers as to what kind of facilities they are using. Most of them are public facilities, followed by accommodation facilities such as hotels and inns. Others included shelters for overnight stays in cars and the use of empty classrooms in shelters.

Since public facilities are owned by the local government, it is assumed that it is relatively easy for the local government to add new shelters as internal adjustments will be made. It is considered to be the factor that the number of public facilities as newly added shelter is the largest. On the other hand, accommodation facilities and private facilities need to conclude agreements to be used as shelters, and it is considered difficult to secure them compared to public facilities. However, accommodation facilities are attracting attention due to the spread of COVID-19 [24]. In order to prevent the collapse of medical care, hotels are being rented and converted into accommodation facilities for the mildly ill.

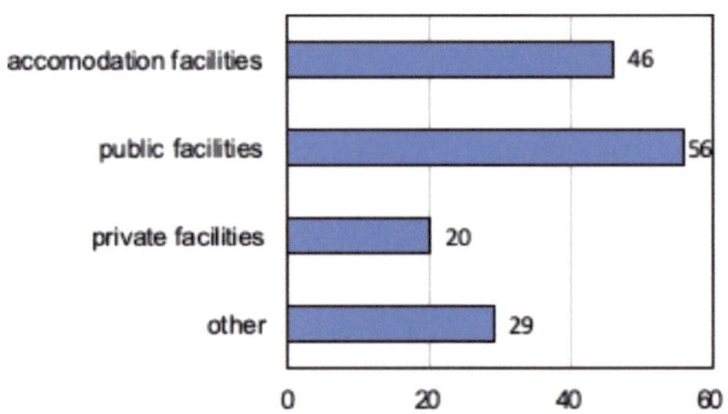

Figure 6.
Details of the newly added shelter.

In addition, it is presumed that a special place was set up for the shelter for overnight stays in the car, as many people stayed in the car during the 2016 Kumamoto earthquake [27].

5. Actual shelter management under COVID-19

5.1 Outline of opening a shelter

Figure 7 shows the shelter opening period under COVID-19. About half of them are opened within 24 hours, and about 90% are opened within 3 days. It can be seen that the opening was relatively short.

Figure 8 shows the total number of evacuees in shelters under COVID-19 per shelter. About half are 10 or less, and the total number of evacuees is small. It also includes cases where evacuees did not come to the shelter even though they opened the shelter. Considering this together with **Figure 7**, it is assumed that the scale of the disaster was smaller than usual.

5.2 Dissemination and collection of information on distributed evacuation

Figure 9 shows whether residents were urged to do distributed evacuation under COVID-19. Here, distributed evacuation is defined as various evacuation that keeps

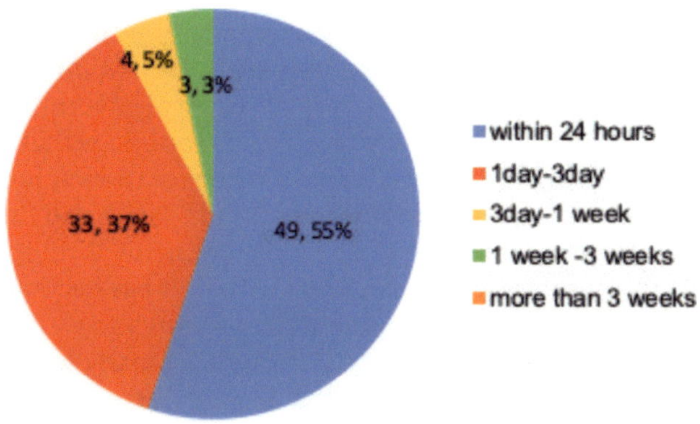

Figure 7.
Shelter opening period under COVID-19.

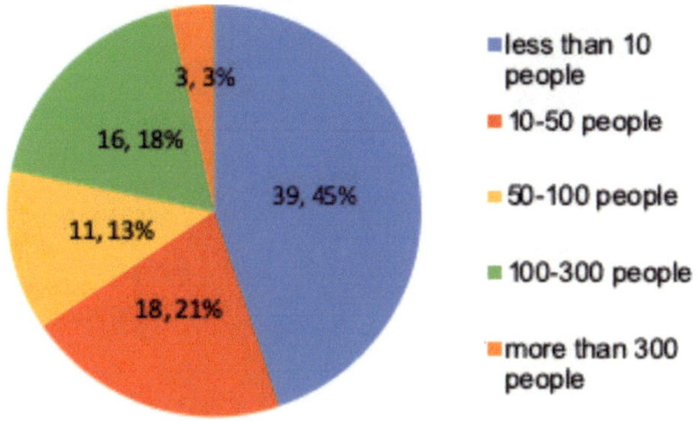

Figure 8.
Total number of evacuees in shelters under COVID-19 per shelter.

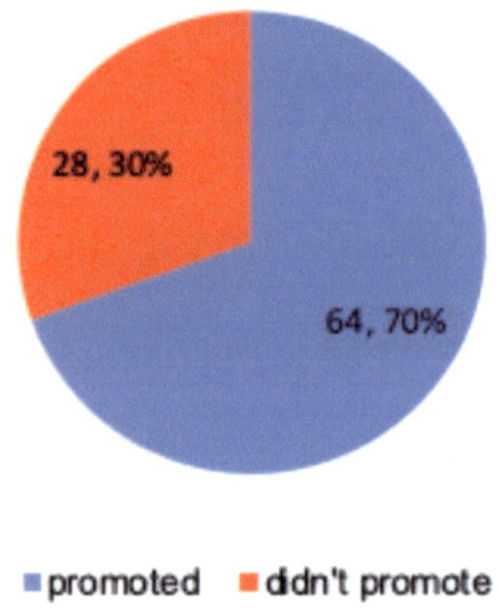

Figure 9.
Whether residents were urged to do distributed evacuation under COVID-19.

a social distance to prevent infection, and in addition to shelters, stay in the car, evacuate at home, evacuate to acquaintances and relatives' homes, and evacuation to accommodation facilities.

As a result of the survey, about 70% of local governments promoted distributed evacuation. Distributed evacuation is effective for preventing infection, but it is different from conventional evacuation methods, so it is important to educate the residents daily so that the residents can correctly understand the meaning and method.

Figure 10 shows the status of grasping evacuees' information in distributed evacuation under COVID-19. Only about 20% of the local governments have grasped it. From the written answers, we received the opinions that "reports from the mayor of each administrative district regarding evacuation at home", "we cannot be grasp unless contacted from residents", and "only grasp the stay in the car in the parking lot of the shelter" It can be seen that many local governments are based on requests from residents to grasp information. It has become clear that it is difficult for local governments to comprehensively grasp evacuee's information.

From **Figures 9** and **10**, it became clear that there are many local governments that have promoted distributed evacuation but have not been able to grasp the information of distributed evacuees. It is expected that the number of evacuees evacuating to places other than shelters will increase, making it more difficult to grasp the information. However, since it is important to know where and how

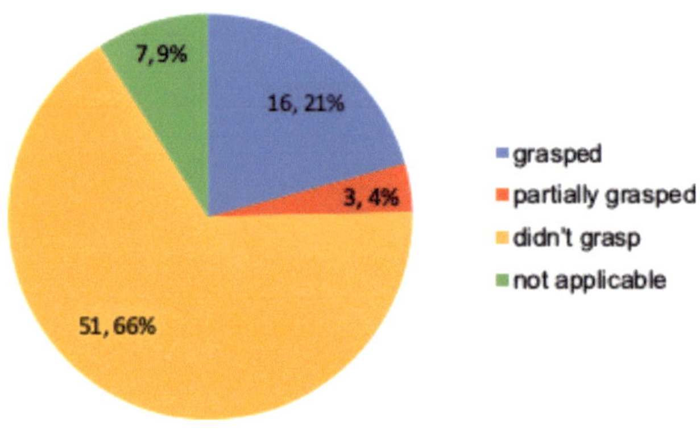

Figure 10.
Status of grasping evacuees' information in distributed evacuation under COVID-19.

many evacuees are in the provision of supplies, it is necessary to consider effective methods. In addition, in order to save people's lives, it's important to grasp where are patients and what medical care is needed, which will lead to effective provision of medical care. Also, these kinds of information should be shared with hospitals or other medical organizations.

5.3 Utilization of proactive measures

Figure 11 shows the utilization status of the shelter management manual under COVID-19. We asked the local government, which had created the manual at the time of the response, about the utilization status. About 95% of local governments answered that they were able to utilize the manual. Specifically, from the written answer, "We were able to install infectious disease control items (hand sanitizers, facility disinfectants, etc.) that had been deployed to shelters in advance at necessary locations such as entrances and exits according to the manual. "I was able to confirm in advance the flow at the time of reception and what to do when a person with poor physical condition appears (separate rooms and flow lines, etc.)" "If a person with poor physical condition occurs, isolate it. The staff members had a common understanding of that points. " Based on these opinions, by creating a manual in advance and using it in the event of a disaster, the flow from setting up a shelter to accepting evacuees can be carried out smoothly, and special measures in the event of an unwell person can be confirmed. It can be said that this led to fostering a common consciousness among the staff. On the other hand, regarding the local governments that answered that the manual could not be used, from the written answer, we obtained the opinions like, "I could not hand over the manual because it was opened at the branch office." "The shelter was opened but there were no evacuees." Although the manual was created, there was a problem that it could not be referred to at the time of opening because it was not on site. It is considered necessary to deliver it in advance so that it can be referred to at each shelter. In addition, it was found that there were cases where the manual was not used because the evacuees did not come to the shelter.

Figure 12 shows the implementation status of shelter management training under COVID-19. As in **Figure 11**, we asked the local governments that were

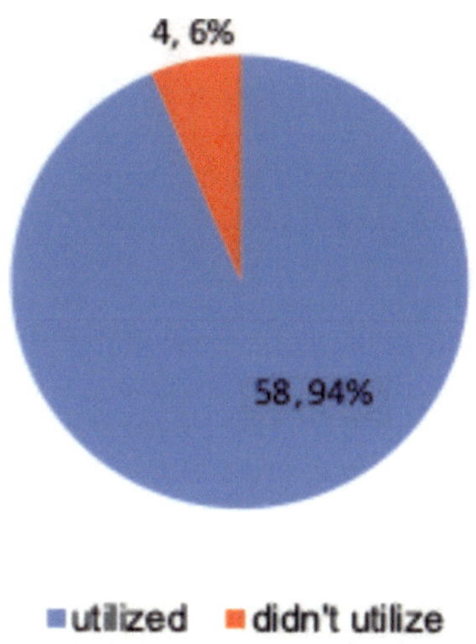

Figure 11.
Utilization status of the shelter management manual under COVID-19.

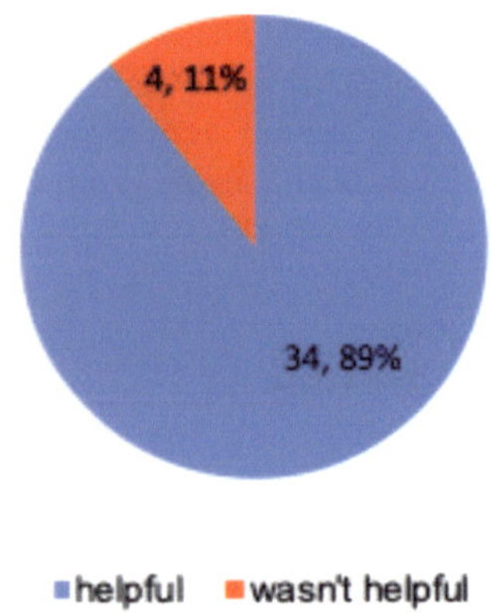

Figure 12.
Implementation status of shelter management training under COVID-19.

conducting the training at the time of the response about the utilization status. About 90% of local governments answered that the training was "helpful". Specifically, from the written answers, there are opinions like, "I think that we were able to operate the shelter with a margin by assuming various situations in advance." "We were able to smoothly set up the venue such as reception and creation of partitions." "The training at the shelter gave me an image of zoning." By conducting the training, shelter operators were able to get an image of the work content and work calmly and smoothly. Unexpected things can happen in the shelter management, but there are many tasks that should always do the same, and the implementation of training could facilitate the movement of the operator for such basic tasks. On the other hand, regarding the local governments that answered that they could not utilize the training, from the written answers, there are opinions like, "because the training was conducted after the typhoon period" and "because the shelter was opened but there were no evacuees". At the time of answering the questionnaire survey, training was conducted, but at the time of opening the shelter, training was not conducted, and as in the case of the manual, there were cases where there were no evacuees and there were no useful situations. It is inferred that it is important to take proactive measures as soon as possible.

5.4 Measures against infectious diseases inside shelters

Figure 13 shows the measures taken at the shelter for COVID-19. Most local governments install disinfectants in various places, and the temperature is measured at the reception desk, regular ventilation is maintained, and social-distances are secured in the evacuation space. There are several new stockpiles needed as a infectious disease countermeasure, but it can be said that many local governments are able to respond to them. In addition, it is said that it is effective to separate the space and flow lines of people who are in good physical condition from those who are in poor physical condition in order to prevent the spread of infection in shelters, but few local governments have taken such measures. It is probable that there was no need to deal with this in the short-term shelter opening like this time because it is not necessary to divide the space and flow line if the person who is in poor physical condition does not come to the shelter.

These measures considered to be helpful not only for COVID-19 but also for other infectious diseases, such as SARS, flu, and norovirus. In the past disasters, there was not much infectious disease control at shelter and nurses or other medical

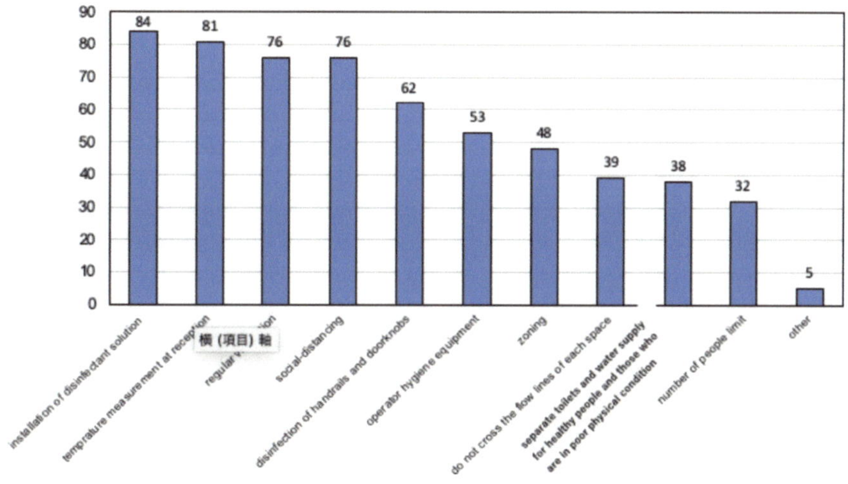

Figure 13.
Measures taken at the shelter for COVID-19.

staff have been dispatched to a shelter to respond. However, like this COVID-19 response, it is considered that local governments should prepare for other infectious diseases or the next pandemic.

5.5 Shelter operator

Figure 14 shows the shelter operator under COVID-19. The number of local governments officials is the largest, and the number of residents is small. It is possible that the residents did not operate the shelter in connection with many people because they were afraid of infection. However, we received the opinions like, "they were very supportive because we were taking measures against infection.", "After taking measures such as wearing a mask, measuring the temperature at the reception desk, and disinfecting, we received an active cooperation from residents based on training." On the other hand, from the local government where the residents did not participate in the operation of the shelter, we obtained the opinions like, "There was no participation of the residents because it was a temporary evacuation and did not proceed to the phase of shelter management by residents. " Based on these opinions, the reason why residents do not participate in shelter management is that the shelter opening period was short as shown in **Figure 7** and there was little need to be cooperated by residents. Also, it is considered that COVID-19 is not much effect.

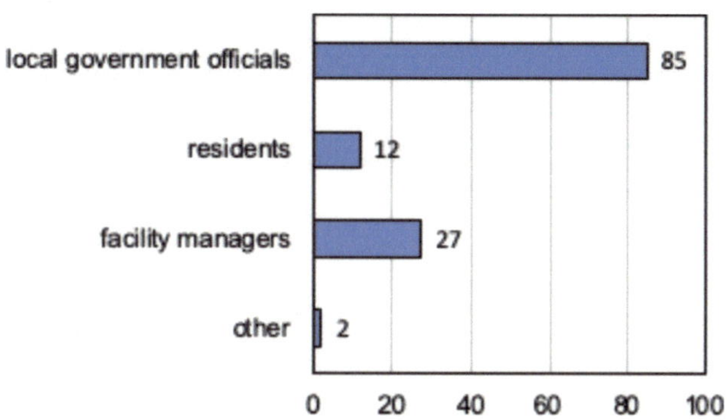

Figure 14.
Shelter operator under COVID-19.

5.6 Difficult tasks and issues

Table 3 shows the difficult tasks and problems of shelter management under COVID-19. The answers obtained were grouped into groups with similar contents, and classified into five: reception, keeping social-distances, zoning, personnel, and responding to residents.

First is the reception. It became clear that work such as temperature measurement, disinfection, and filling out a questionnaire was added as measures against infectious diseases, and the amount of work increased significantly, and it took time. It was also found that congestion was more likely to occur because the time required for reception per evacuee increased. Most of the local governments cited the work related to reception as a difficult work.

Second is work related to keeping social-distances. Measures were taken to install partition panels and corrugated cardboard partitions for each household, but

Reception
• It took time to accept evacuees duo to temperature measurement, etc.
• When accepting evacuees, multiple staff members were required, such as temperature measurement → disinfection → mask distribution → evacuees card → tent guidance.
• It took a long time to receive the test because of the temperature measurement and filling out the questionnaire.
• It took time to set up because it was necessary to separate the reception desks such as pre-reception and secondary reception from those who are not infected and those who are suspected
• It took time to collect information on evacuees (address, name, etc.)
• Since many evacuees came from the beginning of the shelter, the reception was not in time.
• Congestion at reception
Social-distancing
• Preparing to accept evacuees, especially the installation of partition panels. It was for several people in a few hours.
• Installation of cardboard partitions
• There was a shortage of partitions prepared in advance for the number of evacuees.
• Arrangement of evacuation spaces to avoid crowded evacuees
Zoning
• It took time to allocate healthy people, people requiring special care, people with poor physical condition, etc.
• Since information on close contacts cannot be obtained from the public health center, zoning cannot be performed without the declaration of the evacuees.
Management personnel
• Since the number of shelters will be increased, staff cannot be accommodated between each shelter, and the number of shelter response staff will decrease.
• Many shelter management staff are needed
Resident support
• Those who live in the sediment-related disaster warning area and were worried about COVID-19 and had difficulty in giving instructions to those who did not evacuate.
• Even if you ask the evacuees to keep social-distances and refrain from unnecessary contact as a measure against COVID-19, acquaintances approach each other and chat.

Table 3.
Difficult tasks and problems.

the installation was time-consuming. In addition, it was reported that the partition was insufficient because it was not included in the conventional stockpile and was newly prepared.

Third is zoning. In order to prevent the outbreak of clusters and the spread of infection at shelters, evacuation spaces should be provided according to the physical condition of the evacuees, such as those in good physical condition, those requiring special attention who are at high risk of serious illness, close contacts, and those who are in poor physical condition. It was found that there were Issues such as the time required for this allocation and the fact that the evacuees must rely on the evacuees' self-reports because it is the health center that possesses the information on the close contacts necessary for zoning. Even if a manual or training is provided for a large policy, it is not known what kind of physical condition will actually come to the shelter, and it is necessary to respond flexibly on the spot.

Fourth is the management staff. In this survey, shelters were opened in a relatively short period of time, but securing management personnel, which has been an issue in the past, has become an issue. Under COVID-19, some local governments have increased the number of shelters opened to carry out distributed evacuation. In that case, the staffing at each shelter will be different from before, and there is a high possibility that there will be a shortage. In addition, since infectious disease control work has been added, it is considered difficult to handle with the same number of people as before. It can be said that securing management personnel has become a more prominent problem under COVID-19.

Last is the response to residents. It is thought that it is difficult to encourage residents to make correct decisions and take actions in situations where they are exposed to the combined dangers of a COVID-19 and a natural disaster. If you evacuate to a shelter when your home is safe against natural disasters, the risk of infection increases, while if your home is dangerous to natural disasters but you stay at home due to fear of the risk of infection at the shelter, a natural disaster may kill you. It can be said that it is necessary to take the best action to save lives according to the situation each person is placed. In addition, awareness of infectious diseases and their countermeasures is expected to vary greatly from person to person. Therefore, asking people with low consciousness to cooperate with the measures is mentioned as a difficult task.

6. Conclusions

The purposes of this study are i)to clarify the current status of proactive measures regarding the shelter management under COVID-19, and ii) the actual state and issues of shelter management under COVID-19. We conducted a questionnaire survey targeting local governments.

As a result, the findings obtained from this study are as follows.

i. It was found that proactive measures for shelter management under COVID-19, such as the creation of manuals incorporating measures against COVID-19, the implementation of training, and the addition of shelters, are in progress.

ii. It was found that the proactive measures were very useful, and that the shelter was operated with the measures against infectious diseases under COVID-19. However, due to the addition of infectious disease control work, it became clear that it would take time and difficulty at reception, and that it would be even more difficult to identify evacuees with the recommended distributed evacuation.

Proactive measures regarding the shelter management under COVID-19 have progressed considerably, and it became clear that these were also useful in the actual shelter management under COVID-19, reaffirming the importance of proactive measures. In addition, it is considered that this measure will be helpful for other infectious diseases, such as SARS, flu, and norovirus. This is because droplet infection and contact infection are the main transmission routes and basic knowledge of infectious diseases is common.

However, issues have also been raised, and it is thought that improving these will lead to more efficient shelter management.

7. Limitations of this research and prospects

The limits of this study are described.

First, the number of responses from local governments that actually opened shelters under COVID-19 is small. At the time of the survey, the period during which a natural disaster could occur under COVID-19 was about half a year, and few local governments opened shelters there. As the number of cases increases, it is possible that the overall trend will change, and new issues will become apparent.

Second, the scale of the disaster targeted was small. This is fortunate, but the scale of the disaster and the lengthening of the shelter opening period could lead to events different from those revealed in this survey.

In the future, based on the results of this research, we would like to deepen our studies on countermeasures for complex disasters of natural disasters and COVID-19, especially shelter management.

Acknowledgements

We would like to express our sincere gratitude to the people in charge of disaster prevention in local governments nationwide who responded to the questionnaire survey during the difficult period due to COVID-19. Thank you very much.

Author details

Arisa Yasui[1*] and Muneyoshi Numada[2]

1 Department of Civil Engineering, School of Engineering, The University of Tokyo, Tokyo, Japan

2 Interfaculty Initiative in Information Studies, Institute of Industrial Science, The University of Tokyo, Japan

*Address all correspondence to: antant36z@icloud.com

References

[1] WHO, WHO COVID-19virus (COVID-19) Dashboard. Available from: https://covid19.who.int/, [accessed 2021-04-22]

[2] WHO, Cumulative Number of Reported Probable Cases of Severe Acute Respiratory Syndrome (SARS). Available from: https://www.who.int/csr/sars/country/table2004_04_21/en/ [accessed 2021-04-22]

[3] WHO, Middle East respiratory syndrome COVID-19virus (MERS-CoV): Summary of Current Situation, Literature Update and Risk Assessment–as of 5 February 2015. Available from: https://www.who.int/csr/disease/COVID-19virus_infections/mers-5-february-2015.pdf?ua=1 [accessed 2021-04-22]

[4] WHO, COVID-19 vaccines. Available from: https://www.who.int/emergencies/diseases/novel-COVID-19virus-2019/covid-19-vaccines [accessed 2021-04-22]

[5] Kazuko Ueyama et al., "Current situation and future suggestions of Niimi University as an ShelterDue to the heavy rain disaster in July 2018", Bulletin of Niimi University, Vol. 39, pp.185-187, 2018.

[6] Takashi Ito and Hiroshi Kawana, "School as a" designated shelter"in the event of a disaster A case study at an elementary school located in an area affected by the Great East Japan Earthquake", Ibaraki University Faculty of Education Bulletin (Educational Science), Vol. 65, pp. 425-435, 2016.

[7] Mainichi Shimbun, West Japan Heavy Rain 90% of Mabi's dead are too old to go upstairs at home, 2018.7.22, Available from: https://mainichi.jp/articles/20180722/k00/00m/040/106000c [accessed April 22, 2021]

[8] I., K., Kouadio, S., Aljunid, T., Kamigaki, K., Hammad, and H., Oshitani, "Infectious diseases following natural disasters: Prevention and control measures", Expert Review of Anti-infective Therapy, Vol. 10, No. 1, pp.95-104, 2012.

[9] Ken Kimi, Taro Kamigaki, Keiji Mimura, Hitoshi Oshitani, "Survey of infectious diseases in evacuation centers in Miyagi prefecture after the great East Japan earthquake", Japan Public Health Magazine, Vol. 60, No. 10, pp.659-664, 2013.

[10] Kenichi Goto and Fumio Oka, "Infectious gastroenteritis epidemics and countermeasures for infectious diseases at Kumamoto earthquake evacuation centers", Journal of Infectious Diseases, VOl. 91, No. 5, pp.790-795, 2017.

[11] E., L., Yee, H., Palacio, R., L., Atmar, et al, "Widespread outbreak of norovirus gastroenteritis among evacuees of Hurricane Katrina residing in a large" megashelter "in Houston, Texas: lessons learned for prevention", Clinical Infectious Diseases, Vol. 44, pp.1032-1039, 2007.

[12] K., Izumikawa, "Infection control after and during natural disaster", Acute Medicine & Surgery, Vol. 6, pp.5-11, 2019.

[13] T., Kawano, Y., Tsugawa, K., Nishiyama, H., Morita, O., Yamamura, and K., Hasegawa, "Shelter crowding and increased incidence of acute respiratory infection in evacuees following the great eastern Japan earthquake and tsunami ", Epidemiology and Infection, Vol. 144, No. 4, pp.787-795, 2016.

[14] I., Uckay, H., Sax, S., Harbarth, L, Bernard, and D., Pittet, "Multi-resistant infections in repatriated patients after natural disasters: lessons learned from the 2004 tsunami for hospital infection control", Journal of Hospital Infection, Vol. 68, pp.1-8, 2008.

[15] S. Shinoda, "Special issue on infectious disease control of natural disasters," J. Disaster Res., Vol.7, No.6, pp. 739-740, 2012.

[16] M., Ishii, T., Nagata, and K., Aoki, "Japan medical Association's actions in the great eastern Japan earthquake", World Medical & Health Policy, Vol. 3, No. 4, pp.1-18, 2011.

[17] Hideki Kawamura, Koichi Tokuda, Masayuki Kawakami, Toshiaki Arimura, Tatsuya Kawaguchi, Tamano Matsui, Junichiro Nishi, "Kagoshima medical association disaster medical assistance team 2016 Kumamoto earthquake infection control support activities", Environmental Infection Magazine, Vol. 32, No. 5, pp.282-290, 2017

[18] K. Iwata, G. Ohji, H. Oka, <. Takayama, T. Aoyagi, Y. Gu, <. Hatta, K. Tokuda, and M. Kaku, "Communicable Diseases After the Disasters: with the Special Reference to the Great East Japan Earthquake, "J. Disaster Res., Vol.7, No.6, pp. 746-753, 2012.

[19] K. Kaku, "Preparedness for natural disaster-associated infections," J. Disaster Res., Vol.4, No.5, pp. 337-345, 2009.

[20] M., Ishii, "Activities of the Japan medical association team in response to the great East Japan earthquake", Japan Med Assoc J, Vol. 55, No. 5, pp. 362-367, 2012.

[21] H., Kanamori, H., Kunishima, K., Tokuda, and M., Kaku, "Infection Control and Hospital Epidemiology, 32 (8), pp.824-826, 2011.

[22] F. Kasuga, "Special Issue on Understanding Emerging and Re-emerging Infectious Diseases," J. Disaster Res., Vol.6, No.4, p. 371, 2011.

[23] Ayako Kudo, Shihoko Sakuma, Keiko Inatomi, Megumi Ikeda, Seiko Nishina, "Local Governments' awareness and response to infection prevention in the event of a disaster", Environmental Infection Magazine, Vol. 27, No. 3, pp.171-177, 2012.

[24] Cabinet Office, "Manual for securing accommodation facilities for accommodation treatment for mildly ill persons with new COVID-19virus infection (1st edition)", 2020.4.23.

[25] Human and Disaster Prevention Future Center, "Preparation Checklist Ver.2-Guide to Prevent Infection at Evacuation Centers", DRI Special Issue, 2020.

[26] JVOAD, "New COVID-19virus Evacuation Life Useful Support Book", 2020.5.29.

[27] Kotaro Tsuboi, "Study on disaster response in Nishihara Village in Kumamoto earthquake and life reconstruction / health evaluation of victims", Environmental Information Science Academic Research Papers, Vol. 31, pp.77-82, 2017.

Chapter 8

Science-Based Technological Transfer as a Key Tool in Public Health

Alonso Ureta Dumont and Jovanka Trebotich Zúñiga

Abstract

Only a small portion of all the projects that are funded with public grants reaches the market, due to a gap known as "Death Valley" between the public and private source of resources. Know Hub Chile (KH) is a non-profit organization founded to transform scientific research results into goods and services available to the market and for the benefit of society. When the Covid-19 emergency reached Chile, the organization launched the "KH Bridge" a program of proof-of-concept and selected three technologies able to support hospitals in solving their needs. The first one was a smart shift planning platform of medical staff for reducing the virus spreading probability; the second solution aimed to assess the use of masks, and counting capacity and physical distance of patients by using video camera analytic technology in real-time; and the third project selected was an innovative design of personal protection equipment made with copper nanoparticles. All these solutions were piloted and validated into public hospitals for three months with a USD 25.000 budget. The KH Bridge experience has shown that the pandemic scenario has been an opportunity to validate university technologies in real environments and in shorter time frames, contributing to public health operations.

Keywords: Covid-19, Pandemic, Know Hub Chile, Proof of concept program, Know Hub Bridge, OpenBridge Covid-19

1. Introduction

Innovation and technology transfer are a fundamental part of society sustainable growth. In terms of Research and Development (R&D) investment, Chile is still far from OECD countries, being only 0.36% of the Gross Domestic Product (GDP), against an average of 2.4% GDP. Currently, universities are the largest precursor of innovation and technology transferring, capturing 45% of the total investment in research, equivalent to USD 452 million at 2017. Despite this, only 49% of this investment is dedicated to applied R&D activities, with a focus on technology transfer [1].

Between 2015 and 2018, 11 news Transfer and Licensing Offices (TLOs or university technology transfer offices or TTOs) were founded into the universities, which move from 18 to a total of 29. However, the magnitude of this increase on the TLOs was not observed on the transfer indicators, which present a slight increasing (**Figure 1**). This issue could be reelevated to the lack of capabilities on technology transfer and

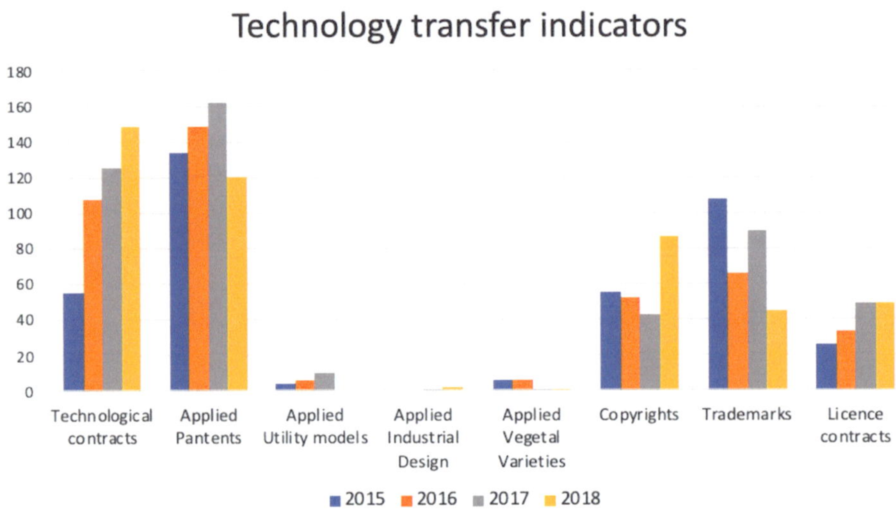

Figure 1.
Technology transfer indicators between 2015-2018.

commercialization inside the TLOs. It is still insufficient open new OTLs, without an additional support on technology transfer and commercialization [2].

In 2009, the World Bank published "Promoting Technology Transfer and Commercialization: Chile" [3] report, pointing out the need to update the national regulatory framework for technology transfer, since it does not achieve international standards. The following needs of the Chilean ecosystem stand out from this report:

- To improve institutions, regulations and practices for an efficient and dynamic intellectual property management system.
- To develop strategic partnerships for science-oriented, science-enhancing Public Technological Institutes.
- To accelerate the creation of technology companies.
- To develop skills and competencies to support these companies.
- To stimulate the universities "third mission": contributing to economic growth.
- To trigger demand for technology and innovation.
- To promote a culture of entrepreneurship and innovation.

In response to these points, various public policies were generated between 2011 and 2015 to develop trained human capital, and to promote technology commercialization or "go to market", in addition to the creation of institutions devoted to facilitate technology transfer processes, and TLOs in universities and research centers.

Towards the end of 2015, a new public policy was designed, the "Technology Transfer Hubs" (three in total). Under this instrument, seven public universities and three research centers created Know Hub Chile in January 2018. Its main objective is collaborating to transform scientific research results of its partners in products, services and start-ups companies for the society benefit. For reaching this objective, Know Hub developed a series of programs to accomplish specific challenges of the Chilean (and Latinoamerican) innovation ecosystem. For instance, Know Hub Bridge program was created at the end of 2019 to close gaps in the development of technologies generated with public funding, and to improve their chances of reaching the market [4].

In parallel, due to the Covid-19 pandemic, the Chilean system of health tried to be prepared to the emergency that already had begun in Europe. Thus, a series of measurements were initiated, such as the purchase of mechanical ventilators, medical supplies for personal protection, reagents for PCR sample analysis, among others. Given the high world demand, there was a shortage of some of these items. In addition, there was a growing need for more effective technological solutions to mitigate the virus spreading, which led to local technological capabilities to meet the needs of health institutions [5].

In this context, from the innovation ecosystem, innovation challenges focused on validating technologies that would help to fight against coronavirus, such as the "Covid-19 Challenge" (TransferenciAP) [6], "SiEmpre initiative" carried out by SOFOFA hub [7] and the "Innovation Challenges for diagnostic kits and personal protection elements", promoted by the Chilean Economic Development Agency (Corfo) and the Ministry of Science, Technology, Knowledge and Innovation (MinCTCi) [8, 9].

In parallel, Know Hub Chile launched its pilot program Know Hub Bridge, to accelerate the validation of technologies that helped Chilean public hospitals to combat Covid-19. The initiative was called OpenBridge Covid-19 and was carried out together with Open Beauchef (University of Chile) and Santander X [10].

In this chapter we will discuss how the Technology Transfer Hubs policy, and specifically how Know Hub Chile established itself in the innovation ecosystem, and how the implementation of the pilot program Know Hub Bridge, under the name of OpenBridge Covid-19, has allowed to closing gaps in Science and Technology Based Companies (STBCs) by transferring their technologies to public hospitals during pandemic times.

2. Technology transfer institutions in Latin America

For some years now, several countries in Latin America have begun to generate the necessary institutions to carry out technology transfer, understanding that these technologies have the potential to impact the quality of life of society. In this sense, LTOs have been the institutions with the greatest development in recent years in Latin America, mainly housed in universities and research centers. In some countries, such as Colombia, Regional Research Results Transfer Offices (OTRI in spanish) have been created, covering various regional demands of the country through five offices -Connect Bogota, Tennova UEE, OTRI Estratégica de Oriente, CienTech and Reddi- [11].

Along with the development of the LTOs and/or technology transfer units, other institutions have also emerged to support and complement the work of these offices or their similes. In this regard, Ecuador through the Secretary of Higher Education, Science, Technology and Innovation (SENESCYT) has generated the Innovation and Technology Transfer HUB (HUB iTT) project in 2018, to "promote the development of innovation, entrepreneurship and technology transfer activities carried out in the country's higher education institutions". Thus, six HUBs iTT have been created throughout Ecuador, grouped to meet regional needs (North, Quito, Central,

Cuenca, Guayaquil and Manabí) [12, 13]. Another country that has created a similar institutional framework is Chile, through the technology transfer HUBs, whose history and results are discussed in more detail in this chapter. It should be noted that this new institutional framework is still incipient in the region, so as success stories are generated with HUBS in Ecuador and Chile, it is highly probable that more countries will generate public policies that support the creation of these institutions.

3. Technology transfer hubs in Chile

3.1 Innovation ecosystem

In 2011, Corfo launched the first Program for the Creation and Strengthening of TLOs. This program was open to universities and technology centers. Eighteen projects were funded, with a budget of USD 7.14 million. Despite this significant investment, it was not enough to maintain the structure of the offices with a sustainable financial model.

In 2015, Corfo launched a second TLO program, which tried to consolidate and to position the offices, hoping to improve transfer indicators. Through this program, 15 TLOs were financed. In addition, in order to consolidate the existing TLOs and strengthen the new ones, a new stage in the specialization of technology transfer in Chile began with the "on campus-off campus" model.

3.2 "On campus - Off campus" model

The "on campus-off campus" model takes into consideration the need to strengthen commercialization and transfer capabilities within universities, considering that the specialization of competencies is the way to achieve successful commercialization with greater probability.

The "on campus" component corresponds to the role played by the TLOs in the identification, follow-up and compilation of research and development results within universities and research centers. The aim is to promote research focused on solving specific problems or needs of the productive sector and society. Similarly, the role of technological asset management is considered, according to the guidelines or capabilities of each institution.

The "off-campus" component is related to entities that have the capabilities and human capital highly specialized in scaling and transferring research and development results generated in universities and research centers. This work itself is oriented to the generation of global business in different industries, with access to support networks in internationalization of scientific and technological enterprises, which involves a decrease in the gap in the capabilities required by the TLOs, performing this activity through two ways: using their own work, or coordinating and intermediating external services (**Figure 2**).

Along with the implementation of the model, the Technology Transfer Hubs were born with the objective of strengthening the transfer capabilities of universities and associated research centers, through the "on campus and off campus" model, focusing on improving the processes of intellectual property, technological development and commercialization, in a joint work with the TLOs [14].

3.3 Origin of technology transfer HUBs in Chile

Technology transfer hubs were created by Corfo as a public policy that sought to close the gap between the generation of technologies in universities and research

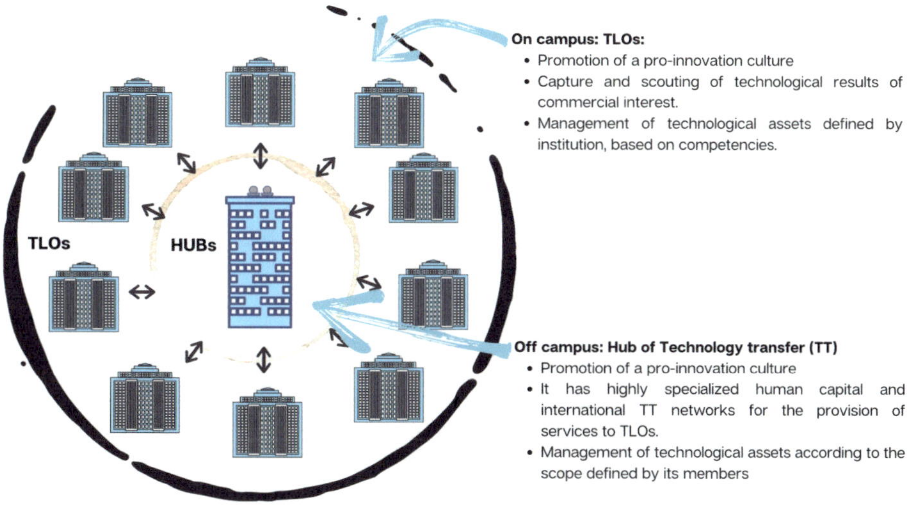

Figure 2.
On–off campus model.

centers and their transference to the market, using the "on campus - off campus" model described above. Hubs are associative organizations comprised by several universities and research centers, which are linked to companies, trade associations, investment and venture capital funds, among others. According to Corfo, "the Hubs should perform functions of technological surveillance and competitive intelligence, intellectual property management, commercialization of licenses, and creation and assistance to spin-offs. It also involves closing capability gaps required by the TLOs, through their own work, or by intermediating external capabilities." [14].

The specific objectives are: [14].

- Implement an associative model with specialization of functions on campus-off campus that achieves the necessary scale for the sustainability of the technology transfer HUBs in the medium and short term.

- Attract and generate human capital specialized in intellectual property management, technology transfer and industry linkage models, such as technology contracts, open innovation, among others.

- Improve the market potential of the technological assets generated by R&D&I projects, adopting international best practices in technology management.

- Increase the creation of technology-based ventures based on R&D results, increasing the amount of private resources invested and boosting access to early-stage venture capital, both nationally and internationally.

- Strengthen the positioning of on campus - off campus technology transfer entities in the national innovation and national entrepreneurship ecosystem."

"The expected outcomes of this new program are: [14].

- Development of a HUB's 10-year strategic plan that considers a governance and business model that allows the achievement of its objectives and sustainability.

- Implementation of an associative model with specialization of functions on campus and off campus.
- Increasing the quantity and quality of the actors' competencies in the innovation system related to management of intellectual and industrial property, technology transfer, links with industry and open innovation.
- Increasing the value of the portfolio of technological assets and innovations, improving the management of disclosures, intellectual and industrial property, and new technological businesses with a global focus.
- Increasing the number and amounts of applied R&D contracts entered into by universities with companies, licenses and university-company collaboration projects in high-impact strategic sectors.
- Increasing the commercialization of Chilean technologies abroad.
- Increasing the number of spin-offs and technology-based companies.
- Increasing the number of technology-based spin-offs by obtaining funds for scaling them and in the amounts of private investment (Venture Capital) for spin-offs and technology-based companies."

To finance the hubs, Corfo launched in 2015 a competitive award to subsidy 80% of the total cost of the project, with a maximum of USD 8,000,000 for 5 years, and a potential extension of a second 5-year period.

"The projects were selected after an international evaluation. Subsequently, an internal Corfo committee reviewed the proposals and decided to fund the three proposed projects: HubTec, Know Hub Chile (KH) and Andes Pacific Technology Access (APTA), each focused primarily on agriculture; health; industrial production, technology and energy and comprised by a group of Chilean universities, companies, research centers and technology centers." [15].

4. Know hub Chile

4.1 History of know hub Chile

Know Hub Chile was born as a non-profit corporation on January 23, 2018 and as part of a public policy discussed previously. Its main objective is collaborating to transformer scientific research results of its partners into products and services available to the market and society, with emphasis on their global impact. In other words, Know Hub Chile collaborates to transform science into innovation.

Know Hub Chile was initially founded by seven universities -Universidad de Chile, Universidad de Talca, Universidad Católica del Maule, Universidad del Bío-Bío, Universidad Católica de Temuco, Universidad Austral de Chile and Universidad de Los Lagos- and three scientific institutions -Instituto de Neurociencia Biomédica, Instituto de Investigaciones Agropecuarias and Centro de Estudios en Alimentos Procesados- mainly from central-southern Chile. At the beginning of 2019, the eleventh member joined: the Universidad Tecnológica Metropolitana.

4.2 Programs of know hub Chile

Initially, Know Hub Chile implemented a working model based on the identification and commercialization of technologies that were in an advanced stage of development and high market potential developed by its associates. Under this model, Know Hub Chile created the first technology portfolio, comprised by more than a hundred research results and technologies that were evaluated by different entities (KIM Global Spain, Genesis Partners and University of California Riverside). The conclusions obtained from this process were the following:

1. Low state of development of the technologies evaluated, since most of them were at Technology Readiness Level (TRL) 3 or 4;

2. Most of the technologies did not have a commercial partner, the customer was not identified and they did not even respond to a specific industry need;

3. Research teams barely committed to the later stages of technology development, and/or lack of funding for further development.

Considering the conclusions, the commercialization potential of Know Hub Chile's first technology portfolio was quite low. For this reason, during the first half of 2019 the foundation decided to modify its strategy.

Firstly, Know Hub Chile's current strategy is based on the design and implementation of programs that respond to gaps in the innovation ecosystem, aiming to bring research results to the market and society. Secondly, the foundation seeks to provide strategic support to its partners, beyond technology commercialization activities, with the objective of improving institutional capabilities in technology transfer. In this way, and thirdly, Know Hub Chile major goal is to contribute to the maturation of the Chilean innovation ecosystem.

Based on this strategy, and in terms of technology transfer, Know Hub Chile designed five programs to improve commercialization opportunities and to accelerate transfer processes focused on international markets. These programs are:

- Know Hub Ignition: strengthening and promoting technologically based entrepreneurship.

- Know Hub Portfolio: identifying, assessing, selecting and managing technologies developed by its associates in order to bring them to market directly or through Know Hub's strategic alliances.

- Know Hub Bridge: reducing technology risk to improve technology of opportunities to international market.

- Know Hub Connect: strengthening the bonds with industry through technology contracts.

- Know Hub Dual-Tech: supporting the creation and acceleration of science- and technology-based companies with civil-military applications.

While three programs were designed for positioning and validating the foundation:

- Know Hub Building: To develop and strengthen the professional and institutional competencies of our partners in issues related to technology-based innovation.

- Know Hub Partnership: Generate national and international public-private alliances to collaborate in initiatives that broaden the scope of technology-based innovation. To expand the scope of their partners' and national ecosystem technology transfer in order to bring technologies closer to society.

- Communications: Strengthen the dissemination and positioning of Know Hub Chile, through its success stories in technology transfer and its value proposition.

5. Know hub bridge program

As previously mentioned, Know Hub Chile is deploying its efforts to transfer Chilean technologies through various mechanisms, such as the creation of programs to reduce the gaps that prevent technologies from reaching the national and international markets effectively.

In this sense, and as part of KH's mapping of the national innovation and entrepreneurship ecosystem, it was observed that there is a lack of integration and cohesion between the different funding sources for R&D and innovation, both public and private. This means that a significant number of technologies in which resources and time have been invested do not manage to overcome the "valley of death" and fail to reach the market.

The "valley of death" concept was initially applied in the field of entrepreneurship by Sthepan Markham (2002), describing the inability of a company to maintain a sustainable business model [16]. This is also a metaphorical concept used to describe the gap between academic-based innovations and their commercial applications in the market. More specifically, the "valley of death" refers directly to the difficulty of maturing TRL 6 to 8 technologies through their demonstration and validation stage due to a series of barriers that prevent them from reaching the market. Among the barriers are high costs associated to carry out demonstration and validation tests, low capital investment, difficulties to obtain certifications, among others. Overcoming the "valley of death" is one of the most expensive stages in the development of an innovation [17]. In the specific case of Chile, an additional barrier is the industry's reticence to technological risk, avoiding innovations to reach the value chain of industries as mining, salmon farming, forestry.

In the specific case of Know Hub Chile's partners, out of more than 120 technologies evaluated by the foundation, 52% have a TRL 4 or lower and more than 65% do not have a commercial partner to support their transfer to the market. These figures are a true reflection of what has been seen in the national innovation and entrepreneurship ecosystem.

In order to improve the transfer chances of the portfolio by increasing their value and mitigating technological risks for the industry, Know Hub Chile has designed Know Hub Bridge. This program promotes the creation of favorable conditions for the maturation and introduction of new technological products or services in the market. Also, the initiative contributes to the development of scientific and technological based companies (STBCs) or technology-based companies (TBCs), by the investment of third parties in them or by licensing the technologies directly to the industry.

To this end, Know Hub conducts a review of other existing programs to formulate its own program.

In this regard, the "Horizon 2020" program of the European Union (EU) - specifically of the European Commission- stands out for implementing the "Innovation Union" strategy. This initiative seeks to create an open environment for innovation that facilitates the conversion of great ideas into products and services that boost EU economy and create jobs. Horizon 2020/Innovation Union has a strong focus on the market [18].

One of the instruments within "Horizon 2020" focuses on small and medium-size enterprises (SMEs) by supporting the technology development, helping to leverage capital for technology development and commercialization, mitigating technological risk and accelerating technology arrival to the market. Since its implementation in 2014, this instrument has managed to raise around USD 3.6 billion of private investment, investing a total of USD 1.5 billion, which means that for every dollar of public money invested, is generated USD 2.83 of private investment. This amount has been increasing over time. They have also supported more than 4,500 SMEs and are expected to reach 6,000 by 2021 [19].

Another initiative is The Research Council of Norways's programme on Commercializing R&D results (FORNY2020), which is a Proof-of-Concept Funding that supports testing, scaling-up and the continuation of research projects to facilitate the commercialization of research results carried out in public research institutions [20].

Finally, the U.S. Department of Defense (DOD) Science and Technology (S&T) program, has two initiatives, "Advanced Technology Development" (ATD) and the "Advance Component Development and Prototypes" (ACD&P), that support the generation of prototype models and their testing in controlled or real operating conditions, allowing the transition from the laboratory to operational use or even being part of the DOD acquisition processes [21].

All these programs -and many others of the Proof of Concept type- have in common that they finance technologies with a high potential to be transferred (TRL 5–6) or commercialized in short or medium term. These technologies come from different areas and need financing to achieve validation under real conditions, scaling up and market launch. In general, funding ranges from USD 25 K to USD 100 K. Finally, these programs not only focus on technologies coming from universities or research centers, but also from STBCs.

All these elements gave rise to the Know Hub Bridge program, whose general objective is to improve the transfer opportunities and terms of negotiation of the research results of KH's partners, by reducing the technological risk for potential licensees and/or investors, through the financing of market viability tests. The specific objectives of the program are as follows:

- To generate an increase the commercial value of the technologies generated by Know Hub Chile's partners.

- To increase the level of technological development of the research results or TRL in a period of 12 to 18 months, at the most.

- To facilitate and accelerate the commercialization of research results and/or technologies developed by Know Hub Chile partners, by mitigating part of their technological risks.

- To increase the number of technological products or services belonging to Know Hub Chile's partners that are ready to be commercialized in national and international markets.

- To increase the number of technological products or services belonging to Know Hub Chile's partners that achieve private leverage in co-investment format.

The Know Hub Bridge program is composed by 3 stages (**Figure 3**):

1. *Identification of research results or technologies with potential to be transferred to the market*. KH Bridge focuses on the maturation of technologies that have a level of development equivalent to a TRL 4 status. Its first element of value is the identification of research results or technologies or inventions with commercial potential developed by professional teams from KH's partners, as well as technologies developed by technology-based companies derived from KH partners. This identification process is carried out through an open call for a determined period of time. The proposals are submitted through an application form, which are submitted to a formal evaluation based on evaluation criteria: amount of investment and increase in value, time to commercialization, team capacity and project design. Then, the selected proposals present their plan of activities and key milestones to be developed during the program.

2. *Execution of activity plan/key milestones.* Proposals supported by the KH Bridge program are challenged to develop a plan of activities and key milestones that will have a duration of 12 months, which may be extended up to 6 additional months (as in the case of projects involving biological cycles). This plan should state activities, milestones with their respective detailed descriptions, budget, time and the people responsible for the team to carry out each of the activities.

3. *Support in the business model and commercialization of research results or technologies*. During the program, Know Hub Chile will actively support the definition of the business model and the raising of private investment for market entry, customer search and/or productive scaling of research results from technology-based companies, as well as in the prospecting of potential licensees and/or companies interested in the development of final stages of research results or technologies, both nationally and internationally.

In general terms, the program consists of supporting the selected teams for a maximum period of 12 months, moving from a TRL 4 to a TRL6.

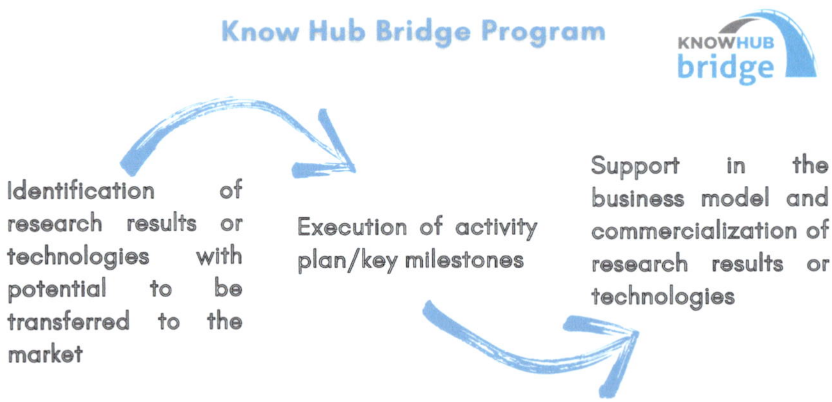

Figure 3.
Stages of know hub bridge program.

5.1 Piloting the program: COVID-19 open bridge experience and results

When the Covid-19 pandemic began in Chile and Latin America, initiatives focused on validating technologies that would help to fight against coronavirus have arisen. At Latin America level, the "Covid-19 Challenge" (TransferenciAP) [22], and Chilean level "SiEmpre initiative" carried out by SOFOFA hub [23] and the "Innovation Challenges for diagnostic kits and personal protection elements", promoted by the Chilean Economic Development Agency (Corfo) and the Ministry of Science, Technology, Knowledge and Innovation (MinCTCi) [24, 25].

In parallel, Know Hub contacted to the National Institute of Geriatrics (Instituto Nacional de Geriatría, INGER) and the Padre Hurtado Hospital. Both health institutions requested to support the generation of spaces for innovators to propose solutions for problems triggered by the pandemic. Know Hub Chile took up this request, allocating resources from the Know Hub Bridge Program to generate a pilot experience to seek innovative solutions related to the health emergency.

In this sense, KH collected, organized and prioritized the requirements of the health centers in three thematic axes: Personal Protective Equipment (PPE); Cleaning, Asepsis and Disinfection Technologies, and Information and Communication Technologies (ICTs). Due to the urgency of the pandemic, the developed technologies must be transferred within three to four months. Know Hub Bridge would finance the feasibility tests in clinical fields.

In order to accomplish the tight deadlines, collaboration was essential. Thus, the Innovation and Entrepreneurship Center of the Faculty of Physical and Mathematical Sciences of the Universidad de Chile, OpenBeauchef joined to the initiative, contributing with its experience in evaluation and incubation, contacts, and links with the Universidad de Chile Clinical Hospital (HCUCH). Thus, the name of the call was OpenBridge Covid-19 and its objective public were groups of researchers, entrepreneurs or graduate students linked to KH's partner institutions.

The international entrepreneurship project Santander X, from the bank of the same name, also joined to the initiative proving resources for another award. The Santander X Award acknowledged ideas from undergraduate and graduate students from KH institutions that were also linked to the three strategic axes of the call.

The Open Bridge COVID-19 call is characterized by the rapid implementation of technologies and/or research results to solve the particular needs of institutions such as INGER, HCUCH and other health institutions, in order to mitigate the effects generated by the pandemic caused by SARS-CoV-2 in these institutions and in the Chilean health system.

To achieve its objective, OpenBridge Covid-19 worked in two parallel fronts.

Firstly, supporting the maturation of technologies that have a level of development equivalent to a TRL 4 status, through the implementation and development of a work plan to be developed in 3–4 months that allows a validation process together with the INGER, HCUCH and/or other health institutions;

Secondly, working with the developers of the technologies in all the elements related to protection strategy, business model and legal aspects related to the creation of companies that are able to perform adequately as potential suppliers of the mentioned health institutions and/or prepared to raise investment.

OpenBridge Covid-19 opened its call for applications on May 6, 2020. After an intense communication and scouting campaign with KH partners, on May 29, 2020 the process close successfully with 43 applications.

After a selection process, where 13 teams passed to the pitch stage, three initiatives were selected to be financed:

- Safe Vision (SV), is a video analytical system for health facilities which is connected directly to the standard cameras of these centers. Its purpose is to process images for metadata analysis in real time. The current system counts capacity and flow of people (patients, companions and health staff), checks masks and other PPE usage, and verifies compliance with social distancing. Safe Vision generates indicators likely to configure alerts to health center personnel. Created by the startup Dual Vision

- Medical Shield Staffing (MSS), is a system which manages health staff time availability, in order to work in different shift settings. This information feeds a dynamic optimization model, which uses stochastic dynamic simulation tools and mathematical programming. The system provides a shift scheme proposal, through a user-friendly interface, which minimizes contagion probability. The principle used by the model is concentrating work shifts on the virus incubation period, assigning medical staff free days to cover up contagion period, in case of infection. Developed by a research team from the Universidad de Chile

- Active Protection (ActPro), is a Personal Protective Equipment (PPE) for health workers. Given the fact that it has copper nanoparticles incorporated – with antimicrobial and antiviral activity– and due to its ergonomic design, it would prevent SARS-CoV-2 contagion, whether in direct contact with infected patients, or during disposal or replacement PPE process. Developed by a research team from the Universidad Católica de Temuco.

These three solutions were piloted for 4 months in public hospitals with a budget of USD 20 K each.

After slightly over more 4 months of design and implementation of pilot experiences with the selected teams, the results obtained within the framework of OpenBridge Covid-19 are the following:

5.1.1 Safe vision

5.1.1.1 Diagnosis

The health centers do not have systems in place to comply the measures established by the health authority related to physical distance, mask use, number of people allowed in facilities and temperature measurement. All control procedures are carried out manually by facility personnel.

5.1.1.2 Proposal

Image analysis system based on artificial intelligence and computer vision, and using the existing camera system to count people, identify mask use and determine physical distancing. The images are processed, obtaining data that are presented on a platform, allowing to visualize data in real time, configure issue alerts, track historical metrics and make decisions to improve compliance with the measures, and resource optimization of health facilities.

5.1.1.3 Results

The Dual Vision's team developed its own recognition algorithms for people counting and for identifying mask use and physical distancing. To do this, they took images from the existing cameras in the healthcare facility and began to train the artificial intelligence system in real conditions. Once the recognition algorithms were developed, system assembly optimizations were made to obtain a packaged product at a lower cost. In parallel, the team worked on the development of an intuitive visualization platform to present the information in real time. In terms of visualization, it was decided to sectorize the metrics to aid decision making, and to include an option to access to historical record.

To implement the solution at INGER, additional cameras were required for installing in strategic spots to check areas of interest. Once the cameras were calibrated, the analytical phase began. To verify the correct functioning of the system, stress tests were performed. The piloting process began with a white run to show the hospital management area the system operating under real conditions. After this experience, the hospital staff provided feedback and requirements, which resulted in improvements to the service. It is expected that the hospital will acquire the technology.

In commercial aspects, the startup team proposed a Software As A Service (SaaS) business model with a one-year contract monthly charged, amortizing the software components and product development,

It should be noted that INGER has expressed interest in continuing to expand the range of analytics beyond the needs of the pandemic. The hospital objective is to obtain relevant information to improve the quality of patient care.

Dual Vision currently has business in the retail area as well. Know Hub Chile team is supporting them to achieve the venture consolidation in a short term.

5.1.2 Medical shield staffing (MSS)

5.1.2.1 Diagnosis

Public health centers in Chile do not have automated systems for staff shifts planning for different medical areas -such as Intensive Care Units or ICUs- in order to obtain the best shift patterns that allow personnel to rest and reduce the probability of getting Covid-19.

5.1.2.2 Proposal

MSS is a system that manages the availability of health personnel to work in different shifts configurations through a dynamic optimization model, which uses stochastic dynamic simulation tools and mathematical programming. The system delivers, through a friendly user interface, a shift planning proposal that minimizes the probability of contagion among personnel.

5.1.2.3 Results

MSS technology was designed, implemented and successfully put into operation at the Hospital Clínico de la Universidad de Chile (HCUCH) and the Hospital Clínico Herminda Martín de Chillán (South of Chile), two facilities that have been the front line fighting against the coronavirus. In the case of HCUCH, a facility that expanded its Critical Patient Unit as a result of the pandemic, MSS contemplated the design of shifts with a lower risk of infection, which at the same time would be adjusted to the available medical staffing: the 2 × 10 and 4 × 4 shift schedules maintain the same number of hours worked for each department and their implementation reduced the risk of infection among hospital workers by 25%. In the case of the Critical Patient Unit of the Hospital Clínico Herminda Martín, MSS was able to reduce the risk of contagion by 9%. Currently, the MSS team is finishing the validation process in another Chilean health institution.

In the commercial aspects, the team expects a business model based on licensing the technology to companies that have the operational capabilities to carry out the MSS service. In addition, the technology can be used in other areas where shift systems are used, such as retail and mining.

5.1.3 Active protection

5.1.3.1 Diagnosis

Personal protective equipment has become unusually important in the current pandemic, so any improvement in its design and materiality is necessary to prevent the infection of medical staff.

5.1.3.2 Proposal

ActPro is a personal protective equipment, specifically a plastic apron, for health staff use. Given the fact that it has copper nanoparticles incorporated –with antimicrobial and antiviral activity– and due to its ergonomic design, it would prevent SARS-CoV-2 contagion, whether in direct contact with infected patients, or during disposal or replacement PPE process.

5.1.3.3 Results

To date, it has been designed a model of protective plastic apron according to the needs of medical staff. The team has had a close interaction with personnel from an specific area of the Hospital Dr. Hernán Henríquez Aravena, in Temuco (South of Chile) and concluded that the health staff requires a PPE easy to put on and to take off for disposal. In addition, the team has carried out several evaluations of the polymer used to manufacture the PPE, occupying different concentrations of copper nanoparticles to generate the antimicrobial property. Currently, an external laboratory is certificating the PPE. It is hoped to scale this pilot project to other areas of the same hospital and validate the design and technology of the material containing copper nanoparticles.

Regarding commercial aspects, the team wants to manufacture and sell the plastic apron directly. They also decided to development other PPEs, such as boots, shoe covers, and full body suits, not only for use in the medical field, but also in the food industry and other areas where personnel need to be protected.

Know Hub Chile has been supporting the teams to carry out their respective pilots, and guiding their commercial aspects, such as defining the value proposition, business model, and strengthening the team in commercial issues. Another important point for Know Hub Chile is that the technologies can be scalable and the scientific-technological based ventures can be sustainable over time, continuing beyond the Covid-19 pandemic. For that reason, the corporation has helped the teams to explore other customer segments where the technology can be applied.

6. Conclusions

In the context of the Covid-19 pandemic, the economic situation has been strongly impacted, especially in Latin American countries that were already in severe recessions and political instability. In Chile, strong public spending has been made to remedy the consequences of the economic activities that have come to a halt, as well as to support the most vulnerable families. In this context of crisis, the generation of scientific knowledge and its transfer become relevant in society by demonstrating the ability to solve concrete problems, such as the generation of new PCR identification kits, treatment of convalescent plasma, and the development of vaccines, among others. In budgetary terms, it is expected that there will be a sharp cut in public spending in the coming years, and one of the budgets that will be impacted is science, technology and innovation. However, with the consolidation of the Ministry of Science, Technology and Innovation, it is hoped that the budgets allocated will increase, and that regardless of the prevailing political climate, a greater contribution of GDP will be allocated to scientific and technological development, and continuity will be given to public policies on technology transfer. In this sense, the ministry has created a new entrepreneurship program called "Startup ciencia", to promote the development of technologies with potential, and the budget for the extension of the Hub project is currently being discussed by the National Agency for Research and Development (ANID), in order to achieve sustainability. It is hoped that this change in the valuation of the contribution of science to society in a transversal way will result in establishing technological development as an engine for sustainable economic growth, using as a basis the scientific and technological knowledge generated by the country's universities and research centers, with Know Hub Chile being a key element in facilitating the arrival of technologies to the market.

The entities that articulate the technology transfer process -as technology transfer hubs and specifically Know Hub Chile- are able to adapt to extraordinary complex circumstances like the Covid-19 pandemic. In this sense, collaboration and flexibility have marked initiatives such as OpenBridge Covid-19, where technologies developed by universities and STBCs were able to assist health centers in their fight against the current pandemic, accelerating and supporting them to "cross" the "valley of death". So, even though the pandemic has been one of the worst issues that humankind has faced last times, there has also been an opportunity for innovator. In fact, the circumstances have pushed to validate technologies in a real environment and in short periods of time, making a concrete contribution to national public health through technologies coming from academia.

The three initiatives supported by OpenBridge Covid-19 achieved the objective of being piloted in a real environment. It should be noted that within the technological risks assumed by KH supporting these technologies, it was expected that despite the successful piloting, some of them would not raise market interest due to very high entry barriers, low scalable technologies, lack of commercial/operational capabilities of the team, among others. In this sense, Safe Vision technology is the one that has made the most progress towards an early market launch, not only in the medical field but also in other areas, such as retail and mining, industries that would need this kind of technologies and beyond the pandemic. This process is supported by the KH team.

There is still a lot of work ahead for these initiatives to achieve sustainability considering that the pandemic will remain an unresolved issue in the coming months or even years. Also, the teams should be able to look beyond and ensure their continuity supporting health institutions in other needs unrelated to the pandemic, such as improving patient care quality.

Acknowledgements

The authors would like to thank the Know Hub Chile team for reviewing and approving the final version of this work, specifically Fernando Venegas, Javier Ramírez and Eliette Angel.

Know Hub Chile is a project financed by the Corporación de Fomento a la Producción (Corfo), through Project code 15 HUBTT 57326.

Conflict of interest

"The authors declare no conflict of interest."

Thanks

The authors and Know Hub Chile would like to thank the health centers and their directors who were part of the OpenBridge Covid-19 initiative: Instituto Nacional de Geriatria, Hospital Clínico de la Universidad de Chile, Hospital Padre Hurtado, Hospital Dr. Hernán Henríquez Aravena de Temuco and Hospital Clínico Herminda Martín de Chillán. We would also like to thank OpenBeauchef and Santander X for their support in the initiative.

Author details

Alonso Ureta Dumont* and Jovanka Trebotich Zúñiga
Know Hub Chile, Santiago, Chile

*Address all correspondence to: alonso.ureta@knowhub.cl

References

[1] MinCTCi, División de Innovación. Boletín Caracterización de los participantes de la Transferencia Tecnológica en Chile [Internet] 2020. Available from: https://ctci.minciencia.gob.cl/wpcontent/uploads/2020/01/20200110-Boletin-transferencia-tecnológica-1.pdf [Accessed: 2021-04-02]

[2] RedGT. Reflexiones en torno a la transferencias tecnológica en Chile: Evolución historica en Chile, escenario actual, desafíos y propuestas, Red de Gestores Tecnológicos [Internet] 2020. Available from: https://media.wix.com/ugd/4cb9cc_af94060c02a046c1a3914c6af5ccd891.pdf [Accessed: 2021-04-02]

[3] World Bank. Fostering Technology Transfer and Commercialization: Chile [Internet] 2009. Available from: http://ctie.economia.cl/wpcontent/uploads/2018/04/Fostering-Technology-Transfer-and-Commercialization-2009.pdf [Accessed: 2021-04-05]

[4] Choupay E. Public policy to promote technology transfer in Chile - Licensing, technology transfer offices and technology transfer hubs: Case study contribution to the OECD TIP Knowledge Transfer and Policies project [Internet] 2019. Available from: https://stip.oecd.org/assets/TKKT/Case Studies/5.pdf [Accessed:2021-04-05]

[5] Hospital Clínico U. de Chile informa “quiebre de stock nacional” de reactivo para PCR y clínicas suspenden examen por “problemas de capacidad técnica” [Internet]. 2020. Available from: https://www.latercera.com/nacional/noticia/hospital-clinico-u-de-chile-suspende-toma-de-muestras-para-pcr-por-quiebre-de-stock-nacional-de-reactivo-de-laboratorio/43RABHW7TZGPBKR6IC5MAZXTHE/ [Accessed: 2021-04-07]

[6] Reto COVID-19 selecciona a sus 8 innovaciones ganadoras [Internet]. 2020. Available from: https://www.redgt.org/post/reto-covid-19-selecciona-doce-innovaciones-finalistas [Accessed: 2021-04-07]

[7] SOFOFA HUB: Fondo Privado de Adopción Tecnológica SiEmpre (CPC) financiará fase de validación preclínica para 5 prototipos de ventilación mecánica [Internet]. 2020. Available from: https://web.sofofa.cl/noticias/fondo-privado-de-adopcion-tecnologica-siempre-cpc-financiara-fase-de-validacion-preclinica-para-5-prototipos-de-ventilacion-mecanica/ [Accessed: 2021-04-08]

[8] Retos de innovación – Diagnóstico COVID19 [Internet]. 2020. Available from: https://www.corfo.cl/sites/cpp/convocatorias/retos_de_innovacion_covid19 [Accessed: 2021-04-09]

[9] Retos de innovación – Elementos de Protección para el personal de salud COVID19 [Internet]. 2020. Available from: https://www.corfo.cl/sites/cpp/convocatorias/movil/retos_de_innovacion_elementos_de_proteccion_covid19 [Accessed: 2021-04-09]

[10] Programa OPEN BRIDGE COVID-19 [Internet]. 2020. Available from: https://knowhub.cl/programa-bridge/ [Accessed: 2021-04-20]

[11] Minciencias. Oficinas de Transferencia de Resultados de Investigación-OTRIS [Internet]. 2021. Available from: https://minciencias.gov.co/viceministerios/conocimiento/direccion_transferencia/transferencia-conocimiento/oficinas-otris [Accessed: 2021-06-01]

[12] Secretaria de Educación Superior, Ciencia, tecnología e Innovación. Programas y Proyectos [Internet]. 2021. Available from: https://www.

educacionsuperior.gob.ec/programas-y-proyectos/ [Accessed: 2021-06-01]

[13] Secretaria de Educación Superior, Ciencia, tecnología e Innovación. Senescyt presenta los HUBs, una red que fomenta la innovación y el emprendimiento. [Internet]. 2018. Available from: https://www.educacionsuperior.gob.ec/senescyt-presenta-los-hubs-una-red-que-fomenta-la-innovacion-y-el-emprendimiento/ [Accessed: 2021-06-01]

[14] Corfo. Bases "Hub de Transferencia Tecnológica". Santiago de Chile: Gerencia de Capacidades Tecnológicas [Internet] 2015. Available from: https://www.dropbox.com/s/uw3c4h6hko61109/Bases-T%C3%A9cnicas-HUB-de-Transferencia-Tecnol%C3%B3gica.pdf?dl=0 [Accessed: 2021-04-06]

[15] Choupay, E. Public policy to promote technology transfer in Chile -Licensing, technology transfer offices and technology transfer hubs: Case study contribution to the OECD TIP Knowledge Transfer and Policies project [Internet] 2019. Available from: https://stip.oecd.org/assets/TKKT/CaseStudies/5.pdf [Accessed: 2021-04-05]

[16] AI Natsheh A, Gbadegeshin S, Ghafel K, Mohammed O, Koskela A, Rimpiläinen A, Tikkanen J, Kuoppala A. The causes of valley of death: A literature review. In: 15th International Technology, Education and Development Conference (INTED2021); 8-9 March 2021; INTED2021 Proceedings; 2021. p.9289-9298

[17] McCrea J, Palumbo G. 21 - Nanocoatings for commercial and industrial applications. In: Whang S, editor. Woodhead Publishing Series in Metals and Surface Engineering, Nanostructured Metals and Alloys. 1st ed. Cambridge: Woodhead Publishing; 2011. p. 663-686. DOI: 10.1533/9780857091123.4.663.

[18] Oportunidades de financiación en Horizonte 2020 [Internet]. 2018. Available from: https://oficinaeuropea.ucm.es/component/phocadownload/category/11-cursos-y-jornadas?download=67:h2020-oportunidades-de-financiacion [Accessed: 2021-04-12]

[19] Innovation Kitchen: Impact through innovation in SMEs with the European Innovation Council (EIC) pilot [Internet]. 2019. Available from: https://ec.europa.eu/easme/sites/easme-site/files/2019-eic-report.pdf [Accessed: 2021-04-14]

[20] Apply for Proof-of-Concept funding (FORNY2020) [Internet]. 2018. Available from: https://www.visinnovasjon.no/2018/06/15756/ [Accessed: 2021-04-15]

[21] Early Stage Research and Technology at U.S. Federal Government Agencies [Internet]. 2017. Available from: https://www.ida.org/-/media/feature/publications/e/ea/early-stage-research-and-technology-at-us-federal-government-agencies/d-8481.ashx [Accessed: 2021-04-15]

[22] Reto COVID-19 selecciona a sus 8 innovaciones ganadoras [Internet]. 2020. Available from: https://www.redgt.org/post/reto-covid-19-selecciona-doce-innovaciones-finalistas [Accessed: 2021-04-07]

[23] SOFOFA HUB: Fondo Privado de Adopción Tecnológica SiEmpre (CPC) financiará fase de validación preclínica para 5 prototipos de ventilación mecánica [Internet]. 2020. Available from: https://web.sofofa.cl/noticias/fondo-privado-de-adopcion-tecnologica-siempre-cpc-financiara-fase-de-validacion-preclinica-para-5-prototipos-de-ventilacion-mecanica/ [Accessed: 2021-04-08]

[24] Retos de innovación – Diagnóstico COVID19 [Internet]. 2020. Available from: https://www.corfo.cl/sites/cpp/convocatorias/retos_de_innovacion_covid19 [Accessed: 2021-04-09]

[25] Retos de innovación – Elementos de Protección para el personal de salud COVID19 [Internet]. 2020. Available from: https://www.corfo.cl/sites/cpp/convocatorias/movil/retos_de_innovacion_elementos_de_proteccion_covid19 [Accessed: 2021-04-09]

Section 2

Responding to Public Health Crises

Chapter 9

Coordination of Public Health Response: The Role of Leadership in Responding to Public Health Emergencies

Peter J. Fos, Peggy A. Honoré and Russel L. Honoré

Abstract

Public health emergencies are becoming more commonplace every year. Naturally occurring public health emergencies, such as hurricanes, typhoons, tsunamis, and floods cause significant devastation to property and people. Although these emergencies are becoming more and more common, response is still very challenging. A root cause of failed response is a lack of coordination between national, regional, and local public health agencies. These failed and unsuccessful responses are seen with naturally occurring public health emergencies, including pandemics. This chapter addresses coordination, its barriers and challenges, with a focus on the role of leadership in response to public health emergencies. Coordination leadership is a critical aspect of successful and effective response to emergencies. Leadership styles will be discussed and examples of effective leadership. Lessons learned will be presented, as well as research findings. Examples discussed include Hurricane Katrina, the tsunami of 2004 in Thailand, the COVID-19 pandemic, and the Sendai Framework for Disaster Risk Reduction, Sustainable Development Goals.

Keywords: leadership, emergency preparedness and response planning

1. Introduction

The nature of public health emergencies demand coordination and collaboration between local, state, regional and national capabilities. Local authorities do not have the capability, alone, to address these catastrophic events. In a Federalism system of governance, such as what exists in the US, the Constitution mandates divisions of power between federal and individual state governments [1]. Consequently, agencies at these different levels are not always naturally aligned to work collaboratively. Other models of government where authoritative territory issues are present also complicates coordination of efforts. A challenging issue is determining who is in charge of the response to emergencies when agencies from different levels are involved. The current COVID-19 pandemic emergency in the US with its lack of national coordination and state testing, consistency in data reporting, and vaccine distribution and public dispensation serves to illustrate this point. To successfully plan, mitigate risk, and respond to the effects of public health emergencies requires leadership to manage the coordination at all levels. This chapter focuses primarily on the role of leadership in planning for and coordinating a response to a public health emergency. Among many other sources, evidence in the chapter is drawn from research conducted by Preparedness and Emergency Response Research Centers (PERRCs) funded through the Centers of Disease Control and Prevention (CDC) in the 2006 Pandemic and All-Hazards Preparedness Act (PAHPA). In the reauthorization process for PAHPA, the US Senate Subcommittee on Bioterrorism and Public Health Preparedness convened a Roundtable to gather recommendations from national experts on how to strengthen US capacity for an all-hazard public health response. Some recommendations by the panel included increases in preparedness and response research funding, development of performance metrics, and implementation of system capacity assessments [2].

Following the events of September 11, 2001, the importance of integrating and coordinating public health resources with first-responding agencies for planning, training, risk mitigation, and response to public health emergencies was formally recognized. However, the disconnect between these agencies resulted in barriers and conflicts culturally and jurisdictional. In an effort to facilitate this integration, in 2003 public health was included as a first-responder agency by the federal government [3]. This effort was less than successful because federal agencies are organized according to federal guidelines, while public health agencies follow state laws and regulations. This disparate organizational structure is a hinderance to coordination and collaboration. This situation begs for strong, effective leadership.

There are two classic examples of the challenges to coordination from which many lessons can be learned. The first is Hurricane Katrina and the second is the COVID-19 pandemic. These events required a high-level of coordination of international (in COVID-19's case), federal, state, and local public health agencies. These events, on the surface, seemed to be similar to those which have occurred in the past, but the enormity of the required public health response was unexpected.

2. Coordination

Coordination can be simply defined as the act of making different people or things work together for a goal or effect [4]. Coordination has been defined in terms of positive and negative. Negative coordination is when decisions are made in one public health agency considering decision of other agencies, while attempting to avoid conflict. Positive coordination involves agencies not focusing on conflicts, but on finding ways to work together in a manner that each agency benefits [5]. Coordination problems usually are due to redundancies and gaps in services across agencies. Positive coordination is preferred because it results in better services.

Strategic coordination is what is needed for public health response. Strategic coordination involves countries through their public health agencies working together based on strategic goals. Examples of such goals can be found in the CDCs Public Health Emergency Preparedness and Response Capabilities developed as National Standards for State, Local, Tribal, and Territorial Public Health [6]. Another is the World Health Organization's (WHO) Joint Evaluation Tool as a mechanism to assess country capacity to implement the International Health Regulations as mandated by the 48th World Health Assembly [7]. A common feature of these goals is to move toward standardization of practices across all jurisdictions for activities such as detecting, preparing and responding to threats, improving the health status of a population, delivering COVID-19 vaccines to the population, or creating a coordinated public health response program [8].

Coordination levels have been delineated in the form of a scale from total independence of top-level decision makers to a very coordinated governmental strategy [9]. It is not common for agencies to be at the top level of the coordination scale, but it does illustrate possible coordinating goals.

3. Leadership theory and styles

Leadership has been defined in several ways. One definition is leadership is a process by which a person has influence over others to accomplish an objective and directs an organization that makes it more cohesive and coherent [10]. Another definition is leadership is a process by which an individual influences a group of others to achieve a common goal [11]. These definitions are describing "process leadership" which is the process of leaders applying their leadership knowledge and skills to situations. Leadership is learned, but it is influenced by leaders' beliefs, values, ethics, and character [12].

It is important that the effects of leadership are sustainable. Sustainable leadership has the following characteristics: sustainable leadership 1) creates opportunities for training and learning, 2) ensures success over time, 3) maintains the leadership of others, 4) develops human resources, and 5) develops diversity and capacity [13]. Sustainable leadership is often characterized by distributive leadership throughout an organization [14]. Successful leaders facilitate people's learning from other's diverse practices. Other's practices and approaches may be enlightening and informative [15].

Several theories have been postulated concerning leadership. Bass' Theory of Leadership states: a) personality traits lead people into leadership roles, b) events cause people to rise to the occasion, c) people can choose become leaders, and d) people can learn leadership skills [16]. Behavioral theories have stressed the role of how leaders' behavior impact their effectiveness and followers [17]. Behavioral leadership theory styles are autocratic, democratic, and laissez-faire. Behavioral theory states that leaders adopt one of these styles and that leaders are made and not born [18]. Contingency theory suggests that a leader' behavior is dependent on the situation. This theory is based on the proposition that successful leaders must align their approach to the specific situation, and there is no one optimal approach to leadership [19].

Transactional leadership theory states that a two-way relationship between a leader and followers is essential in meeting success. This theory is based on rewards and incentives for followers [20]. The servant leadership theory suggests that leaders serve first, then lead. The theory advocates patience, kindness, humility, respectfulness, honesty, and commitment. Following this theory, the leader must overcome self-interest to serve others [21]. Dominant leadership theory posits influencing others by being assertive and using one's power and formal authority [22]. Research has shown that dominant leaders are preferred in times of uncertainty. This is based on the assumption that dominant leaders are decisive and action oriented [23].

There are two major leadership styles, directive and participative. Directive leadership style involves giving clear directions, expectations, and objectives to followers. This style is most effective when a situation is complex, novel, or unexpected. Leaders using the directive style making decisions independent of input from subordinates [24]. Using this style leaders have a tendency to control discussions, dominate interactions, and direct tasks to their completion [25]. Directive leaders motivate subordinates to act to support the leader's strategy to address situations [26]. A result of directive leadership is achievement of high levels of performance by providing clear goals [27]. Directive leadership has shown to improve exchange and processing of knowledge, which is another result for performance improvement [28].

Participative leadership is the process of jointly making decisions by a leader and subordinates [29]. The focus of this leadership style is on interpersonal behavior and interactions This leadership style has been shown to be beneficial for effective overseeing of teams [30]. Participative leadership allows for sharing of knowledge, and professional development of team members [31]. Studies have shown that participative leadership increases team members' commitment, and allows for acceptance of change and effectiveness [32]. This style is associated with improved team motivation and attitudes toward the tasks at hand [33].

Leadership has a profound effect on managing the response to routine public health events, as well as those that are catastrophic. Weak leadership can magnify the effects of public health emergencies. Strong leadership will significantly reduce the effect of emergencies [34]. What is often the case, strong and effective leadership is not seen because its success reduces the awareness of its effect [35].

4. Coordination challenges/barriers

Public health emergencies require coordination, but challenges exist. In fact, coordination is a fundamental problem for public health agencies. A challenge for public health agencies is to work with new partners, as well as the challenge to work differently with regular partners. Beginning with the events of 9–11, in addition to providing health services on a routine basis, the federal, state, and local public health agencies are expected to be prepared for natural disasters, terrorist attacks, and pandemics. Public health agencies are well prepared to respond to recurring events, such as food-borne outbreaks. The same can be said for seasonally occurring infectious disease outbreaks of flu and pneumonia Both of these outbreaks have serious health outcomes, but their occurrence is expected and strategies to manage them are programmable. Once these outbreaks are identified, public health agencies mobilize personnel, following well-established and longstanding plans and procedures, to stop the outbreaks and coordinate treatment of those who may have been affected.

Hurricane Katrina has been identified as the worst natural disaster to ever occur in the United States. To classify it as a major disaster is an understatement. Hurricane Katrina attacked the United States over a five-day period, from August 25th to August 29th in 2005. The storm first struck Florida, then intensified and made landfall in Louisiana. Its devastation was spread over several Gulf Coast states, but its primary affect was felt in the City of New Orleans. The failure of the levees in New Orleans resulted in floodwaters over 80% of the city and over 1,500 deaths [36].

Shortly after Hurricane Karina passed through New Orleans and downgraded to a sub-tropical disturbance, it became clear that the storm had overwhelmed public health agencies. Lt. Gen. Russel Honoré testified to the U.S. Senate that Hurricane Katrina "beat us" [37]. A coordinated response was not implemented at first, because of the lack of communications, which were eliminated by the storm. Coordinated responses required command and control functions, which did not exist in the first few days after Hurricane Katrina made landfall. Results of this included: delayed and duplicate efforts by public health and governmental agencies, uncoordinated search and rescue efforts, confusion over delivery of needed supplies, lack of clarity as to who was coordinating hospitals' evaluation of patients, lack of local police protection, and confusion over who was in command [38].

The absence of command and control was the greatest challenge for the Hurricane Katrina response because it is essential for emergency management. Again, in his testimony to the US Senate, Lt. Gen. Honoré stated that the art of command is to arrive at a situation and unconfuse the people [37]. The effects of the storm eliminated local command centers, either due to facility destruction or loss of communications. Successful coordination occurs when there is a singular command and effort, as well as a well-defined chain of command. There must be one person in command with a clearly defined line of command and control. The different federal, state, and local agencies must be guided by a jointly agreed set of objectives. Coordination is manifested by all agencies working to achieve the same objectives.

To alleviate many of the outcomes of Hurricane Katrina, a Joint Task Force Katrina (JTF-Katrina) was quickly established and lead by Lt. General Russel Honoré, a co-author of his chapter. JTF-Katrina consisted of federal and state military, local law enforcement, and federal, state, and local agencies. Establishing JTF-Katrina resulted in regaining command and control. JTF-Katrina assisted federal, state, and local agencies to provide immediate assistance in search and rescue, emergency medical care, evaluations, restoring infrastructure, damage assessment, and resupplying food and water. The assistance was successful due to a high level of coordination and collaboration.

On January 6, 2021 insurgents rioted and assaulted the US Capitol and American democracy. This insurrection was fueled by falsehoods of unfair election processes and ultimate confirmation of the Electoral College votes for President and Vice President of the US. Uncharacteristically, security at the US Capitol was overwhelmed and resulted in significant property damage and six deaths. Speaker of the House of Representatives, Nancy Pelosi, appointed Lt. Gen. Russel Honoré to lead a review of US Capitol security. A significant part of Lt. Gen. Honoré's review will be to evaluate the coordination of the various federal and local law enforcement agencies with respect to command and control [39]. The reason for his selection was based on past successful leadership in coordinating public health emergency response.

The COVID-19 pandemic is the worst public health emergency in the world since the Influenza Epidemic of 1918. The Influenza Epidemic lasted two years and resulted in 500 million infections worldwide (one-third of the world's population at that time) and 50 million deaths. Nearly 25% of the US population was infected and 675,000 people died [40]. COVID-19 first emerged in late 2019 in Wuhan, China and, at first, seemed to be a problem far away for the other parts of the world. In early January 2020, China announced that Wuhan and other cities were locked down in attempt to stop the spread of the virus. Many countries, including the US, deemed it a China problem and travel to and from China was prohibited. It was thought that this would reduce the risk that the COVID-19 would not become a problem outside of China. This assumption was based on historical information from the severe acute respiratory syndrome (SARS) pandemic of 2003. SARS is a coronavirus which caused respiratory illness, and cases were first seen in Asia. SARS spread to more than 12 countries. In total, across the world, 8,000 people showed symptoms, and 774 of the symptomatic patients died. In the United States eight people who had traveled to infected areas became ill. However, there was no community spread in the United States [41]. But, despite travel restrictions, it soon became evident that the COVID-19 differed from SARS and was spreading throughout the world.

As was seen with Hurricane Katrina, the COVID-19 pandemic found the world unprepared to address its rapid, deadly, and wide-spread effects. An infectious agent with such high levels of infectivity, pathogenicity, and virulence was never seen before across the world. Majority of COVID-19 deaths (80%) in China was observed in people 60 years of age and older. Early in the pandemic, most deaths in the United States (80%) occurred in individuals 65 years of age and older, with the highest percentage in those 85 years of age and older [42]. Hospitalization rates were high in the United States, to the point of overcrowding of intensive care units. Hospitals were challenged because they had not planned for the bolus of severely ill patients, and rapid modification of strategic and business plans were mandated. Elective surgeries were eliminated and re-assignment of surgical staff to intensive care units resulted. Additionally, supplies and resources acquisition and supply-chain management was a challenge [43].

In March 2020, the Italian National Healthcare Service in COVID-19 hotspot areas was overwhelmed. This was due to years of budget cuts and fragmentation of services. The National Healthcare Service is regionally organized and as a result the national government had little control. This led to no coordination between national, regional and local agencies [44]. For example, in Milan the COVID-19 pandemic response was based on a rapidly developed algorithm for identification of cases and referral for treatment. The algorithm consisted of determining individual's residence, if they had been in close contact with cases or suspected cases, and close contact with anyone with respiratory symptoms who had traveled to Asia. Individual who were screened were triaged to a hospital or home for isolation. The algorithm is continually outdated to align with local directives. This algorithm is now used nationally [45].

The response to the COVID-19 pandemic in Spain also faced many challenges. Spain has been one of the worst affected countries in the world. There was a lack of pandemic preparedness. Spain had insufficient surveillance systems, inadequate supplies of personal protection and critical care equipment. Poor coordination among national and regional agencies resulted in delayed response and slow decision making. The lack of preparedness was also evident in nursing homes [46].

5. Lessons learned

Coordination is a major problem because of the complexity of health-related activities. The lack of evaluations to assess capacity to meet strategic goals, lack of coordinated resources and infrastructure including essential data, and disasters lacking the necessary attention of interagency coordination are major barriers. A systematic focus on public health emergencies and the understanding of the need for managing resources and information must be similar across agencies. Establishing a timely and rigorous evaluation process is needed to have successful continuous quality improvement. Leadership is the essential ingredient for successful coordination. Public health response varies based on the events, so leadership needs to have the ability to be flexible. Command and control must be agile to adjust to the changing circumstances within, and across, public health events [47]. Leaders must be decisive, while being flexible. Leaders also must be a) knowledgeable in public health practice, b) able to maintain situational awareness, c) provide continued situational assessment, d) inspire trust, e) coordinate diverse members of the response team, and g) lead and manage effective, timely communications [48].

Because hurricanes are annual events, federal, state, and local agencies have an opportunity to develop a unified plan. In Louisiana, federal and state military have established a coordination plan in the event of a major storm. The plan consists of: establishment of a pre-event united command and control organizational structure, pre-positioning of unified disaster assessment team, designation of a single point of contact for the federal coordinating officer to coordinate activities, implement a local or state employee disaster clause to reassign personnel to fill disaster support gaps, pre-position interoperable communication systems, identify external sources to mitigate common resources shortfalls, pre-assign space in state emergency operations center for integration of federal agencies, develop a plan to sustain governmental operations, pre-arrange support contracts for needed resources, acquire an uninterrupted power supply, and collaborate with industry to receive commitments to re-establish critical services post-storm. This coordination plan requires a dominant and directive leadership style to be successful.

The effects of a pandemic have similar response needs. Coordination is essential to successfully address pandemics. Decentralized and fragmented public health agencies need better coordination and establish a plan for command and control. Capacity for surveillance must be increased to a level at which the magnitude of pandemics do not take countries by surprise. Coordination between private, public, and governmental agencies must be formalized. An example is the initial distribution of the COVID-19 vaccine in the US, which has been less than successful. This is due, in part, to the decentralized, state-controlled distribution strategies, which differ from state to state. Agreements among these entities, as well as industry, must be developed and maintained. Adequate and appropriate resources, including human resources, must be planned and financed for long-term periods. Consistent command and control arrangements are requisite, as well as a firm commitment from political leaders to sustain preparedness over time. It is essential that coordination leadership must be participative, while being decisive, but flexible at the same time, due to the uncertainty of the COVID-19 pandemic.

The National Association of County and City Health Officials summarized the proposed response to pandemics [49]. The response recommended the following measures: isolation of infected and exposed individuals, travel restrictions, prohibiting social gatherings, school closures, rationing of medical supplies, and cancelation of elective surgeries. These recommendations were prophetic because these same measures are being used in the COVID-19 pandemic. An important adjunct to this response is community engagement, which is included in the coordination effort to address the effects of pandemics. Preparedness, response, and recovery capacity on the community level can help to optimize pandemic contingency planning [50].

The United Nations has developed a disaster risk reduction model that aims to align policies across the world. The Sendai Framework for Disaster Risk Reduction, Sustainable Development Goals is a global agreement to assist in risk reduction efforts. The Sendai Framework's core priorities are a) understanding disaster risk, b) strengthening disaster risk governance, c) investment in disaster risk reduction, and d) enhancing disaster preparedness [51]. The Sendai Framework's goal is to reduce the loss of life, injury, health impacts, and the effect of the social determinants of health.

6. Research findings

The PERRCs, presented in the Introduction of this chapter, were created specifically by US Senate authorization to conduct public health systems research for preparedness and response purposes [52]. A sample of significant findings from the research conducted at nine university-based centers included:

- ensure surge capacity through mutual aid agreements between jurisdictions for epidemiology and surveillance functions

- build community leadership capacity capable of coordinating mental health and psychological needs

- increase capacity for communicating information during emergencies to vulnerable residents and health care providers

- communication inequities hamper the ability to sufficiently prevent and respond to disasters, and

- assess inter-organizational coordination to assure a resilient public health system during disasters.

In summary some of the most important findings are the need for adequate surge capacity, communication and information sharing, and closing inequity gaps. Communication is a basic element of coordination and is dependent on strong working relationships between agencies. Research studies have found that institutional relationships are not enough; personal relationships and trust enable effective communication and coordination [53]. Information when responding to public health emergencies is ever-changing, resulting in fragmentation and misalignment of response resources and an absence of coordination. Information must have integrity to adequately assist decision making and coordination. Another study found that stable, accurate, and consistent methods of communication and information sharing is essential [54].

In a case study of challenges in sharing and coordinating information the researcher learned that sharing is dependent on agency, community, and individual factors. Individual responders have been found to be more willing to receive information than to share information with others. This has been related to information overload among those individuals who are responding to the effects of a public health emergency [55]. The following strategies have been proposed to enhance information sharing: a) establishment of institutional incentive mechanisms for interagency information sharing, b) ensure fair distribution of benefits from interagency information sharing, c) knowledge of the operations of other agencies will improve information sharing, d) establish agency norms and standards for information sharing, f) establish an inter-agency information sharing system, and g) integrate the inter-agency information sharing system into the daily operations of agencies [56].

A study of the tsunami disaster of 2004 in Thailand evaluated the response of the health care system [57]. Study findings included that the most factors important for disaster response is: information flow, overall coordination, and leadership. The information flow is critical between public health and governmental agencies, and the population. The study learned that information flow between agencies was not consistent, and was the cause of ineffective response activities. Coordination during the response was adequate, but the health care system was not prepared for the magnitude of the event. Leadership was effective at most levels, except for hospitals were physicians made the decisions without quality information.

It is important not to overlook those who are most severely affected by public health emergencies. Populations, and subpopulations, that are most vulnerable are affected disproportionately. As was mentioned above, one of the foci if the Sendai Framework is to reduce the effect of the social determinants of health. Those that are poor, uneducated, living in substandard housing, lacking access to transportation are the most vulnerable [58]. Those who are vulnerable are marginalized in society [59]. During naturally occurring public health emergencies minority groups in the US experience the greatest negative impact [60]. Poor coordination among governmental agencies, non-profits, and private sector entities, as well as unequal disaster risk, worsens the effect within these vulnerable populations [61]. Health equity issues, created by unjust governmental and health policies, cause unequal negative impacts, as have been seen with the COVID-19 pandemic [62].

Public health, particularly in the US, has established policies and procedures to prepare leaders to respond to public health emergencies. The Association of State and Territorial Health Officials (ASTHO) published preparedness policy and position statements [63]. In preparedness guiding principles, ASTHO recognizes the role of state and territorial agencies in preparation and response to public health emergencies. The guiding principles include a) prevention, mitigation, resilience, and recovery; b) sustained funding; c) optimal preparedness for all populations; d) preparedness science and recognition of emerging emergencies; e) importance of partnerships; f) continual evaluation of preparedness. ASTHO outlines the importance of a collaborative national preparedness response, as well as the roles of federal, state, local, territorial, and tribal agencies.

Healthy People 2020, as a response to the COVID-19 pandemic, created policies for preparedness [64]. The National Health Security Strategy (NHSS) guides objectives for preparedness focused on community resilience, public health emergency response systems, capabilities, and resources. Five strategic objectives are the hallmark of the preparedness policy. Community resilience is the first objective and focuses on local coordination of health and public health agencies. The second objective is the development of countermeasures to address public health emergencies of all types, including infectious disease epidemics. The third objective is focused on continual situational awareness for early detection and coordinated response. The fourth objective establishes the importance of coalitions, and partnerships, of public health and emergency management agencies. The final objective involves global health security. This objective is focused on world-wide public health emergencies, specifically the COVID-19 pandemic.

7. Conclusions

Leadership is essential in coordination of response to public health emergencies. Work leadership is not only ineffective, it results in worsening of the effects of public health emergencies. A characteristic of public health emergencies is uncertainty. In uncertain situations dominant and directive leadership is required. Due to the ever-changing nature of public health emergencies, the dominant and directive leader must be flexible to adjust to changes. Effective leadership is dependent on quality data-sharing and communications. Public health response must be carefully and thoroughly planned, considering the need for managing resources across all responding agencies, public and private.

Acknowledgements

Support for development of this chapter was funded, in part, by the National Institute of Minority Health and Health Disparities of the National Institutes of Health under grant S21MD1007136.

Conflict of interest

The authors declare no conflict of interest.

Author details

Peter J. Fos[1]*, Peggy A. Honoré[2] and Russel L. Honoré[3]

1 Minority Health and Health Disparities Research Center, Dillard University, USA

2 LSU Health Sciences Center, School of Public Health, School of Medicine, USA

3 U.S. Army Retired, USA

*Address all correspondence to: pfos@dillard.edu

References

[1] Cornell Law School. Federalism. [Internet]. 2020. Available from: https://www.law.cornell.edu/wex/federalism

[2] Statement of Peggy A. Honoré Before the United States Senate Subcommittee on Bioterrorism and Public Health Preparedness Roundtable on Public Health Preparedness in the 21st Century. March 28, 2006. Available from: http://web1.sph.emory.edu/PHSR/PHF_Archive/Senate/HonoreSenateRoundtable.pdf

[3] The White House. December 17, 2003. Homeland Security Presidential Directive/Hspd-8. Available from: http://www.whitehouse.gov/news/releases/2003/12/20031217-6.html

[4] Your Dictionary [Internet]. Available from: www.yourdictionary.com/coordination

[5] Sharpf FW. Games real actors could play: positive and negative coordination in embedded negotiations. Journal of Theoretical Politics. 1994;6:27-53. DOI: 10.1177/0951692894006001002

[6] Centers for Disease Control and Prevention. Center for Preparedness and Response. Public Health Emergency Preparedness and Response Capabilities. National Standards for State, Local, Tribal, and Territorial Public Health. [Internet]. 2019. Available from: https://www.cdc.gov/cpr/readiness/capabilities.htm

[7] World Health Organization. Joint External Evaluation Tool – 2md Edition. IHR 92005) Monitoring and Evaluation Framework. [Internet]. 2018. Available from: https://www.who.int/ihr/publications/WHO_HSE_GCR_2018_2/en/

[8] Peters BG. The challenge of policy coordination. Policy Design and Practice. 2018;1(1):1-11. DOI: 10.1080/25741292.2018.1437946

[9] Metcalfe L. International policy coordination and public management reform. Internal Review of Administrative Sciences. 1994;60:271-290. DOI: 10.1177/002085239406000208

[10] Sharma MK, Jain S. Leadership principles, models, and theories. Global Journal of Management and Business Studies. 2013;3(3):309-318. Available from: https://www.ripublication.com/gjmbs_spl/gjmbsv3n3spl_14.pdf

[11] Northouse G. Leadership theory and practice (3rd ed.). Thousand Oaks, New Delhi, Sage Publications, Inc. 2007.

[12] Jago AG. Leadership perspectives in theory and research. Management Science. 1982; 28(3):315-336. DOI: 10.1287/mnsc.28.3.315

[13] Hargreaves A, Fink D. The seven principles of sustainable leadership. Educational Leadership. 2003;61(7):8-13.

[14] Spillane JP, Halverson R, Diamond JB. Towards a theory of leadership practice: A distributed perspective. Journal of Curriculum Studies. 2004; 36(1):3-24. DOI: 10.1080/0022027032000106726

[15] Capra F. Creativity and leadership in learning communities. A lecture at Mill Valley School District [Internet]. 1997. Available from: http://lebendig.org/creativity.pdf

[16] Bass BM. From transactional to transformational leadership: Learning to share the vision. Organizational Dynamics. 1990;18:19-32. DOI: 10.1016/0090-2616(0)90061-5

[17] Bolden R, Gosling J. Leadership competencies: Time to change the tune?

Leadership. 2006;2(2):147-163. DOI: 10.1177/1742715006062932

[18] Ayman R, Korabik K. Leadership: Why gender and culture matter. The American Psychologist. 2010; 65:157-170. DOI: 10.1037/a0018806

[19] Verkerk PJ. Fiedler's contingency model of leadership effectiveness: Background and recent developments. OCTO-Report, 9002. 1990. Eindhoven University of Technology.

[20] Yahaya R, Ebrahim F. Leadership styles and organizational commitment: Literature review. Journal of Management Development. 2016;35(2):190-216. DOI: 10.1108/JMD-01-2015-0004

[21] Wooi CT, Salleh LM, Ismail IA. Lessons from the major leadership theories in comparison to the competency theory of leadership practice. Journal of Business and Social Review in Emerging Economies. 2017;3(2). DOI: 10.26710/jbsee.v312.86

[22] Kiazad K, Restubog SLD Zagenczyk, TJ, Kiewit C., Tang R. In pursuit of power: The role of authoritarian leadership in the relationship between supervisors' Machiavellianism and subordinates' perceptions of abusive supervisory behavior. Journal of Research in Personality. 2010;44:512-519. DOI: 10.1016/j.jrp.2010.06.004

[23] Hemant K, Sirvanathan N. When the appeal of a dominant leader is greater than a prestige leader. In: Proceedings of the National Academy of Sciences of the United States, 2017;114(26):6734-6739. DOI: 10.1073/pnas.1617711114

[24] Mroz JE, Yoerger M, Allen JA. Leadership in workplace meetings: The intersection of leadership styles and follower gender. Journal of Leadership and Organisational Studies. 2018;25(3):1-14. DOI: 10.1177/1548051817750542

[25] Clark KD, Waldron T. Predictors of leadership behavior in early career white-collar professionals: The roles of personal characteristics and career context. Journal of Leadership and Organisational Studies. 2016;23(1):37-38. DOI: 10.117/1548051815587759

[26] Haar SV, Koeslag-Kreunen M, Euwe E, Segers M. Team leader structuring for team effectiveness and team learning in command-and-control teams. Small Group Research. 2017;48(2):215-248. DOI: 10.1177/104649641789897

[27] Ceri-Booms M, Cureu PL, Oerlemans LAG. Task and person-focused leadership behaviors and team performance: A meta-analysis. Human Resources Management Review. 2017;27(1):178-192. DOI: 10.1016/j.hrmr.2016.09.010

[28] Burke CS, Stagl KC, Klein C, Goodwin GF, Salas E, et al. What type of leadership behaviours are functional in terms? A meta-analysis. Leadership Quarterly. 2006;17:288-307. DOI: 10.1016/j.leaqua.2006.02.007

[29] Benoliel B, Somech A. The health and performance effects of participative leadership: Exploring the moderating role of the big five personality dimensions. European Journal of Work and Organisational Psychology. 2014;23(2):277-294. DOI: 10.1080/1359432X.2012.717689

[30] Newman A, Rose PS, Teo ST. The role of participative leadership and trust-based mechanisms in eliciting intern performance: Evidence from China. Human Resource Management. 2016;55(1):53-67. DOI : 10.1002/hrm.21660

[31] Buengeler C, Homan AC, Voelpel SC. The challenge of being

a younger manager: The effects of contingent reward and participative leadership on team-level turnover depend on leader age. Journal of Organizational Behavior. 2016;37:1224-1245. DOI: 10.1002/job.2101

[32] Fatima T, Safdar S, Jahanzeb S. Participative leadership and employee creativity: Moderating role of need for achievement. International Journal of Business and Management. 2017;12(1):1-14. DOI: 10.1108/LODJ-07-2019-0319

[33] Bouwmans M, Runhaar P, Wesselink R, Mulder M. Fostering teachers' team learning: An interplay between transformational leadership and participative decision-making? Teaching and Teacher Education. 2017; 65:71-80. DOI: 10.1016/j.tate.2017.03.010

[34] Kweit MG, Kweit RW. A tale of two disasters. Publicus. 2006;36(3): 375-392. Available from https://www.jstor.org/stable/4624754

[35] Kapucu N, Van Wart M. (2008). Making matters worse: An anatomy of leadership failures in managing catastrophic events. Administration & Society. 2008;40(7):711-740. DOI: 10.1177/0095399708323143

[36] Shrum W. What caused the flood? Controversy and closure in the Hurricane Katrina disaster. Social Studies of Science. 2013;14(1):3-33. DOI: 10.117/0306312713498654

[37] U.S. Senate Committee on Homeland Security and Governmental Affairs. Hurricane Katrina: The Defense Department's role in the response. February 9, 2006.S. Hrg. 109-813.2007. Available from: https://www.govinfo.gov/content/pkg/CHRG-109shrg27028/pdf/CHRG-109shrg27028.pdf.

[38] U.S. Congress. House of Representative Report 109-377 (2006). A failure of initiative final report of the select bipartisan committee to investigate the preparation for and response to Hurricane Katrina. 2006. Available from: https://www.congress.gov/109/crpt/hrpt377/CRPT-109hrpt377.pdf

[39] Kavi A. New inquiries into the Capitol assault aim to address security lapses before Biden's inauguration. The New York Times, January 16, 2021. Available from: https://nyti.ms/3swcPVh

[40] National Archives. National Archives News. The flu pandemic of 1918. [Internet]. 2021. Available from: https://www.archives.gov/news/topics/flu-pandemic-1918

[41] Centers for Disease Control and Prevention. SARS basic fact sheet. [Internet]. 2021. Available from: https://www.cdc.gov/sars/about/fs-sars.html

[42] Centers for Disease Control and Prevention. Severe outcomes among patients with coronavirus disease 2019 (COVID-19): United States, February 12 – March 16, 2020. Morbidity and Mortality Weekly Report. 2020;69(12):343-346.

[43] Ehrlich H, McKenney M, Elkbuli A. Strategic planning and recommendations for healthcare workers during the COVID-19 pandemic. American Journal of Emergency Medicine. 2020;38(7):1446-1447. DOI: 10.1016/j.ajem.2020.03.057

[44] Armocida B, Formenti B, Ussai S, Palestra F, Missoni E. The Italian health system and the COVID-19 challenge. The Lancet Public Health. 2020;5(5). DOI: 10.1016/S0468-2667(20)30074-8

[45] Spina S, Marrazzo F, Migliari M, Stucchi R, Sforza A, Fumagalli R. The response of Milan's medical system to COVID-19 outbreak in Italy. The

Lancet, 2020;395:e49-e50. DOI: 10.1016/S0140-6796(20)30493-1

[46] Garcia-Basteiro A, Alvarez-Dardet C, Arenas A, et al. The need for an independent evaluation of COVID-19 response in Spain. The Lancet, 396, August 22, 2020. Available from: https://www.thelancet.com.

[47] Wise CR. Organizing for homeland security after Katrina: Is adaptive management what's missing? Public Administration Review. 2006;66(32): 302-318. DOI: 10.1111/j.1540-6210.2006.00587.x

[48] Deitchman S. Enhancing leadership in public health emergencies. Disaster Medicine and Public Health Preparedness. 2013;7(5):534-540. DOI:10.1017/dmp.2013.81

[49] National Association of County and City Health Officials. Local health department guide to pandemic influenza planning. [Internet]. 2006. Washington, D.C.: NACCHO. Available from: http://www.naccho.org/topics/infectious/influenza/documents/NACCHOPanFluGuideforLHDsII.pdf

[50] Schoch-Spana M, Franco C, Nuzzo JB, Usenza C. Community engagement: Leadership tool for catastrophic health events. Biosecurity and Bioterrorism: Biodefense Strategy, Practice, and Science. 2007; 5(1). DOI: 20.1089/bsp.2006.0036

[51] Reifels L, Arbon P, Capon A, Handmer J, Humphrey A, Murray V, Spencer C, Wong DF. Health and disaster risk reduction regarding the Sendai Framework. Australian Journal of Emergency Management, 2018;33(1). Available from: https://knowledge.aidr.org.au/resources/ajem-jan-2018-health-and-disaster-risk-reduction-regarding-the-sendai-framework/

[52] Leinhos M, Qari SH, Williams-Johnson M. Preparedness and Emergency Response Research Centers: Using a Public Health Systems Approach to Improve All-Hazards Preparedness and Response. Public Health Reports. 2014;129(6-Supplement 4):8-18. DOI: 10.1177/00333549141296S403

[53] Waugh WL, Streib G. Collaboration and leadership for effective emergency management. Public Administration Review. 2006; 66: 131-140. Available from: https://www.jstor.org/stable/4096577

[54] Comes T, Van de Walle L. The coordination-information bubble in humanitarian response: Theoretical foundations and empirical investigations. Production and Operations Management. 2020;29(1): 2484-2507. DOI: 10.111/poms.13236

[55] Mendonca D, Jefferson T, Harrald J. Collaborative adhocracies and mix-match technologies in emergency management. Communications of the ACM. 2007;50(3):45-49. DOI: 10.1145/1226736.1226764

[56] Bharosa N, Lee J, Janssen M. Challenges and obstacles in sharing and coordinating information during multi-agency disaster response: Propositions from field exercises. Information Systems Frontiers. 2009;12: 49-65. DOI: 10.1007/s10796-009-9174-z

[57] Peltz R, Ashkenazi I, Schwartz D, et al. Disaster healthcare system management and crisis intervention leadership in Thailand: Lessons learned from the 2004 tsunami disaster. Prehospital and Disaster Medicine. 2005;21(5): 299-302. Available from: http://pdm.medicine.wisc.edu

[58] Ferreira RJ, Buttell F, Ferreira SB. Ethnical consideration for conducting disaster research with vulnerable populations. Journal of Social Work Values and Ethics. 2015;12(1):29-40. Available from: https://www.

researchgate.net/profile/Reggie_Ferreira/publication/277596673_Ethical_Considerations_for_Conducting_Disaster_Research_with_Vulnerable_Populations/links/556e09c308aefcb861db972e/Ethical-Considerations-for-Conducting-Disaster-Research-with-Vulnerable-Populations.pdf

[59] Gaillard JC. Vulnerability, capacity, and resilience: Perspectives for climate and development policy. Journal of International Development. 2010;22(2):218-232. DOI: 10.1022/jid.1675

[60] Cupples J, Glynn K. The mediation and remediation of disaster: Hurricanes Katrina and Felix in/and the new media environment. Antipode. 2014;46(2):359-381. DOI: 10.1111/anti.12060

[61] Collins TW. Marginalization, facilitation, and the production of unequal risk: The 2006 Paso del Norte floods. Antipode. 2010;42(2):258-288. DOI: 10.1111/j.1467-8330.2009.00755.x

[62] Fos PJ, Honoré PA, Kellum KP. The relationship of diabetes and COVID-19: A health disparity. Diabetes & its Complications. 2020;4(1):1-5. DOI: 10.33425/2639-9326.1065

[63] ASTHO. Policy and position statements: Preparedness guiding principles. 2017. Available from: http://www.astho.org/Policy-and-Position-Statement/Policy-Statement-on-Preparedness

[64] HHS Office of Disease Prevention and Health Promotion. Healthy People 2020: Preparedness. 2020. Available from: https://www.healthypeople.gov/2020/topics-objectives/topic/preparedness

Chapter 10

Building Interdisciplinary Teams in Emergency Care to Respond to National Emergencies: Addressing the Opioid Epidemic

Erick Guerrero, Jemima A. Frimpong, Angelique Hearn, Veronica Serret, Welmoed K. van Deen, Howard Padwa, Rebecca Trotzky-Sirr, Michael Menchine and Daniel L. Howard

Abstract

This study responds to the gap in knowledge in translating team members' interdisciplinary knowledge to address wicked problems. We use qualitative methodology to understand the team-building process and response to the opioid epidemic in emergency care. We collected data through direct observation of nine health system science researchers and thought leaders as they performed in team-building activities and semi-structured interviews. The cultural exchange framework informed our selection and assessment of team-building activities, and the science of team science (SciTS) framework informed our understanding of promoting interdisciplinary collaborations. We identified six themes representing three areas: (1) Knowledge Building and Strategy Development (need for interdisciplinary understanding of substance abuse and mental health in the emergency department (ED); interdisciplinary approaches to fight the opioid epidemic in the ED); (2) Team Demographics and Collaboration (prescribing and collaboration; the role of interdisciplinary team composition and effectiveness in the ED); and (3) Identity and Relationship Building (role of professional identity in contributing to interdisciplinary research; building effective organizational relationships in the ED). Members' personal and professional connections are fundamental for developing nuanced interdisciplinary strategies to respond to the opioid epidemic in the ED. We discuss implications for strategies that promote team building and improve treatment practices.

Keywords: team building, interdisciplinary collaboration, emergency care, opioid epidemic, implementation science

1. Introduction

There is growing interest in leveraging the knowledge, expertise, and skills of teams of experts from different disciplinary backgrounds to respond to wicked problems affecting our society. Wicked problems are problems that require insight from experts who cut across multiple disciplines, in order to address the problem [1]. The interconnected aspect of such problems highlights their complexity. However, it is still unclear how team members from different disciplines can effectively leverage their unique knowledge to develop innovative solutions to harmful epidemics, such as the opioid epidemic faced by the United States. Interdisciplinary team approaches, those that involve applying the knowledge and skills from different academic disciplines or subjects that are normally regarded as distinct, to the same issue [2] are gaining visibility in translation, dissemination, implementation, and improvement research. In this research study, we seek to understand and develop strategies that facilitate the formation and sustainability of interdisciplinary teams and improve health-care delivery in crisis situations [3]. We focus on opioid epidemic crisis in the United States and how EDs respond to the opioid epidemic, within the context of interdisciplinary teams. EDs are dynamic settings where interdisciplinary teams, in which collaborators can be located at different departments or institutions, endorse different ideologies, or rely on different methodologies, but share the common goal of addressing a problem, are necessary to developing cohesive and insightful solutions to the opioid epidemic in the United States.

2. Interdisciplinary teams in the emergency department to respond to the opioid crisis

2.1 Team building conceptual framework

Building on conceptual work on multi and interdisciplinary teamwork in translational science [3, 4], this study examines how team building interactions and phases affect [5] team members' response to initiating opioid use disorder (OUD) treatment for patients in the ED. We relied on the science of team science (SciTS) framework to explore the key challenges and solutions to promoting interdisciplinary collaborations (see **Table 1**). SciTS seeks to understand barriers and facilitators of collaborative and team-based research efforts and identify conditions, understand processes, and achieve outcomes associated with team objectives [6]. Barriers and facilitators are at different levels, including intrapersonal (own knowledge and competencies brought to the team), interpersonal (communication, connection and shared knowledge among team members), physical environment (structure of communication, collaboration, execution and problem solving), societal and political (community norms, political discourse), and technological (communication, connection, description). Understanding interactions and interdependencies between these factors can lead to a better understanding of the process of how team becomes effective in addressing critical issues. Furthermore, using SciTS to understand how to develop and support interdisciplinary collaboration may lead to effective translation of research findings into practice [6, 7].

We rely on a cultural exchange approach (see **Table 1**), which centers on sharing of ideas and knowledge between group members representing different professional systems, to help us understand the transaction of knowledge, attitudes, and practices that occurs during interactions [8]. During this process, we evaluated a series of discrete activities and document aspects from team science (space, communication, knowledge) to identify how team-building exercises ultimately enhanced problem-solving. This method consisted of evaluating four conditions through team building activities: 1) groups' accessibility to one another; 2) a sense of mutual respect; 3) creation of a shared language; 4) willingness to compromise/accommodate the needs

Framework	Components
Science of Team Science (SciTS) Framework • To explore the key challenges and solutions to promoting interdisciplinary collaborations • Important for effective translation of research findings into practice	• Intrapersonal (own knowledge and competencies brought to the team) • Interpersonal (communication, connection and shared knowledge among team members) • Physical environment (structure of communication, collaboration, execution and problem solving) • Societal and political (community norms, political discourse) • Technological (communication, connection, description)
Cultural Exchange Approach • To select team building activities that meet specific criteria	• Group accessibility to one another (e.g., interaction activity - bowling) • A sense of mutual respect (decision making activity- ESCAPE room) • Creation of a shared language (e.g., health-systems experts meeting) • Willingness to compromise or accommodate each other needs (e.g., consensus group) to develop interdisciplinary approaches to respond to wicked problems.

Table 1.
Frameworks.

of others [8]. These activities are essential to bridging and merging diverse perspectives and transcending disciplinary boundaries.

This study focuses on assembling a interdisciplinary team of scholars (Social Work, Nursing, and Medicine) at a research University and undertaking a team-building process so as to build interdisciplinary approaches to 'wicked problems' [9]. We implemented team-building activities and assessed the process of becoming an interdisciplinary team while conducting a research study addressing ED responses to the opioid epidemic (IRB # RC010001). The efficacy of ED responses to the opioid epidemic can be considered a 'wicked problem' requiring a interdisciplinary approach, because such responses are influenced by contradictory and changing conditions and are seemingly intractable for any given discipline [9]. Our findings may inform strategies for constituting and preparing interdisciplinary teams to effectively respond to challenging issues, and to understand transformational experiences that may support the achievement of their common goals.

3. Methods

3.1 Sample and procedures

The sample included one team of nine researchers: four researchers from USC Social Work, two researchers from nursing, a researcher from the Keck School of Medicine, and an ED practicing physician from the Los Angeles County + University of Southern California (LAC + USC) Medical Center. We constituted a team with members from disciplines that have been shown to be important to improving care delivery in emergency departments. Each team members also had experience in opioid use disorder research or care delivery in the ED, but mostly from a disciplinary lens.

We began our research by drawing from the literature on team building to develop a curriculum of team-building activities informed by the cultural exchange framework. During the course of the study, we introduced participants to team-building activities that match their disciplinary knowledge and strategies and shown to promote multidiscipline approaches for ED treatment of individuals with OUD. We selected activities that met the Palinkas et al., criteria [8] and accessible to study participants: 1) group accessibility to one another (e.g., interaction activity - bowling); 2) a sense of mutual respect (decision making activity- ESCAPE room); 3) creation of a shared language (e.g., health-systems experts meeting); 4) willingness to compromise/accommodate each other needs (e.g., consensus group) to develop interdisciplinary approaches to respond to wicked problems.

3.2 Data collection

We collected data through three different approaches and settings: direct observations during structured team building activities with the full team of nine members followed by semi-structured interviews of five members; direct observation from a scientific presentation; and a focus group and consensus session with six members (see **Figure 1**). We sought to elicit interdisciplinary insight, as a fundamental mechanism for translating team-effective practices and generate innovative frameworks, methodologies, and policies toward solving identified problems [5, 10]. Our data collection was guided by the cultural exchange framework (identification of team building activities) and the SciTS framework (identification of barriers and facilitators to collaboration).

3.3 Team building activities

During 2016 and 2017 the team development activities were both virtual and in-person. These structured activities included 1) interacting in a bowling activity to promote communication and mutual respect through positive competition, and 2) engaging members in an iterative problem-solving team-building activity to promote brainstorming, develop a shared language and compromising, and accommodating the needs of others in the pursuit of solutions. We used ESCAPE rooms for this activity, where the goal is to work as a team to figure out clues and escape the room within a pre-determined time. We relied on direct observation during and semi-structured interviews after team building activities with individual team members to identify their awareness of their own team-building process and the team's responses. The deliberative sessions, following team activities, allowed us to develop shared goals based on the interdisciplinary work and understandings of the potential paths to achieve these goals, and ultimately increase the cooperation as a team as suggested in Hall et al. [5].

3.4 Focus group

We used a focus group and a deliberative session to discuss iterative findings from original research (findings from survey research on the ED). The focus group comprised of six participants (social work researchers, social work research assistants and a project coordinator, a social worker/clinical psychologist, research assistants, and a physician), all of whom participated in various team-building activities. Our scripted questions focused on understanding the problems and solutions to the ED response to the opioid epidemic, with consideration for the diverse background, education, and training of participants. We also interviewed ED physicians from the LAC+USC Medical Center. This allowed us to frame the problem and

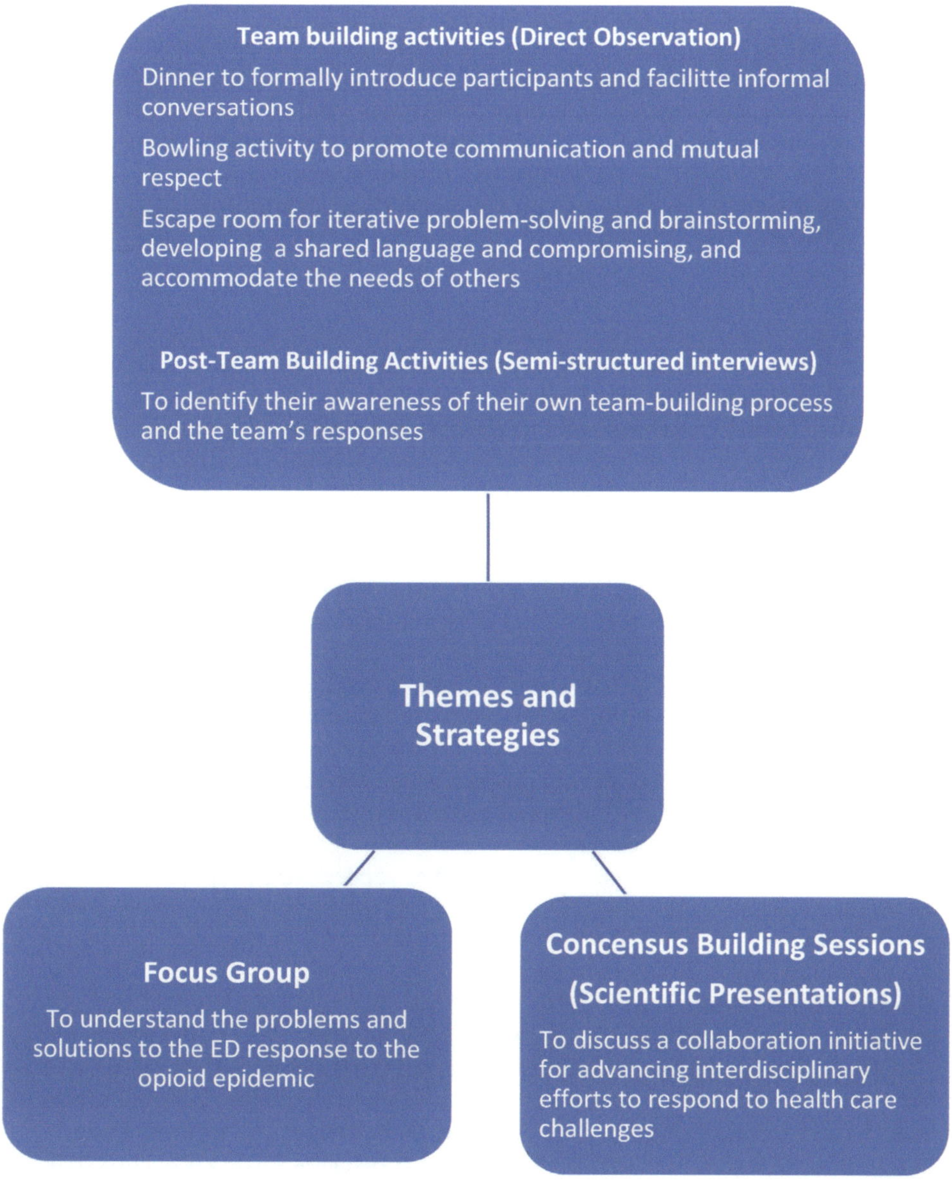

Figure 1.
Data collection schema.

solutions from different interdisciplinary perspectives and find ways to integrate these different perspectives into an innovative, coherent, and potentially effective approach to the problem.

3.5 Consensus building sessions

In line with findings showing that time and space are key elements for creating interdisciplinary research collaborations [11], the team (5 to 9 members) met in-person once per month for 1–2 hours for 8 months at different locations. These meetings included a scientific meeting and a consensus meeting, where we brought together leaders from academic and health-systems backgrounds to discuss a collaboration initiative for advancing interdisciplinary efforts to respond to health care challenges, including the current opioid epidemic. Each meeting was structured to give members the opportunity to communicate their disciplinary perspectives and experience, highlight common ground, and create shared language and knowledge. Given research suggesting that off-campus meetings, i.e., off-sites, were helpful in the implementation phase to minimize distractions while assessing study progress [5], we held several in-person meetings and activities in an off-campus location. This approach provided information and context regarding individual and team problem solving.

We conducted additional analysis of transcripts from an interdisciplinary symposium, referred to as the health systems science meeting. This allowed us to integrate organization and implementation science and understand how these sciences can form a foundation for an institutional response to the opioid epidemic. The goal was to focus on areas shown by research to be associated with team science, identify barriers and facilitators, and use learnings to develop team interdisciplinarity.

We also created a database using reports written retrospectively by team members working together on a pilot study for assessing the process of becoming interdisciplinary when responding to ED actions for addressing the opioid epidemic. This qualitative analysis outlines the experiences and observations the team members had in participating in a series of activities that progressed from unstructured to structured activities.

The goals of assessing the team building process were to: 1) qualify the collaboration between social work, nursing and medicine (for example, we assessed team members' perception of the process of moving toward a interdisciplinary approach. We relied on semi-structured interviews to examine perceived change in exchanging disciplinary knowledge and contributing toward the research goals), and 2) record group activities that successfully contributed and those that did not contribute to team progress (we compared direct observation reports of team building activities such as team bowling and analysis of semi-structured interview data).

3.6 Analytical strategy

To study team processes, two Ph.D.-level researchers and a doctoral student observed and documented team interactions. These included in-person meetings and activities, phone conversations, and e-mail exchanges. All interviews and focus groups were recorded and professionally transcribed. Data was kept strictly confidential based on the original (2016) and revised human protection protocol (IRB # RC010001). Two doctoral level and one graduate level raters analyzed transcripts with InVivo software using template analysis, a set of techniques for thematically organizing and analyzing textual data via thematic codes that are defined a priori as critical to study questions and inductively through the coding process. The research team identified the most common and prominently expressed codes and themes that emerged from the interviews. When these codes and themes were not clear, raters discussed them and reached consensus on the best description. Themes were validated with outside social work and medicine researchers.

3.7 Results

Our findings emphasize the contributions of interdisciplinary teams toward ED response to the opioid epidemic, after exposure to processes that facilitate and promote the formation and effectiveness of a more integrated interdisciplinary team. The process of team building developed in this study was engaging and fostered professional relationships in a setting outside of work. Participants reported that the three iterative team-building activities—dinner, team bowling, and escape rooms—were valuable to team building in that they were critical to the team's connection and knowledge-building experiences. Dinner introduced participants to each other, bowling helped them become more acquainted, and the escape rooms taught them problem solving and interdependence. Participants were motivated to meet new team members and become more familiar with those they already knew. Through these encounters, teammates were able to discuss with each other the details of their projects related to the opioid crisis and opportunities for collaboration that will foster improved care practices for opioid use disorders.

Data from focus groups, team building activities, and scientific presentation provided two perspectives on the response to the opioid epidemic problem. The focus group provided a point of view that is more implementation-based, while the Health Systems Science and interdisciplinary symposium perspective provided a multi-theoretical explanation of how systems can be implemented at different organizational levels. Throughout the transcripts, six overarching themes emerged that provide insight on the challenges practitioners in the ED and organizations face, while dealing with the opioid epidemic (see **Figure 2**). These themes were: need for interdisciplinary understanding of substance abuse and mental health; interdisciplinary approaches to fight the opioid epidemic; prescribing opioids and collaboration; the role of interdisciplinary team composition and team effectiveness; the role of professional identity to contribute to interdisciplinary research; and building effective organizational relationships.

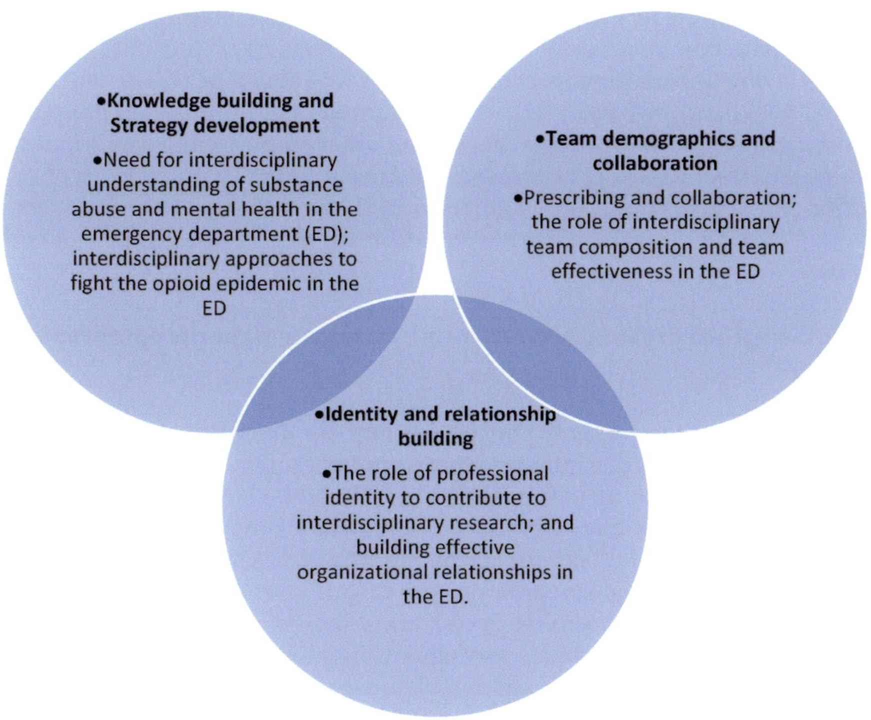

Figure 2.
Interrelated themes.

4. Knowledge building and strategy development

4.1 Interdisciplinary understanding of substance abuse and mental health in the ED

Participants from different disciplines express to different degrees that the complexity of substance abuse and mental health disorders is not always properly understood in the ED. One participant explains the importance of having other experts in the ED to understand brain chemistry and social conditions by noting, "addiction is now understood as a brain disease for which we have brain medication." She further elaborates that "conversations need to be had with ER physicians to emphasize drug addiction as the underlying problem to the presenting issue." Another participant explains that some "patients who have substance use and mental health issues also have current life devastation issues, like they have no friends anymore because they alienated everybody. So now [they're] here in the ER. They will come in the ER every other day for no other reason other than opioids." Substance abuse is a complex issue that requires more time than can be provided in an ED visit.

One participant explains that other experts can help ER physicians "understand all the different components of substance abuse". This participant further explains that ED practitioners "don't care about reasons that contribute to the problem. I think, they think, if they can see the person, treat the person and get them out and now they are not causing harm but helping them."

ED physicians may also have distorted expectations when treating someone with an opioid addiction. One participant explains that opioid treatment outcomes have to be "clear, relevant and realistic… Physicians want to see 100% of patients who start buprenorphine do so when completely sober. And you're like that's just not a realistic thing." The ED physician supports this claim, stating, "if physicians believe that patients cannot get better there is hopelessness of engaging in other options." Having unrealistic expectations of how well someone will do when treated with MAT goes hand-in-hand with not being familiar with the science of opioid addiction, coupled with the mental health and other co-occurring conditions that challenge the effectiveness of treatment. Enhancing physician knowledge of opioid addiction and related conditions, supported by the availability of practitioners from other specialties, is therefore an important aspect of addressing the opioid epidemic.

4.2 Interdisciplinary teams, networks and training to fight the opioid epidemic in the ED

A running theme throughout the focus group discussions is the value placed on being part of an interdisciplinary team or network. One participant said that she "extremely values being part of the team." She adds that she is "very big on collaboration. I think no one knows everything and when people come together with their different level of experience of expertise you see the best results whether it's implementing new policy or the care of an individual." Some participants noted how interdisciplinary education should be part of the curriculum in medical school. As an example, participants highlighted the interdisciplinary curriculum of the geriatric program, which incorporates dental services, occupational therapy, physical therapy, social work, and physicians. Oncology was cited as another interdisciplinary field, with one participant noting the value of social work in it: "I think that's also true in palliative care. They really value the social worker."

Although working together in an interdisciplinary team appears to make sense, one participant said that such a perspective is often lost in medical school, where medical doctors may not learn how to work with other to have the most impact on health ..."So maybe we should bring in that model [to medical school] of interdisciplinary and the social work theory of empathy, active listening, and put them together in a class, presentation or workshop."

The dual benefit of interdisciplinarity was also highlighted. That is, conversations should be initiated with ED providers or seize the opportunities in the ED to demonstrate that interdisciplinary teamwork benefits both the patient and the ED prescriber. The ED prescriber's network may also help ED practitioners increase their understanding of the opioid problem. According to the presenters describing the process of seeking advice, "It depends on the qualities of the expert, the quality of their expertise, how accessible they are to you, it depends upon your needs as an advice seeker, and a lot of it depends on accessibility." These networks can be defined "in terms of physical proximity, social proximity, or history of prior relationships." Findings from the scientific presentation suggest that quality of expertise and accessibility to the expert were significant indicators when predicting the presence, absence, or a tie of a network formation. Furthermore, the presenters noted that "faculty experts and supervisors were more likely to be new sources of advice for clinicians over time. Also, being in the same organization and being from the same discipline were significant predictors of the tie formation." Participants also highlighted the effectiveness in working across disciplines and departments. Every participant has had an opportunity to work with colleagues from other disciplines, and clearly acknowledge how the depth and quality of conversations are enriched by collaboration.

5. Team demographics and collaboration

5.1 ED practitioners' prescribing and collaboration

Participants highlight that the ED is a major player in the prescribing of opioid medication and would benefit from greater collaboration from other disciplines. For example, one participant investigated whether differences in belief systems exist among ED practitioners, affecting how often they prescribe opioids. The participant noted that ED practitioners rely on a set of values to determine when to prescribe, with ED doctors "making decisions in a different way" when treating patients who show in the ED seeking opioid prescriptions. ED practitioners may assess the deservedness of patients, based on their race, language, complaint, etc.

One participant offered a physician's perspective, explaining that "most doctors do not confront patients about their opioid use, and have a conversation about other options. Almost never happens, it requires too much energy. Doctors have two easy ways out, kick them out of the ED or give them the pills."

ED practitioners may have continued the problem by refilling narcotics prescriptions. "That has been our response to this problem," one participant states. One ED leader reports that opioids and antibiotics are prescribed 80% of the time when pain is the chief complaint. Participants say that in many instances ED providers "feel they don't have the background or the experience" to prescribe opioids. They further state that "right now we don't have a current approach to prescribing opioids that includes providing incentives to [ED providers]." One participant suggests working collaboratively with other professionals on "the process and structure and referral to treatment, rather than attempting to change prescriber behavior." "Doctors want to solve the problem and they wonder about the result." This participant explains that even when prescribing an opioid like hydrocodone, physicians focus on the number of pills prescribed, usually prescribing a lower number of pills, "12 pills from 20-30." This participant also feels that "there is a sense of helplessness around responding to addiction requiring other professions to improve treatment effectiveness." This suggests ED practitioners' need for interdisciplinary approach to support each other and help improve treatment.

Moreover, this participant explains that providing Medication Assisted Treatment (MAT) requires an interdisciplinary team effort, but currently is disjointed because "ED doctors' structure of work is in shifts. They go away!" ED physicians and ED practitioners understand there is a real opioid abuse problem; however, they do not have the time, energy, or even the incentive to treat ED patients from start to end. Creating dialog with ED providers seems to be key to educating them and changing their opioid diagnostics and prescribing behavior. Moreover, ED providers need to be engaged carefully otherwise "they get really defensive and it's not a very productive conversation." The consensus among participants was that by creating dialog between ED practitioners and interdisciplinary experts on opioid addictions and treatment, ED prescribers can move away from refilling prescriptions to focusing on treating and resolving some of the underlying issues of substance abuse.

Participants described several ways in which interdisciplinary collaborations can help ED practitioners improve their opioid prescriptions. One expert physician noted that one traditional approach is to become familiar with the state of the science regarding opioid addiction and treatment, coaching prescribers and telling positive stories. By understanding current methods of opioid addiction treatment, ED prescribers will gain confidence in their ability to properly treat opioid addiction, rather than continue to refill opioid prescriptions. One participant explained "coach[ing]" a senior ED attending physician through the decision process when a patient presented to the ED with opioid withdrawal symptoms. "Telling positive stories" of how ED practitioners saved their patients' lives by providing the opioid treatment they needed. This participant explained that "[ED practitioners] come on board once they see that it works or when they are shown evidence or support. Then it makes them a little more open." Participants suggested disseminating these types of success stories visually, perhaps through documentaries that retell the struggles and success of opioid addiction.

However, some participants noted that there is pushback against having ED practitioners initiate individuals with chronic opioid abuse on MAT. When they discussed poignant findings from an exploratory survey in the ED, "33% strongly agreed or agreed while the rest were uncertain to initiate MAT for OUD." In some instances, the hesitation to start MAT is based on not knowing if the patient will "follow up with treatment" or the provider being uncertain if treatment "will cause harm." But, as one participant stated, "if [they] read the papers and the science behind it, the ED doctors should all be like of course we're going to do this life saving treatment [initiate MAT in the ED]."

The lead presenter in the health systems science meeting explained that organizations can respond to change. They "can be proactive in basically having the systems in place to respond to that change in terms of leadership, management practices, [and] structures." The presenters further explain that:

Based on the systems approach, organizations are made up of the sub-systems and it is important that we engage these different sub-systems, so in the case of hospitals, of course, management vs. clinical, a lot of the cultural competency work started more on the clinical side and often times, the management was not engaged. It is important to have those two components together.

Overall, behavioral change among ED practitioners will take much effort, including changing the institutional culture to be less siloed and more based on collaboration, supported by dissemination of information on evidence-based treatment practices. At the institutional level, changing the ED prescriber's behavior may happen through the collaboration among professionals to adopt frameworks of change, such as the "Causal Model of Organizational Performance and Change." Although the focus has been on the behavior of the ED prescriber, the overall responsibility of fostering change should also be at the institutional level.

5.2 Team composition and effectiveness in the ED

Working in interdisciplinary teams in healthcare was deemed instrumental to new treatment implementation and the health outcomes of patients. However, teams were required to have certain characteristics in order to be effective. According to one participant in the interdisciplinary symposium, teams are described as bounded: "who's on the team and who's off the team." Teams are also interdependent: "there's a reason to be together and work together." The presenters further explained teams as having "some stability to the membership over time, norms of conduct, and some authority for executing work processes so they can't just be mindless in terms of just executing what leadership, and some process for them to determine how to do the work."

Team size was also considered important, especially for teams in healthcare. The presenters explained that "how large the team is can affect its effectiveness or affect the implementation of best practices. When teams become too heterogeneous it can be challenging for teams." Similarly, the presenters explained that too much diversity in the team is associated with worse outcomes for team functioning. The presenters also noted that "when professional identities are too disconnected, it's hard to find a common ground." Moreover, connections between teams, team climate, relational coordination, and psychological safety can influence the effectiveness of the team. The presenters suggested that if healthcare teams are structured appropriately, "they can yield all the things we want: implementation of evidence-based practices, the effectiveness of these practices, and improved patient care." Participants also noted that team science suggests that feedback should be provided to teams so as to make them more effective. In healthcare, patient instant feedback from a survey is not generally enough to determine team effectiveness. Overall, the impact healthcare teams have on implementation and patient care is highly dependent on the membership composition and purpose. Additionally, feedback loops, rather than a linear approach to providing feedback should be a part of efforts to improve how effective teams are in providing treatment.

6. Identity and relationship building

6.1 Professional identity and contributions to interdisciplinary research in the ED

Professional identity was discussed among the participants as it relates to the work they are doing and that needs to be done. Participants describe themselves as social workers, nurses, researchers, and physicians. They describe how their prior training and experiences help them effectively function in their current capacity. For instance, a participant who currently functions as a researcher describes formally working as a therapist and "dealing with a lot of clients seeking services for mental health needs." He acknowledges that mental health disorders are prevalent among those with substance abuse disorders. The same participant bridges the science of social work with the service provided. He states, "we know the research. We know what people need. We know certain things don't work. So, let's try to get involved in that."

The participant's perspective highlights the extent to which discipline-specific training informs knowledge and the conceptualization of one's role in the care delivery process, and within teams. These views are directly related to their value and contributions to an interdisciplinary approach to opioid addiction treatment. As a social worker, he understands how and where he fits into the spectrum of service delivery and treatment. Other participants in the field of social work share similar views. They have a "deep concern for not only understanding but solving issues that affect the most vulnerable. I try to do that through research, through understanding and through interventions." Another participant also in the field of social work adds that she "provides the best services possible to our consumers by being able to connect them with resources, housing, medication, case management therapy and everything." In general, social workers seem to have a genuine sense of service for those in need.

Interestingly, one participant who is a physician by training identifies as a physician only at work and endorses a different view of health care or special populations elsewhere. She states, "I don't really feel like that's my identity outside of work. I'll be like, oh, I work at a hospital, but as a physician at work, I guess, I have mixed opinions." She further highlights the characteristics of taking a non-traditional role as a physician by explaining, "I think of myself more as like an implementer, operation person and trying to take the tools and the knowledge of research and put that into practice, and trying to build a connection between research and what actually happens in real life." She understands that she can use her position as a physician to influence the desired change. She states that "there is a lot of opportunity for leadership and what I consider the right thing to do." She further explains that as a physician she cannot be the solution, but instead part of the solution, reiterating the importance of an interdisciplinary team approach.

7. Building effective organizational relationships in the ED

Building organizational relationships across disciplines has proven to be challenging on two fronts. First, individuals do not always know how to effectively build relationships across professions or disciplines. The importance of building relationships is not always fostered or even emphasized in medical school, for example. One participant explains, "I don't think we're given a lot of tools to understand how to build relationships. And then when you go to medical school it is very much a competitive thing as opposed to a collaborative thing. And I think that's changing slowly overtime, but it's one that the admission process seeks out to identify. I think you are studying with a baseline of students who tend to be like the gunner student in the class whose studying at four in the morning as opposed to building relationships."

Second, building relationships takes a significant amount of time. Even when a relationship is established with key figures, those individuals have to be willing to support new ideas. As the above participant notes, staff "wanted to do this [team building] three or four years ago, but I didn't know the pharmacy director. I didn't know people. To be like, hey, don't you think this would be cool? I think right now it's working and I think we're right at the point where I could give a lecture and the receptive 33% audience member says they're going to call me next time they have a case. And they called me the next time they had a case and we treated and they saw the miracle that happened when you actually treat substance abuse." Building relationships may be easy for some but challenging for others. In health care, workers are interdependent. Having the emotional intelligence to navigate different personalities can be as important as having the medical knowledge to save lives.

Another participant further explains that even after relationships are built, the relationships must be continuously nurtured. Individuals must build credibility among their colleagues, especially among those who are more resistant to changing the way they work. The presenters explain that "effective leadership can help build effective collaborations through influence and expert guidance." But it takes time to develop the leadership necessary to influence relationships. At the ED, building effective organizational relationships requires leaders who cultivate relationships over time and by gradually gaining buy-in from employees. "It is a trickle-down effect from top manager's leadership to direct service providers" and rely on this and other networks to improve their work. One presenter stated that "social networks are important for implementation, because these ties are conduits for information, for expertise, for social influence. A lot of different implementation strategies leverage these social networks. We try to find an opinion leader and have them exert their influence within an organization or a champion." One participant illustrates how their team is already doing this.

> *Isn't that kind of what we are doing? I mean how we have built a relationship with two leaders in the ED, a physician and a head nurse who are very involved in the ED and very passionate about this topic. It kind of helped us get in so we could build relationships with other nurses and physicians. They see us when we are going on Sundays. They say, hey you guys are here again, let me get some people for you. So, kind of just making ourselves present there so they get more comfortable knowing that we are there because we care about this topic. And then I'm sure they'll want to see us later and we can present it to them. I think we kind of started that and can continue building on it. "Building organizational relationships will facilitate the overall implementation of MAT. Over time, these relationships will be instrumental in influencing not only ED practitioners, but will have a greater influence at the organizational level."*

8. Discussion

The opioid epidemic poses several challenges for health professionals and health service delivery systems. The current study sought to understand the team process necessary for researchers to be more effective in tackling this wicked problem. From a systems perspective, the opioid epidemic can be ameliorated through a number of approaches that require high-level coordination and execution among teams. These include changing the way opioids are prescribed, how substance abuse is defined and treated, how collaborations across disciplines take place, the composition and effectiveness of healthcare teams, understanding professional identity, and building organizational relationships to improve collaboration and health outcomes (see **Table 2**). These are the themes identified in this study, but also consistent with the National Institute on Drug Abuse (NIDA) priorities to combat the opioid epidemic [12], as well as the NIDA's three-prong approach—reducing prescriptions, enhancing access to treatment and preventing overdoses—to address this epidemic [13]. Inherent in these priorities are interdisciplinary team approaches to effectively responding to the opioid epidemic.

The team-building activities undertaken in this study supported the key aspects of the cultural exchange framework, and are aligned with evidence informed approaches. These were 1) accessibility to one another; 2) a sense of mutual respect;

Themes	Strategies
Need for interdisciplinary understanding of substance abuse and mental health	Enhance physician knowledge of opioid addiction and related conditions, embed practitioners from other specialties who allow for a holistic approach to addressing the opioid epidemic
Interdisciplinary approaches to fight the opioid epidemic	Create an environment for collaborations fosters depth and high quality of conversations
Prescribing opioids and collaboration	Develop and implement institutional level policies and practices
Role of interdisciplinary team composition and team effectiveness	Determine the optimal mix of diversity in a team, and put in place feedback loops, rather than a linear approach to providing feedback
Role of professional identity to contribute to interdisciplinary research	Create a culture where problem solving, and professional identities are framed within the context of interdisciplinarity (professional identities are a key part of addressing operational problems)
Building effective organizational relationships	Provide opportunities for building leadership skills, and developing emotional intelligence

Table 2.
Themes and strategies.

3) creation of a shared language; and 4) willingness to compromise/accommodate the needs of others [8]. These activities increased access for all team members to discuss a variety of issues related to ED responses to the opioid epidemic. Team leaders created a sense of mutual respect across disciplines, and activities promoted the co-creation of language to define challenges and solutions for the ED to diagnose and treat OUD. The structured problem-solving activities, as well as the scholarly presentations and consensus group, allowed members to compromise with each other and accommodate new information to lead an effective interdisciplinary collaboration.

Member interactions ranged from building personal connection, sharing world views, to professional and scientifically focused detailing of strategies to break down the problems into different components. These team interactions helped identify barriers and facilitators to using the Science of Team Science framework. For instance, it was clear that physicians, nurses and social workers have and bring unique knowledge and competencies to the team (intrapersonal) that could either disconnect or expand the team knowledge. Yet, communication, connection, and shared knowledge among team members improved greatly with exposure to the team building activities (interpersonal).

8.1 Limitations

We should note limitations of the present study. The study used a small sample of researchers from different disciplines to obtain a deep understanding of how team building may enhance problem solving. Although derived from a small sample, the qualitative data were not intended to be representative of interdisciplinary teams, or researchers in ED systems. However, the themes that emerged from this work are consistent with concerns in the field [12, 13]. Furthermore, the comprehensive and multimethod approach to data collection used in this study is consistent with other research in behavioral health [14, 15]. Our results did not provide information about concrete outcomes, but rather to team building process generally, as intended. The physical environment was a barrier to team building – traveling in a large metropolis reduces interactions. The societal and political norms were however not evident. Participants discussed them in terms of hospital policies that prevented new medications from being included in prescribing schedules. Finally, technological issues were important in improving connection. Using video communication and presentations as well as text messaging reinforced the initiative. Future studies can build on our results and address these limitations by examining how each of the team building strategies we implemented influence the quality of decision making and effectiveness of problem-solving abilities of the team, and ultimately opioid use disorder treatment practices.

8.2 Conclusions and implications

This study highlighted the importance of building teams from a personal and general skill level to a more refined disciplinary knowledge and competencies. The team-building process appeared to be significant in building knowledge and connecting members at personal, professional, and disciplinary levels. Participants appreciated this level of connection to support their understanding and problem solving of the opioid epidemic. Health care systems should consider investing (i.e., funding, rewarding, structuring) in team building among experts from different disciplines to improve ways in which the ED can reduce risk of opioid use. Findings from this study have implications for investing in team-building activities to improve interdisciplinary approaches to wicked problems. In this process, it is important that each member of the team is meaningfully included, as well as empowered by the team process and to contribute their unique disciplinary approach. This is especially conducive to developing solutions to pressing issue of building ED capacity to respond to the opioid epidemic.

Acknowledgements

We would like to acknowledge the meaningful participation of colleagues at the Emergency Department at LAC + USC, as well as the research support from the Integrated Substance Abuse Treatment to Eliminate Disparities research team. This study was partly funded by USC Suzanne Dworak-Peck, School of Social Work and Research to End Healthcare Disparities Corp.

Conflict of interest

The authors declare no conflict of interest.

Abbreviations

ED	Emergency department
LAC + USC	Los Angeles County + University of Southern California
MAT	Medication assisted treatment
OUD	Opioid use disorder
SciTS	Science of team science

Author details

Erick Guerrero[1*], Jemima A. Frimpong[2], Angelique Hearn[1], Veronica Serret[1], Welmoed K. van Deen[3], Howard Padwa[4], Rebecca Trotzky-Sirr[5], Michael Menchine[5] and Daniel L. Howard[6]

1 I-Lead Institute, Research to End Healthcare Disparities Corp, Los Angeles, CA, USA

2 Social Science Division, New York University, Abu Dhabi, UAE

3 Cedars-Sinai Center for Outcomes Research and Education, Los Angeles, CA, USA

4 Integrated Substance Abuse Programs, University of California, Los Angeles, CA, USA

5 Emergency Department, Los Angeles County + University of Southern California, Los Angeles, CA, USA

6 Department of Psychological and Brain Sciences, Texas A&M University, University Station, TX, USA

*Address all correspondence to: erickguerrero454@gmail.com

References

[1] Head BW, Alford J. Wicked Problems: Implications for Public Policy and Management. Administration & Society 2015; 47: 711-739.

[2] Oxford University Press (OUP). INTERDISCIPLINARY | Definition of INTERDISCIPLINARY by Oxford Dictionary on Lexico.com also meaning of INTERDISCIPLINARY. *Lexico Dictionaries | English*, https://www.lexico.com/definition/interdisciplinary (accessed 27 June 2021).

[3] Guerrero EG, Moore H, Pitt-Catsouphes M. A Scientific Framework for Social Work Doctoral Education in the 21st Century - Erick G. Guerrero, Hadass Moore, Marcie Pitt-Catsouphes, 2018, https://journals.sagepub.com/doi/abs/10.1177/1049731517709077 (accessed 27 June 2021).

[4] Guerrero EG, Hahn EE, Khachikian T, et al. Interdisciplinary dissemination and implementation research to advance translational science: Challenges and opportunities. J Clin Transl Sci 2017; 1: 67-72.

[5] Hall KL, Vogel AL, Stipelman B, et al. A Four-Phase Model of Transdisciplinary Team-Based Research: Goals, Team Processes, and Strategies. Transl Behav Med 2012; 2: 415-430.

[6] Stokols D, Hall KL, Taylor BK, et al. The science of team science: overview of the field and introduction to the supplement. Am J Prev Med 2008; 35: S77-S89.

[7] Emmons KM, Viswanath K, Colditz GA. The role of transdisciplinary collaboration in translating and disseminating health research: lessons learned and exemplars of success. *Am J Prev Med* 2008; 35: S204-S210.

[8] Palinkas LA, Aarons GA, Chorpita BF, et al. Cultural Exchange and the Implementation of Evidence-Based Practices: Two Case Studies. Research on Social Work Practice 2009; 19: 602-612.

[9] Chin A. Tackling Wicked Problems: Through the Transdisciplinary Imagination Valerie A. Brown, John A. Harris & Jacqueline Y. Russell (Eds). Journal of Natural Resources Policy Research 2011; 3: 417-418.

[10] Choi BCK, Pak AWP. Multidisciplinarity, interdisciplinarity and transdisciplinarity in health research, services, education and policy: 1. Definitions, objectives, and evidence of effectiveness. Clin Invest Med 2006; 29: 351-364.

[11] Austin W, Park C, Goble E. From interdisciplinary to transdisciplinary research: a case study. Qual Health Res 2008; 18: 557-564.

[12] Volkow ND, Frieden TR, Hyde PS, et al. Medication-assisted therapies--tackling the opioid-overdose epidemic. N Engl J Med 2014; 370: 2063-2066.

[13] Volkow ND. Director's Page. *National Institute on Drug Abuse*, https://www.drugabuse.gov/about-nida/directors-page (2017, accessed 27 June 2021).

[14] Aarons GA, Green AE, Palinkas LA, et al. Dynamic adaptation process to implement an evidence-based child maltreatment intervention. Implementation Science 2012; 7: 32.

[15] Palinkas LA, Holloway IW, Rice E, et al. Social networks and implementation of evidence-based practices in public youth-serving systems: a mixed-methods study. Implementation Science 2011; 6: 113.

Chapter 11

Artificial Intelligence (AI) in Evidence-Based Approaches to Effectively Respond to Public Health Emergencies

Lap Yan Wong, Chun Kit Yip, Dao Shen Tan and Wai Lim Ling

Abstract

Artificial intelligence (AI) techniques have been commonly used to track, predict early warning, forecast trends, and model and measure public health responses. Statistics have traditionally been used to track public health crises. AI-enabled methods, such as machine learning and deep learning–based models, have exploded in popularity recently, complementing statistical approaches. A wide range of medical fields have used various well-developed deep learning algorithms. Surveillance of public health emergencies is one region that has gained greatly from AI advancements in recent years. One of the examples of effectively reacting to public health emergencies is the need for developing AI evidence-based approaches to public health strategies for the scientific community's response to the COVID-19 pandemic.

Keywords: Artificial Intelligence AI Public Health Emergencies

1. Introduction

In the first two decades of the twenty-first century, two big deadly epidemics posed a global public health challenge. Infectious disease known as serious acute respiratory syndrome (SARS) cases first appeared in 2002, and a novel coronavirus (SARS-CoV-2) was reported as the etiologic agent in coronavirus disease 2019 (COVID-19), with the start of a new outbreak at the end of 2019. SARS spread to five continents, prompting the World Health Organization (WHO) to declare the outbreak was caused by a novel pathogen, a member of the coronavirus family that had never been seen before in human history [1]. In 2019, a mysterious pneumonia outbreak occurred in Wuhan, China, which the WHO classified as a pandemic in March 2020 [2]. Globally, cases have been recorded in over 20 nations, regions, or territories across five continents [3].

The world is in the midst of a time of recurrent crises, and conventional crisis management models are struggling to cope with today's dynamic crises. The new crisis management system should be converted from a passive crisis response to a dominant crisis management system. It is essential to develop a modernization management system for effective crisis response, which should include the immediate implementation of basic preventive measures against emergencies, as well as accurate and rapid diagnosis for containment and clinical management. Furthermore, new developments in disease-related applied research and technology would be needed to slow the COVID-19 pandemic's spread.

The fields of medicine, research and development, and public health are all being transformed by artificial intelligence (AI) [4]. AI has taken over some routine tasks in the last decade, and its effect on repetitive tasks has already begun. We have all witnessed the information revolution, which in just a few decades has totally transformed the way people operate. The AI era has also resulted in the creation of intelligent advanced solutions for different aspects of life: AI can be used to optimize quantitative activities on a wide scale; it can be used to measure and practice a planned action or project under various conditions; and it can be used to assist in job optimization processes in various industries.

AI has reached a crucial juncture in its growth and implementation. Artificial neural networks, machine learning, and deep learning are examples of AI systems that have made substantial progress. In several tasks, AI algorithms have been able to mimic or even outperform the human brain. Machine learning, as opposed to traditional statistical analysis methods that use a predetermined equation as a model, can account for all interactions among variations and integrate new data to update algorithms [5]. Due to their important information processing properties in terms of nonlinearity, high levels of parallelism, noise and fault tolerance, as well as learning, generalization, and adaptive capabilities, AI systems are advantageous [6]. AI is not only a tool for assisting humans with all types of technological and mental tasks, but also an extension of their senses and abilities.

There is an immediate need for safety assurance and cost efficiency in the management of public health crises as a result of the recent global epidemic. Public health surveillance has benefited greatly as a result of recent AI advancements. There is an increasing body of knowledge in the field of AI-enabled and AI-enhanced public health monitoring research [7]. AI is becoming increasingly important in evidence-based approaches to efficiently respond to public health emergencies.

2. Public health emergency

2.1 Definition of public health emergency

Public health emergencies are a subset of public emergencies that are related to health incidents and have an inclusion and exclusion arrangement with public emergencies. The Emergency of Public Health (Emergency of Public Health) is described as "mainly including infectious diseases, mass diseases of unknown origin, food safety and occupational hazards, animal epidemics, and other events that seriously affect public health and life safety" in the "China National Overall Emergency Plan for Public Emergencies" promulgated on January 8, 2006.

2.2 Overview of AI application in public health

2.2.1 The stage of crisis recovery is important in the management of public health crises

The recovery phase in public health crisis management refers to the stage during which the crisis is gradually alleviated and eliminated. The flow of factors that trigger disasters has slowed, and public health emergencies have been effectively addressed. The government's goal at this time is to reduce the impact of public health crises, contribute to social and economic recovery, summarize crisis management flaws, and improve the experience of managing public health emergencies in crisis.

It is critical to use AI and other technologies to promote the resumption of work and development in order to ensure sustainable and stable economic growth. Intelligent network systems have been used in China [8] to carry out online workplace, online teaching, and other activities. Companies must "not close" during the epidemic, and schools must "suspend classes without suspension." During the nationwide "war epidemic," AI networks such as WeLink, DingTalk, and Tencent Conference were widely popularized in order to minimize the losses incurred by shutdowns and output shutdowns, which played a positive role in reducing crowd gathering and reducing the risk of cross-infection while going out [9]. On the other hand, using a big data platform to analyze the migration and traffic situation in each region, as well as AI technology to prevent the epidemic from resuming, and to genuinely achieve safe resumption of work and development. Manually processing these data makes it difficult to ensure the data's validity and timeliness. Experts use AI to assist them, collect crisis-related data, and determine the type of crisis [10]. Moreover, AI calculates the severity of the crisis' effects and analyzes the causes of the crisis. Furthermore, AI allows for early detection of a problem, allowing for more time to deal with it.

2.2.2 The use of AI to predict the results of public health emergencies

The period in which the crisis will break out in the crisis management of public health crises is referred to as the preparatory stage of crisis management for public health emergencies. Since the onset of public health emergencies is uncertain and unpredictable, it is important to track and alert them. For this stage, improving the ability to monitor and respond to public health emergencies is the main focus of the government's work. The preparatory stage of crisis management for public health emergencies consists of two parts: crisis early warning, crisis training and exercises [10].

Early notice of public health crises is a vital task in the planning stage of disaster prevention. When a crisis occurs, successful early warning will significantly speed up the organization's response time. To develop an infectious disease outbreak early warning system, governments of various countries currently depend primarily on conventional surveillance methods (collaboration of medical institutions at all levels, disease prevention and control centers, and influenza-like case monitoring sentinel hospitals, and medical institutions diagnose and record clinically diagnosed and confirmed cases of influenza). However, there are some disadvantages of this monitoring system: the data collected is from a single source, and there is no comparison or correction of data from other sources; the data acquisition process of daily sampling and weekly summary, the data results are comparatively lagging; the monitoring consumes a lot of manpower and material resources, and the monitoring covers the entire country; the monitoring consumes a lot of manpower and material resources, and the monitoring covers the entire country. The accuracy of the data would be affected by an error in any node in the network [10]. The use of AI to perform infectious disease forecasting and early warning work, as well as monitoring social media, online news posts, and government reports for signs of infectious disease outbreaks, can significantly assist relevant government agencies in keeping track of the epidemic, rationally allocating medical resources, and improving advances. The cost of national disease prediction and infection prevention and control is reduced by the success rate of prevention.

By scanning foreign language news stories, animal and plant disease reports, and various official statements, the AI system provided alerts to its customers, recognizing the first foreign alert of the epidemic at an early stage. Machine learning has been used to track, locate and report on infectious spread. It provides alerts to a wide range of clients, including health care, government, industry, and public health organizations. It also serves as an alert about the existence of a new coronavirus [11]. In several aspects of the global battle against the epidemic, AI has already played a valuable but fragmented role. Screening, contact tracing, contact alerts, diagnosis, automatic deliveries, and laboratory drug discovery are only a few of the applications. AI has already played a useful but fragmented role in many aspects of the global fight against the epidemic. It has been widely used in screening, contact tracing, contact alerts, diagnosis, automated deliveries, and laboratory drug discovery [11]. It also predicts whether or not a person is infectious in advance, as well as the seriousness of the infection. By doing some general data analysis, one can significantly reduce waiting time, determine whether or not one has come into contact with virus carriers, and prevent the virus from spreading. Systematic planning and drills are an important way to enhance emergency response in the event of a disaster. Knowledge map technology can be used in public health emergency training to combine and link all of the information in the knowledge base and create a bottom map that covers all knowledge and records the connections between knowledge and knowledge, significantly increasing the scope and depth of training. The use of AI technology to perform public health emergency simulation exercises, build public health emergency simulation scenarios, deduce public health emergency handling protocols, and summarize the effects of public health emergency crisis exercises. It will help the government assess the epidemic's condition, develop decision-making and deployment capabilities for epidemic prevention and control, and test a range of mature response plans in simulation, setting the groundwork for potential rapid response and precise policy implementation in actual combat in the future [18].

Is it a Cough or a Covid? COVID-19 Detection Using Artificial Intelligence from Cough Sounds.

Increased disease screening and early warning capabilities can help to dramatically delay the spread and effect of a disease. Recent progress in developing deep learning AI models to classify cough sounds as a COVID-19 prescreening tool has shown early promise. Cough-based diagnosis is a non-invasive, cost-effective, and scalable method of diagnosing COVID-19 that, if approved, could be a game-changer in the battle against the virus. Cough sounds have recently been tested as a preliminary diagnostic or a prescreening technique for Covid-19 identification in asymptomatic individuals by AI researchers [11]. This is advantageous because the virus can trigger subtle changes in the body that can be identified by complex algorithms combining audio signal processing and machine learning, even though no symptoms are present. This technology may also be more efficient than the standard strategy of prescreening for COVID-19 based on temperature, especially in asymptomatic patients.

2.2.3 AI accelerating healthcare outcomes

AI expands data access. AI's predictive ability is based on the volume and variety of data available; optimizing emerging tools requires extensive data access across the healthcare ecosystem. To prevent gaming of findings and prejudice, data scientists must commit to robust research over several parameters. AI allows for more concentrated collaboration. Thousands of inputs must be incorporated by scientists and technologists in collaboration with clinical specialist physicians, including lab results, vital signs, drug administration, prescription doses and durations, length of stay in hospital, and patient and hospital demographics, to name a few. Clinicians can participate in the validation process and feature engineering for each organ- or condition-specific version of an AI surveillance system so that the solution can produce customized, actionable risk scores that clinicians will use. Moreover, transparency in clinical surveillance is aided by AI. These surveillance solutions can enable clinicians to apply their own clinical judgment to the performance by offering a visual representation of how and why AI made the predictions. Any AI-enabled tool should do the same thing to promote clinician buy-in and the requisite change management for widespread adoption.

2.3 AI aids decision-making by simulating a real-life epidemic

The government's approaches or policies to combat the outbreak are unquestionably important in effectively controlling the virus's spread. AI can be used to help them make the best decision possible.

Key parameters that define the characteristics of the spread, such as the transmission rate, incubation time, population density in the region, and so on, can be used to create a simulated model that mimics the actual environment of pandemics.

Following the development of the environment simulator, Reinforcement Learning can be used to determine the best strategy for achieving our aim of preventing virus spread while minimizing economic costs.

2.3.1 The SIR models

A simple compartmental model in epidemiology, known as the SIR model, is commonly used to simulate the spread of disease [12]. S represents the number Susceptible/Healthy individuals, I represents the number of Infectious individuals and R represents the number of Recovered individuals. It can be modeled by the below set of ordinary differential equations:

$$\frac{dS}{dt} = -\frac{\beta IS}{N} \tag{1}$$

$$\frac{dI}{dt} = \frac{\beta IS}{N} - \gamma I$$

$$\frac{dR}{dt} = \gamma I,$$

where N is the total population, β is the probability of disease transmission in a contact between a susceptible and an infectious subject. γ is the probability of an infectious individual being recovered in dt.

2.3.1.1 The agent-based model

The SIR model is a fundamental model for studying individual flow between compartments, assuming that all individuals within a compartment are homogeneous. An Agent-Based Model is developed to simulate the behavior of heterogeneous individuals, taking into account their characteristics [13, 14].

We may, for example, identify various types of agents, such as individuals, families, businesses, and governments, and then enable them to communicate with one another. Each type of agent may have different attributes, such as age, location of the person, location of the house/business, and wealth of the agents. Different activities, such as going to work, going home, or making business connections, can be simulated at different times.

Different social, epidemiological, and economic parameters, such as individual mobility, incubation, transmission, recovery time, income, and GDP, must be specifically defined by domain experts, using empirical evidence, or designed by the author to simulate the attributes and actions of agents. During simulation, the economic impact and pandemic statistics, such as individual wealth and the number of active cases, can be generated for evaluation.

2.3.1.2 Reinforcement learning

Reinforcement Learning (RL) is an area of machine learning that focuses on learning strategies or sequential decisions in order to optimize long-term reward in the defined environment.

A basic reinforcement learning model is shown in **Figure 1** [15]. It involves an Agent who interacts with the environment in each time steps by taking different actions. At time t, the agent will receive the current State S_t of the environment and the current Reward R_t. The agent will perform Action A_t based on the *policy* and S_t . Then, the environment will move from current State S_t to the next State S_{t+1} and the associated "reward" R_{t+1} will be output. The state S_{t+1} and reward R_{t+1} will be fed back to the agent. The process iterates until the terminal state is reached. The goal of the model is to learn the *policy* which optimizes the cumulative reward.

To train the RL model and learn the optimal policy, one way is to use Monte Carlo Tree Search, which is a searching algorithm to determine the best moves. It repeated the process of "Selecting → Expanding → Simulating → Updating" to update the nodes in a tree (**Figure 2**) [16]. Each node in the tree represents the action we can take, with a node value which can be the probability of winning or the expected reward. At "Selecting" stage, we select the path by the value of the node until we reach the leaf node at the end of the branch. At the leaf node, we "Expand" by randomly choosing the action from the action space. Then, we "Simulate" the complete rollout, until the terminal state and obtain the final cumulative reward. The reward will then be backpropagated to update the values in each node along the path.

RL, in combination with the Agent-Based Model and the SIR model, will help the government make the best decision possible to combat the pandemic [17]. The state and the environment in RL can be simulated by the Agent-Based Model and SIR Model.

The reward function can be designed based on the pandemic statistics and economic statistics generated from the Agent-Based Model. The trained RL model will

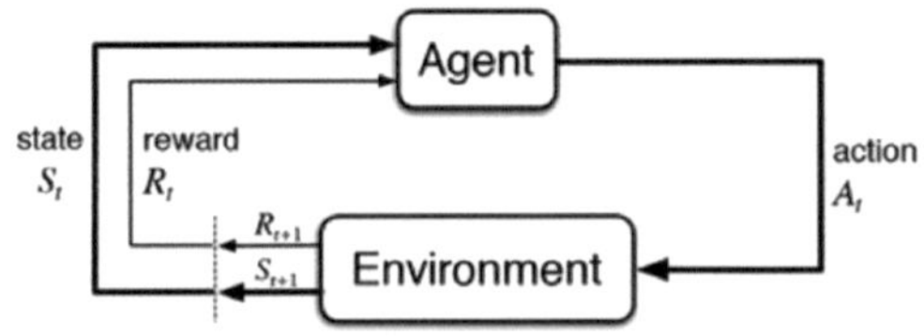

Figure 1.
Basic reinforcement learning model.

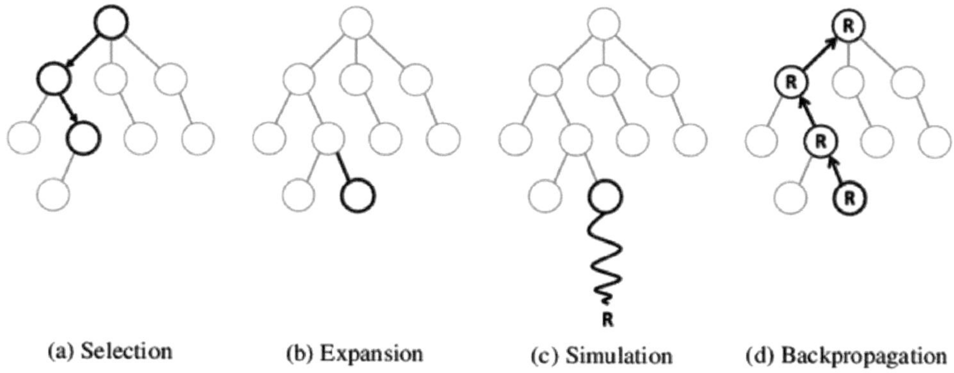

Figure 2.
Phases of the Monte Carlo tree search algorithm. A search tree, rooted at the current state, is grown through repeated application of the above four phases.

be able to advise the government on the best course of action to take at various stages of the pandemic and scenarios in order to contain the pandemic with the least amount of economic effect. The agent is to be trained with empirical demographic data, pandemic data and economic data in pandemic time to simulate the impacts of policies conditioned with the predicted pandemic data. An Action space can be defined. Social distancing, lockdown, company and school closures, wearing a face mask, doing nothing, public hygiene promotion and so on. The impact of policies can be highly dimensioned vectors and subject to execution error. However, all these attributes can be inputs of the simulations and the prediction error can be reduced by more data input.

With the numerous simulations, government can have a full profile of impacts of policies to be taken in different scenarios by making assumption on the parameters of the effectiveness of policy, say the shut-down of schools reduce the younger age group infection by {38.2%, 50%, 61.8%}, and the impact of this reduction can be propagated to other age groups through a trained Boltzmann Machine which depict the dynamics of infection rate between the age groups. The fidelity of the simulations is correlated with the complexity of model and number of data used to train the model.

The reward functions can deviate across regions; however the reward function can be designed based on the pandemic statistics and economic statistics generated from the Agent-Based model. The trained RL model would allow the government to select the optimal policy and evaluate the drawbacks before the policy is implemented.

2.4 Public health emergencies accelerate the implementation of AI

Many AI technologies, such as robots assisting in hospital transportation, have accelerated as a result of the epidemic's social isolation. One of the most contentious examples is contact tracing. Many countries around the world have successfully developed contact tracing systems, allowing them to efficiently monitor the epidemic's spread. This strategy, however, is seen as an infringement of privacy in the United States, Europe, and other countries. Although it has a bright future, there are challenges in the areas of privacy, data processing, ethics, and social issues. When it comes to medical information, these questions must be seriously addressed in the light of public health or personal health. During a public health crisis, the government must strike a balance between citizens' rights and the need for effective prevention and control measures to efficiently control disease transmission until the outbreak is over, and then return to normal.

No one wants to replicate the epidemic's mistakes. AI will be used in the future to prevent epidemics from arising and spreading. Hospitals will make effective use of sensors and wearable devices to collect outbreak data and report possible hazards in a timely manner, allowing them to properly respond to the crisis and avoid losing control again. Inevitably, privacy concerns would arise in the former. There are some notable inconsistencies between privacy rights and the requirements of machine learning. Although privacy security necessitates as little data sharing as possible, machine learning necessitates as much data as possible. Many countries are concerned that misuse of contact tracing could compromise privacy, so they have developed and implemented a variety of privacy security technologies. AI techniques, processes, and technology are being used to develop health care and programs. The good news is that they can coexist, and AI is a double-edged sword that can help to foster global governance and cultural change.

2.4.1 AI enables and promotes medical reform and public health emergencies by speeding up their incorporation into the medical system

Deep learning has the ability to process multidimensional data at high speeds while also facilitating the recognition of unique features, making it one of AI's most far-reaching applications. Deep learning and deep neural networks have already been widely used in a variety of medical applications, including medical image recognition, drug design, decision support, and predictive analytics, to deliver accurate and rapid algorithmic interpretation [18]. A straightforward blueprint for how AI will be infused into health care as a result of the pandemic. The most accurate insights into health and disease can come from all of the world's results. AI will assist us in being adequately prepared for the next pandemic, efficiently responding to public health monitoring and emergencies, and advancing global healthcare systems.

2.4.2 AI-enhanced data analysis for outbreak detection, early warning and flow adjustment

In order to enhance the timeliness and accuracy of outbreak detection and early warning approaches, public health researchers continuously analyze and explore sensor data and indicators to and from the physical world, including health, environmental, social, financial, and economic aspects, among others. Deep learning has been used to identify multiple infectious disease outbreaks. A dynamic neural network model was created to predict the probability of infectious disease outbreaks in the United States, such as Zika virus (ZIKV). Decision-makings can easily modify the risk of an indicator, the risk classification system, and the forecast window for prediction based on their own unique needs [19]. Support vector machine (SVM), gradient boosting machine, and random forest (RF) were applied to simulate the global distribution of infectious diseases. To train the models, multidimensional and multidisciplinary datasets were qualified and quantified, such as social variables, incident medical records, high-risk areas, and cyberspace data. The suitability of the temperature has been stated to have the best discriminatory power among variables, and random forest (RF) is known to obtain the highest area under curve (AUC) value [20]. Each bootstrap sample was fitted with an unpruned decision tree. The risk maps were accurate in over 80% of the observed risk ranks falling within the 80% prediction interval, according to random bootstrap samples drawn from the results [21]. The use of data from the cyberspace, such as keyword google searches, Key Opinion Leaders' blogs, and social media networking messages, has taken significant effort. Machine learning has been used for sentiment analysis and text classification from social media data for surveillance purposes. In India, a social media-based early warning system for mosquito-borne disease has been proposed [18].

2.4.3 What are the latest effects of intelligent early detection of infectious diseases, and what does this mean for the global battle against the epidemic in the future?

There are a number of major effects: For instance, there was no intelligent big data research in the past. The network accounts of various hospitals could not be compared after a single patient was diagnosed with an infectious disease. Now, using AI's dynamic perception, the device may display an outbreak or cluster of infectious disease under uncommon conditions in real time via case reports. Second, the use of AI technology to evaluate the infectious case's time, space, and meteorological factors may have an effect on the local agricultural product market and economic conditions. Third, disease patterns can be forecast and early alerts for key ties can be issued using infectious disease data and local environmental monitoring. While AI's dynamic models of infectious diseases are consistent, the neural network model of experts must be introduced because infectious diseases have different epidemics in different regions.

2.5 Suggestions for accelerating AI-enabled public health emergency crisis response

2.5.1 Strengthen scientific research

The AI industry should concentrate on core technology research and development in order to address technological challenges. Overall, the application of AI technology for disease prevention and control is still in its early stages of growth. Furthermore, AI also has an inexplicability that prevents it from being fully incorporated into the epidemiological system. The use of AI technology in disease prevention has been hampered by the lack of timely data collection and integration capabilities. As a result, play a bigger role in command. Epidemic modeling can be used to perform theoretical research on interpretability and improve the processing of large multi-dimensional data to this end.

2.5.2 Expand AI application scenarios

AI has been commonly used in the medical field as a result of continuous optimization of medical data and algorithm models. AI has achieved a great improvement in work efficiency in a subversive way, particularly during this special time of the new crown epidemic, and has spawned new demands. The use of AI has demonstrated quick landings, a wide range of effects, and major effects. However, AI in disease prevention and control is still in its early stages of research, and there are still flaws and issues in many areas. The use of AI in disease prevention and control should be thoroughly investigated, and a set of creative and reliable AI approaches should be used to aid in the detection and treatment of epidemics, as well as to minimize the risk of staff cross-infection. Improve disease management and control effectiveness, and provide strong scientific and technical support for winning the fight against epidemic prevention and control.

3. Using AI to solve the issue of public health emergencies

AI models have been applied to detect outbreaks of infectious diseases. Researchers have a long history of successfully developing a global outbreak surveillance approach using Internet-based approaches. Internet-based disease tracking approaches have provided a real-time alternative to conventional indicator-based public health disease surveillance [22, 23]. Internet-based monitoring systems use a range of open-source Internet data, including online news and social media, as well as other Internet-based data sources, to detect early warning signals of threats to public health. AI techniques have played a significant role in a series of data processing and analysis activities. AI techniques have recently become popular for completing tasks in highly dynamic, complex, and data-rich environments. In the modern age of public health approaches, it is critical and important. Machine learning and deep learning as AI core technologies are among the most important, methodologically, for fundamental and increasing interests, intense research activities in the interdisciplinary field of AI. Despite the impressive list of achievements already achieved, AI technologies in the sense of public health and public health monitoring are still in their early stages of growth, with a lot of potentials yet to be realized. Outbreak identification, early warning, trend prediction, and public health evidence-based approaches effectively response modeling and assessment are among the core tasks of public health surveillance and response, particularly in light of the current COVID-19 pandemic.

3.1 Using AI to deal with public health emergencies

By pinpointing specific demographics or geographies where population health issues exist, AI and machine learning can help to target and precisely implement education and treatment programs and reduce spending waste. AI enables computers to mimic the cognitive function of human minds, and machine learning gives computers the ability to learn without being explicitly programmed. By using AI and machine learning to review vast sets of real-time data, health experts can identify at-risk populations for any number of diseases, from diabetes to heart disease. Throughout the coronavirus pandemic, the industry has witnessed the power of clinical surveillance. With a broad array of discrete tests that can identify a COVID-19 infection, health systems and public health authorities have needed a way to interpret and track the patients with infections.

3.1.1 Connecting the data with surveillance

Data is at the heart of clinical surveillance. When data is combined with evidence-based clinical decision support, a single source of reality can be created that connects the disease's related symptoms, allowing for the discovery of how quickly a disease is progressing and what lab tests reveal. Keeping up with the latest advances in medical terminology and the related diagnosis and procedure codes is critical for recognizing clinical patterns as well as securing support, funding and reimbursement. Many health systems have transitioned to finding out the patterns in COVID-19 and better predicting respiratory and organ failures associated with the virus, despite being reluctant to implement technology in the past.

When the pandemic struck, healthcare providers immediately shifted their focus to include COVID-19 updates in their clinical surveillance activities. Hospitals and healthcare systems have been able to proactively monitor patient status for earlier interventions and broaden data flow in significant ways with a centralized, global view of COVID-19 cases coupled with real-time alerting. Age, where the disease was possibly contracted, if the patient was examined, and how long the patient was in the ICU are only a few of the important patient measurements that have been monitored. Patients' pre-existing conditions were taken into account during surveillance. This data trail assists providers in developing a constantly evolving coronavirus profile and provides key data points for reporting to state and local governments and public health agencies. Clinical monitoring now brings together information from various areas of the hospital and clinics into a centralized view of COVID care, such as lab results, patient data, co-morbidities, mortality, and drugs, since there are no other ways to put together seemingly fragmented information.

3.1.2 COVID-19 accelerated AI advancements

COVID-19 puts people at risk of sepsis, so they wanted to identify those who were most at risk. Many AI-powered fast-tracking techniques were put to the test. This health epidemic shows what can be done to anticipate and avoid a variety of chronic health concerns. This technology can then be used to save lives and money in cases where prevention has proven to be ineffective. To achieve those savings, it is necessary to refine the use of AI for clinical surveillance; 2) extend access to everything from electronic health records (EHR) to knowledge that exists outside of direct clinical settings, ranging from the omics to social determinants of health; and 3) differentiate AI hype from solutions that offer proven, actionable insights for specific clinical concerns.

3.1.3 The future of AI's prospects in clinical emergencies

Though COVID-19 appeared to be a test ground for machine learning and AI, the industry had been focusing on harnessing technology's power for healthcare-associated infections (HAI) for some time. According to publicly available reports, HAIs cost the US healthcare system up to $45 billion a year [24]. On any given day, about one out of every 31 patients will be infected with at least one HAI [25]. One example is *C. difficile* infections (C. diff). C. diff raises the risk of inpatient death and duration of stay, putting hospitals at risk of financial penalties. Machine learning, on the other hand, will predict which patients are at risk for C. diff infection, allowing physicians to treat patients more effectively and avoid the spread of the infection in hospitals. Hundreds of thousands of variables that may lead to C. diff, as well as how those factors interact, are analyzed using machine learning. It is always learning and incorporating new data and information. Machine learning, when used in a clinical surveillance system, may identify at-risk patients before their infection progresses, adding variables that physicians frequently find difficult to detect when handling several patients, as well as conditions that are outside of their normal scope of practice.

Rules-based systems are less effective for these "edge" scenarios, as researchers know, since each new data feature necessitates a new rule. AI at warp speed will help hospitals and communities respond to complex cases like COVID-19, C. diff, and even sepsis until clusters, outbreaks, or critical medical emergencies worsen. Clinical surveillance based on AI can monitor when relevant factors arise in a specific way and understand how timing plays a role in interactions. Time is difficult to incorporate, but recognizing when the white blood cell count has increased or decreased, for example, is crucial to make reliable C. diff predictions.

These types of forecasts can make a huge difference in clinical emergencies like brain injury, heart arrest, and respiratory failure in healthcare organizations all over the world - cases where minutes can mean the difference between life and death. Clinical surveillance with AI has the ability to provide next-generation decision-support resources that incorporate powerful technology, public health's preventive emphasis, and clinicians' diagnosis and treatment expertise. As a result, surveillance has the potential to play a key role in achieving the quality and cost goals that our industry has long pursued.

4. Conclusion

Overall, the use of AI technology for disease prevention and control is still in its early stages of investigation; there is an inexplicability about AI that prevents it from being effectively incorporated into the epidemiological system, and data collection and integration capacity building is still lacking. Due to lag and other problems, AI technology has been largely restricted from playing a larger role in epidemics prevention and control. To that end, disease modeling should be used for theoretical interpretability analysis, and large multi-dimensional data processing capacities should be enhanced to compensate for the corresponding technological flaws. However, it is important to understand and acknowledge the weaknesses and potentially major prejudices associated with public health big data, and there is still space for improvement. To comply with social ethics and norms, intellectual properties in algorithm methodologies and interpretability, as well as privacy security, should be given serious consideration. AI-enabled and –enhanced evidence-based public health monitoring and response, as seen in various AI applications in the medical sector, has real potential, but there are major challenges ahead.

Acknowledgements

We would like to thank Dr. Zheng Xiang from the University of Hong Kong for his support in the literature review.

Conflict of interest

The authors declare no conflict of interest.

Author details

Lap Yan Wong*, Chun Kit Yip, Dao Shen Tan and Wai Lim Ling
ALOM Intelligence Limited, Hong Kong SAR, China

*Address all correspondence to: drwongleo@gmail.com

References

[1] Ksiazek T, Erdman D, Goldsmith C, et al. A Novel Coronavirus Associated with Severe Acute Respiratory Syndrome. N Engl J Med. 2003;348: 1953-1966. DOI: 10.1056/NEJMoa030781

[2] Velavan P and Meyer G. The COVID-19 epidemic. Trop Med Int Health. 2020;25(3): 278-280. DOI: 10.1111/tmi.13383

[3] European Centre for Disease Prevention and Control. COVID-19. Available from: https://www.ecdc.europa.eu/en/geographical-distribution-2019-ncov-cases

[4] Huang C, Xiang Z, Zhang Y, et al. Using deep learning in a monocentric study to characterize maternal immune environment for predicting pregnancy outcomes in the recurrent reproductive failure patients. Frontiers in Immunology. DOI: 10.3389/fimmu.2021.642167

[5] Waljee A, Joyce J, Wang S, et al. Algorithms outperform metabolite tests in predicting response of patients with inflammatory bowel disease to thiopurines. Clin Gastroenterol Hepatol. 2010;8(2):143-150. DOI: 10.1016/j.cgh.2009.09.031

[6] Basheer I and Hajmeer MN Artificial Neural Networks: Fundamentals, Computing, Design, and Application. Journal of microbiological methods. 2001;43:3-31. DOI: 10.1016/S0167-7012(00)00201-3

[7] Zeng D, Cao Z and Neill DB. Artificial intelligence–enabled public health surveillance—from local detection to global epidemic monitoring and control. Artificial Intelligence in Medicine. 2021;437-453. DOI: 10.1016/B978-0-12-821259-2.00022-3

[8] The State Council of the People's Republic of China. Available from http://www.gov.cn/jrzg/2006-01/08/content_150878.htm

[9] Guo Z, Zhu C, Xia J, et al. Considerations on the Future Development of Smart City Under the "Examination of Epidemic Situation". Designing Techniques of Posts and Telecommunications. 2020;(2):5-8

[10] Zhang Y and Yang Y. The Research on the Response Methods of the Government Network Public Opinions Crisis Based on 4R Crisis Management Theory. Journal of Modern Information. 2017; 37(9): 75-80, 92. DOI: 10.3969/j.issn.1008-0821.2017.09.011

[11] Wired. Covid-19 Will Accelerate the AI Health Care Revolution [Internet]. 2020. Available from: https://www.wired.com/story/covid-19-will-accelerate-ai-health-care-revolution/

[12] Alanazi S, Kamruzzaman M, Alruwaili M, et al. Measuring and Preventing COVID-19 Using the SIR Model and Machine Learning in Smart Health Care. Journal of Healthcare Engineering. 2020; vol. 2020, Article ID 8857346, 12 pages. DOI: 10.1155/2020/8857346

[13] Vyklyuk Y, Manylich M, Škoda M, et al. Modeling and analysis of different scenarios for the spread of COVID-19 by using the modified multi-agent systems - Evidence from the selected countries. 2020. DOI: 10.1016/j.rinp.2020.103662

[14] Silva P, Batista P, Lima H, et al. COVID-ABS: An agent-based model of COVID-19 epidemic to simulate health and economic effects of social distancing interventions. Chaos, Solitons & Fractals. 2020. arXiv:2006.10532v2 [cs.AI]. DOI: 10.1016/j.chaos.2020.110088.

[15] Sutton R and Barto A Reinforcement Learning An Introduction. MIT Press; 2018. ISBN 9780262193986.

[16] James S, Konidaris G, Rosman B. An Analysis of Monte Carlo Tree Search. In: Proceedings of the Thirty-First AAAI Conference on Artificial Intelligence (AAAI-17); 2017; USA. https://ojs.aaai.org/index.php/AAAI/article/view/11028

[17] Kompella V, Capobianco R, Jong S, et al. Reinforcement Learning for Optimization of COVID-19 Mitigation Policies. 2020. arXiv:2010.10560 [cs.LG]

[18] Baldi P. Deep Learning in Biomedical Data Science. Annual Review of Biomedical Data Science. 2018. Vol. 1:181-205. DOI: 10.1146/annurev-biodatasci-080917-013343

[19] Akhtar M, Kraemer M, Gardner L. A dynamic neural network model for predicting risk of Zika in real-time. BMC Med. 2019;17:171. DOI: 10.1186/s12916-019-1389-3

[20] Ding F, Fu J, Jiang D, et al. Mapping the spatial distribution of Aedes aegypti and Aedes albopictus. Acta Trop. 2018;178:155 62. DOI: 10.1016/j.actatropica.2017.11.020

[21] Ong J, Liu X, Rajarethinam J, et al. Mapping dengue risk in Singapore using Random Forest. PLoS Negl Trop Dis. 2018;12(6). DOI: 10.1371/journal.pntd.0006587

[22] Jain V, Kumar S Effective surveillance and predictive mapping of mosquito-borne diseases using social media. J Computat Sci. 2018;25:406 15. DOI: 10.1016/j.jocs.2017.07.003

[23] Anno S, Hara T, Kai H, et al. Spatiotemporal dengue fever hotspots associated with climatic factors in Taiwan including outbreak predictions based on machine-learning. Geospat Health. 2019;14(2). DOI: 10.4081/gh.2019.771

[24] Stone PW Economic burden of healthcare-associated infections: an American perspective. Expert Rev Pharmacoecon Outcomes Res. 2009;9(5):41422. DOI: 10.1586/erp.09.53

[25] Centers for Disease Control and Prevention. Available from: https://www.cdc.gov/hai/data/portal/index.html

Chapter 12

Management of Healthcare Waste in Healthcare Emergencies

Julius Manjengwa

Abstract

Proper management of waste in healthcare emergencies is key to preventing spread of infections within an emergency. The risks of poor waste management are varied with the risks of spreading infectious diseases being the most important to consider. Chemical pollution should also be considered as water sources can easily be polluted. Careful thought and planning including a risk assessment should be carried out and the results should be publicized to create a common understanding of the problem at hand. This will also inform the methods to be used for the management of waste. Training of healthcare workers is key to creating common understanding of the problem at hand. The different types of waste to be generated should be well understood and methods to manage it should be well thought out before implementation. The decision on the different methods used to manage waste should be informed by the risk assessment and the available resources. However effectiveness to deal with the waste produced should be considered above all factors. Proper healthcare waste management is imperative to preventing further infections that might not be part of the original healthcare emergency. Planning to manage waste is a process that requires information before implementation.

Keywords: Waste management, Risk Assessment, healthcare emergency, infections, chemical pollution

1. Introduction

Correct disposal of waste is critical in public health and even more critical in healthcare emergencies to improve safety. Existing collection and disposal systems can also be disrupted when there are unexpected volumes of certain types of health care waste as a result of healthcare emergencies. In some cases like, non-healthcare settings (quarantine centers, holding areas, designated hotels, households and refugee camps for displaced people) there might not be any provisions for managing healthcare waste. If healthcare waste is not dealt with quickly and appropriately enough it has the potential to worsen the situation. Waste from healthcare settings can be varied and includes used needles, syringes, soiled dressings, body parts, dead bodies, pharmaceuticals, medical devices, and laboratory related waste.

In order to better manage healthcare waste strict segregation is key as the bulk of the waste is non-infectious waste that can be managed by simpler methods. Poor segregation might lead to an increase in the volume of infectious waste as once mixed you cannot separate the waste and all the waste will now be treated as infectious. In general non-infectious waste constitute 75–90% of all healthcare waste while only 10–25% of the waste is clinical waste. The focus is on the 10–25% of the waste produced that is infectious. Depending on the type and cause of health care emergency the clinical waste can be sharps, chemicals, radioactive waste, genotoxic waste, pathological waste, pharmaceutical waste and dead bodies.

Healthcare emergencies as a result of an infectious diseases outbreak can lead to increased amount of infectious waste. In the event of a disease that is of a respiratory nature (like TB and COVID-19) surgical masks will be needed to reduce human to human transmissions in everyday life as well as to reduce infections from patients to healthcare workers. The disposal of the face masks in non-healthcare settings requires a different perspective as the waste is now being generated even at household level. Use of latex or plastic gloves can also be encouraged in cases where diseases are spread by contact. This also significantly rises the amount of waste produced outside of healthcare settings. How this waste is managed needs special attention and strong policies. In order to better manage this level of waste production it is important to make sure that new lines of waste management are also opened beyond the usual hospital set up.

In non-emergency situations, the amount of waste produced is stable and easily managed with usual routes and methods. The integrated management of healthcare waste that comprises segregation, collection, storage, transportation and treatment should be significantly enhanced when there is a healthcare emergency. The entire chain should be adequately monitored in order to secure the waste at all stages. In order to better manage the waste introduction of mobile treatment facilities use of microwaves, steam disinfection can be used as innovations. The best available waste treatment technologies should be selected together with transitional methods that can be used to manage healthcare waste on an interim basis. However incinerations remains one of the most important ways of managing waste.

1.1 Risks of poor waste management

In emergency situations the major issues are generation of high volumes of healthcare waste in healthcare settings or generation of health waste in non-healthcare settings. This can overwhelm the existing settings leading to improper management of waste.

The immediate effects of improper healthcare waste management is visual nuisance and serious smells. Healthcare waste is known to be a source of contamination and forms a part of the transmission routes of certain diseases through

i. Direct contact: this can result in needle stick injuries, direct ingestion. The risk with needle stick injuries is the transmission of Hepatitis B, C and HIV which are the most commonly transmitted blood borne pathogens. Injection drug users who do not normally have access to sterile needles can end using any sharps they find in their way leading to transmission of diseases. In areas where people scavenge waste sharps, drugs and other disposables can end up being repacked and being resold. Depending on the route of transmission and type of healthcare emergency other pathogens also become important. During the Ebola outbreak management of dead bodies became key as contact with dead bodies became a significant route or transmission further exacerbating the healthcare emergency. Corona viruses are known to survive outside of the body for days.

ii. Transmission by air: smoke emissions containing pathogens ad hazardous by products like carbon monoxide, dioxin, furans heavy metals and more specific chemicals when expired drugs are burnt.

iii. Pollution of water and environment: Untreated waste can contaminate surface and ground water from pathogens and chemicals. Organisms like Hepatitis A virus, clostridium tetani, polio viruses and fecal coliforms survive in water and soil.

iv. Contact via vectors: Flies carry diseases from one place to another and poorly managed waste can be a source of the pathogens that will be carried by the flies. There are also animal vectors like rodents who carry dangerous pathogens like yersinia pestis (Plague), tularemia and Lassa fever viruses among others [1].

It is important to avoid creation of another healthcare crisis as a result of poor management of waste. Some of the diseases like cholera, plague and Lassa fever have epidermic potential making it important to prioritize healthcare waste management. This chapter explores available methods of managing healthcare waste in healthcare emergencies. The efficacy of the different methods of managing waste are described fully.

2. Preparing to manage waste

In order to protect the environment the waste management hierarchy is a useful tool in guiding how waste is managed. In healthcare emergencies however, it is not always possible to follow this hierarchy. Disposal becomes a common way of dealing with health care waste in healthcare emergencies as either the waste is produced in non-healthcare settings or the amount of waste overwhelms the usual healthcare settings (**Figure 1**).

The modern methods of medicine are such that it is not possible to completely prevent the generation of waste. It is very important that the generation of waste be minimized to the lowest possible level. The types of waste generated most healthcare settings are described below.

2.1 Categories of waste

Waste can be categorized as follows:

Management of waste is highly dependent on knowing the type of waste that is being generated. It is important that facilities take time to evaluate the type of waste that is being generated and to create the necessary awareness about the waste being produced.

The advent of a healthcare emergency should call for a comprehensive risk assessment that Is all encompassing. This needs to be carried out by competent health and safety professional together with other health care professionals.

2.2 Risk assessment

Healthcare emergencies present with risks of exposures to different types of health hazards. It is recommended that a full risk assessment be carried out and all possible exposure scenarios assessed and controlled. The exposure analysis should focus on healthcare workers, waste handlers, the public and the environment.
All types of healthcare waste should be assessed (refer to **Table 1** above) and best ways of handling it described. In some cases a waste needs assessment might be useful [3].

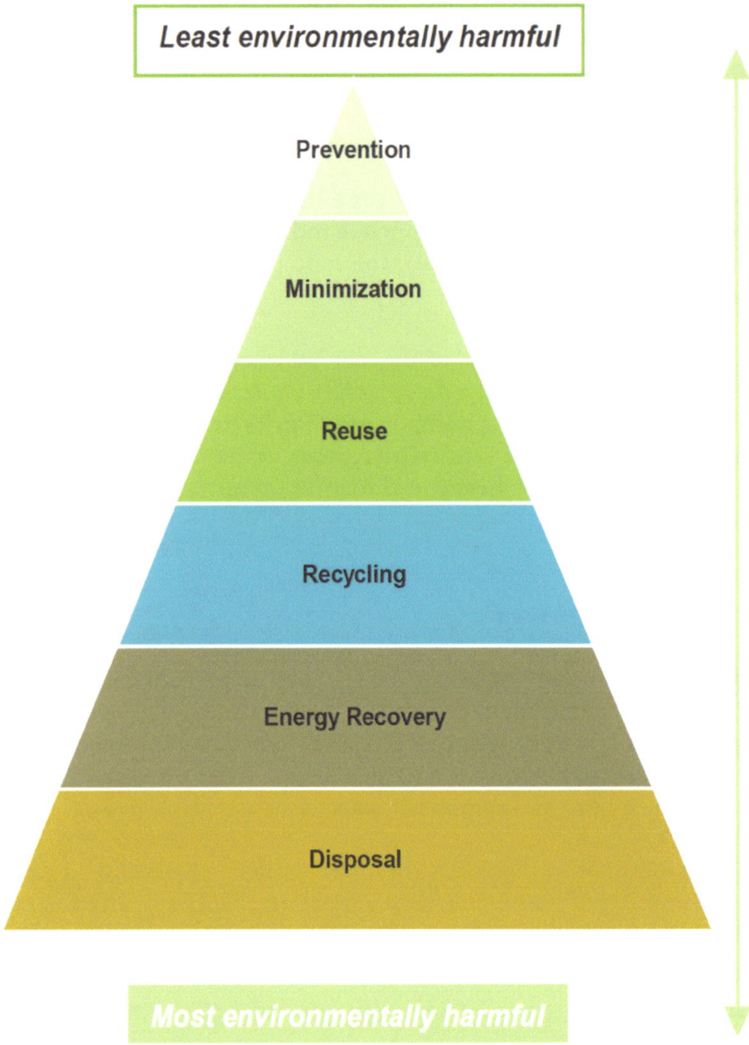

Figure 1.
Waste management hierarchy [2].

The results of the risk assessment should be publicized. If big gaps are identified, waste handling policies and procedures need be updated to adequately address the risks identified. Risks assessments are an important part of anticipating dangers and preventing any accidents and exposures before they happen. Risks assessments are key in elevating awareness and ownership of the waste management procedures in health care emergencies. In most cases the existing policies and procedures might not be able to cover all the types of waste that come with emergencies.

A risk assessment typically involves risk identification, risk quantification, control, implementation and verification. It is recommended to carry out a risk assessment whenever conditions change in facilities and this can cover increased waste production, outbreaks, new procedures and new personnel.

Data to inform the risk assessment can be collected through:

- Interviewing key informants in the healthcare emergency: this helps to get relevant information about the existing healthcare waste management processes and procedures

- A walk through the health facilities, camps, quarantine centers and all places used to manage the health care emergency helps with the familiarization with the physical context of the situation at hand

- Processes involved can be mapped to visualize the situation and this will be complemented by spot checks to verify

2.3 Creation of awareness of the different types of waste being produced

In order to better manage waste in the healthcare emergencies it is critical that everyone involved in the production and eventual management of the waste is aware of the type of the waste that is produced by the healthcare activities. Creating awareness is critical in making sure that everyone is aware of the methods of managing waste that will be used the manage the waste. In healthcare emergencies the most sophisticated and usual methods of managing waste might not be available hence the need to define the available methods.

The awareness can be created by short training sessions, development of SOP's and illustrative job aids on how to manage the waste. Due to the fact that waste is managed by people of different professional backgrounds the trainings need to be in language that is easily understood by everyone who is involved in the management of the waste. Training in vernacular language will be encouraged. Depending on the situation handwritten instruction can suffice.All these interventions can be informed by the risk assessment.

2.4 Training of health care workers and waste handlers

Formal training on waste handling can become a necessity to all healthcare workers in emergencies as it facilities and managers try to avoid transmission of

Category	Waste
Category 1	Human Anatomical Waste (human tissues, organs, body parts)
Category 2	Animal Waste (animal tissues, organs, body parts carcasses, bleeding parts, fluid, blood and experimental animals used in research, waste generated by veterinary hospitals, colleges, discharge from hospitals, animal houses)
Category 3	Microbiology & Biotechnology Waste (Wastes from laboratory cultures, human and animal cell culture, infectious agents from research and industrial laboratories, wastes from production of biological, etc)
Category 4	Waste Sharps (needles, syringes, scalpels, blade, glass, etc. that may cause puncture and cuts. This includes both used and unused sharps)
Category 5	Discarded Medicines and Cytotoxic drugs (Waste comprising of outdated, contaminated and discarded medicines)
Category 6	Soiled Waste (Items contaminated with blood, and body fluids including cotton, dressings, soiled plaster casts, linens, bedding, other material contaminated with blood)
Category 7	Solid Waste (Waste generated from disposable items other than the sharps such a tubing, catheters, intravenous sets etc.)
Category 8	Liquid Waste (Waste generated from laboratory and washing, cleaning, housekeeping and disinfecting activities)
Category 9	Incineration Ash (Ash from incineration of any bio-medical waste).
Category 10	Chemical Waste (Chemicals used in production of biologicals, chemicals used in disinfection, as insecticides, etc.)

Table 1.
Healthcare waste categories.

infections within the healthcare settings. It is however important to train further the waste handlers as they are integral in the management of waste. They are mostly recruited as general hands in the healthcare facilities. It is important that they get training on the management of the different classes of waste that might come in the facilities, Trainings in most cases should emphasizes the risks involved with the different types of waste and how that can protect themselves from the different exposures. The level of technical depth need to be adjusted appropriately to aid comprehension. in most cases local languages are recommended.

3. Available methods to manage healthcare waste

The results of the formal risk assessment forms the basis of interventions. The report should detail identified risks and mitigation measures put in place. Mitigation measures should be revaluated for effectiveness. The identified risks should also inform training of the health care workers and waste handlers. Following careful consideration of the risks and the type of waste that is being produced different ways of managing it need to be described. According to the waste management hierarchy it is important minimization is the first step towards managing the waste. The management of healthcare waste is contextual and should be guided by relevant legislations, regulations, available technology, costs and environmental and occupational health and safety factors [4].

3.1 Minimization

The reduction of waste at point of production should be applied to the furthest extent possible. It includes rational and risk-based PPE's usage, choice of materials with minimal packaging, unpacking at areas of low risk of contamination with infectious agents. Use of materials that can be cleaned or disinfected can greatly reduce amount of healthcare waste [2].

3.2 Segregation

Healthcare activities produce different types of waste. It is always safe to assume that only waste produced in administrative areas is considered non-hazardous. A risk assessment however should inform how you manage the waste throughout the emergency setting. The table below shows a typical color coding of bags under normal non-emergency settings. If these waste management and treatment options are available in emergency situations they should be adopted (**Table 2**).

The three-bin system is the most commonly used and segregates waste into three categories namely general waste, infectious waste and sharp waste. This also simplifies the work of the waste handlers as they will only deal with a small number of waste types. However it is not always the case all the waste can easily be categorized into these three categories (**Figure 2**).

Based on information obtained in the risk assessment the more categories might be needed as per the first table. In emergency situation this might be adequate depending on the type of waste predominantly being produced.

3.3 Collection transportation and storage

After generation and segregation of the waste it needs to be transported from the point of generation either the final disposal point or the temporal holding place. All infectious waste should be collected in clearly labeled lined containers and sharp

Color	Type of Container	Waste Category	Treatment options
Yellow	Plastic Bag	Categories 1, 2, 3 & 6	Incineration deep burial
Red	Plastic Bag	Categories 3, 6, 7	Autoclaving/Micro-waving Chemical Treatment
Blue/White Translucent	Plastic Bag/ puncture proof containers	Categories 4, 7	Autoclaving/Micro-waving/ Chemical Treatment & Destruction / shredding
Black	Plastic Bag	Categories 5, 9, 10	Disposal in secured landfill

Table 2.
Color coding of waste bags.

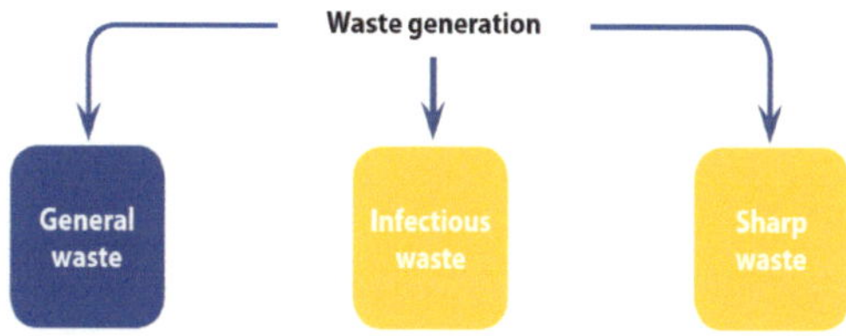

Figure 2.
Three bag waste segregation [5].

waste in sharp boxes. In cases where people are in quarantine centers, holding centers, camps and other non-healthcare settings, waste like used masks, tissues, and other non-biodegradable waste is collected in double bagged red bags. It will be ideal to have the bags sealed and labeled with a date and time.There is no need to treat these materials with disinfectant first but tying and wiping the outside with 0.5% chlorine should be sufficient as an additional measure to reduce spread of diseases. The collection of the waste should take place at times that are least busy to prevent exposure to people from the carts that might be used to transport the waste. Full PPE should be provided to the waste handlers. Transportation of hazardous and non-hazardous waste should always be done separately using the principle of clean to dirty places with hygienically sensitive areas being the areas to start from followed by the other places.

Waste holding areas should be designated wherever possible. When new building are being built it should be incorporated in building design. The size of the holding areas should be according to the amount of waste that is anticipated to be produced. The holding areas should be totally closed off and separated from essential areas like supply areas or food preparation rooms and only authorized staff should have access to that space. The floor of the holding area should be of material that is easy to clean like vinyl.

Waste that is highly infectious like waste contaminated with blood and other bodily fluids, microbiological cultures, stocks of infectious agents from laboratory, swabs,bandages, medical devices and pathological waste must be selected sealed to allow easy disinfection and need to be identified as infectious waste area using the biohazard sign. The time from generation of waste to treating it should not exceed 24 hours in the warm climate areas in the summertime. In temperate climate 72 hours can be allowable in winter and 48 hours in summertime. Refrigerated storage if available can allow for waste to be stored for up to a week. This might be relevant where pathological waste involved. Pathological waste is considered biologically active and gas production might be expected in storage.

If pharmaceutical waste is to be stored it should be separated from other waste. In general pharmaceutical waste can be hazardous and non-hazardous in solid and liquid form. Local and international regulations should be followed to better manage this waste. If chemical waste is anticipated the characteristic of the waste need to be considered in terms of the reactivity of the chemicals. Under normal circumstances this should be a different area from the other waste. In emergency settings there might significantly differences as there might not be all these different spaces to hold waste.

The staff who handles the waste should be given the appropriate personal protective equipment like thick Gloves, boots and aprons. In addition, appropriate training should also be offered. The waste holding centers should be easy to clean, safe and locked up, well ventilated and most importantly protected away from animals, rodents and insects.

When the waste is to be transported offsite the labelling on the waste should be non-washable, the date and time of production should be clear, the name of the person sending other waste should be clearly stated, the category of the waste, and the contact details of a person in case of emergency.

3.4 Treatment

This waste should be treated on site before safe disposal. If the waste is to be moved off-site it is critical to understand where and how it be transported, treated and disposed. Waste should be treated prior to final disposal if non-combustion methods of disposal are to be used. The preferred methods include This can be useful in places where it is difficult or expensive to have an incinerator.

3.4.1 Autoclaving

Use of combination of steam, heat, and pressure to disinfect waste and equipment. The combined effect of saturated steam under pressure and heat kills microorganisms. To guarantee that the process is working well chemical and biological indicators need to be added to be process on a regular basis or with every autoclaving cycle. In combination with shredding, grinding, mixing the volume of the waste can be significantly reduced. Autoclaves can also be easily moved to sites they are needed depending on size in the process increasing access to waste treatment to the different sites for this method of disposal.

3.4.2 Microwaving

This is a recent technology in healthcare waste management. Microwaving technology heats the water in the waste. Some microwaving devices include transformation devices like shredders or blenders. It is however not suitable in waste that might contain metallic items like surgical equipment. It can be done in batches or in a continuous manner (an automated process). However microwaving might not be suitable for all types of waste like anatomical waste. Chemical disinfection should be considered depending on circumstances [6].

3.4.3 Chemical disinfection

The most common and readily available method of chemical disinfection is use of hypochlorite solution. It has oxidizing properties and removes most of the microbial burden in the waste.

3.5 Destruction of the waste

Incineration is the commonest way of destroying most healthcare waste. If it available especially in formal healthcare settings is the most commonly used method of getting rid of the healthcare waste. Incineration involves a high temperature (850–1100 degrees Celsius) dry heating process that reduces organic and combustible waste to inorganic incombustible matter. It highly efficient in reducing weight of the waste. However it produces toxic emissions if the equipment is not well functioning. Dioxins and furans are generated by the combustion process which contains chlorine. They are highly toxic and bio accumulative. They can cause reproductive developmental problems, damage to the immune system, interference with hormones, and also can be mutagenic [6].

It is costly to have the High temperature incinerators. Incinerators use high heat to destroy waste. The De Montfort Incinerators can be rapidly deployed to emergency settings as they are small. In some cases single-chamber drum and brick incinerators can be designed to meet the healthcare emergency needs where resources are limiting. Transition to more sophisticated incinerators can be planned depending on the length of the healthcare emergency. Depending on setting, mobile incinerators can also be availed to add to the waste management strategies in the developed world in response to healthcare emergencies.

More sophisticated types can be deployed with time as they offer the option of polluting the environment less. The sophisticated ones include the dual chamber incinerators, and the co-incinerators. Dual Chamber incinerators burn waste at temperatures as high as 850 degrees Celsius in the primary chamber. The temperatures are maintained by multiple gas and oil burners with the vapors from the primary chamber being directed to the secondary chamber with one or more burners that raises the temperatures to 1100 degrees Celsius. Flue gas treatment is recommended to reduce air pollution. Other incinerators can also allow for multiple types of waste to be dealt with at the same time [6].

The incinerators must be ideally located approximately 61 meters away from habitable buildings, 46 meters from water sources and 300 meters from agricultural site. The waste management site should always be enclosed. In urban settings these waste management centers should be offsite. The ash from the incinerators should be removed safely from the site and appropriately disposed in a pit.

In most healthcare emergencies it might not be possible to have the incinerators in all possible places where healthcare waste is being produced. In addition, the available incinerators are easily overwhelmed due to the increased volumes of waste produced during emergency settings.

4. Other alternatives in healthcare emergencies

4.1 Onsite burial of waste

Onsite burial of waste can be considered in cases where the resources are limiting, and the amount of waste produced is also small and also if it is for a limited of time. The pit should be 1–2 meters wide and 2–5 meters deep. The bottom of the pits should be 2 meters above the ground water level to avoid contamination of ground water (**Figure 3**).

A fence should be constructed around the pit to stop wild animals and people from gaining access to the pit. Alternatively the waste can be burnt to reduce the volume of the waste.

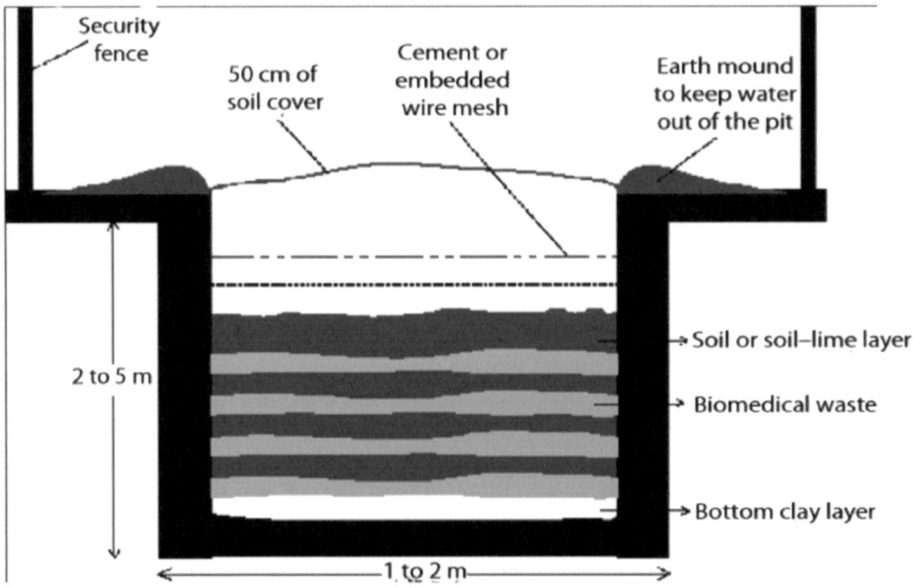

Figure 3.
Waste disposal pit [7].

In cases where pathological waste is also being produced placenta pits can also be used to dispose to dispose pathological waste. These placenta pits need to be located in specific places with the view of avoiding contamination of ground water. Natural degradation and draining of liquid into subsoil will greatly reduce volume of waste.

Sharps need to be disposed in concrete lined pits after decontamination (**Figure 4**).

4.2 Washing, cleaning and disinfection

Existing cleaning and disinfection procedures for healthcare settings should be followed consistently. In most cases 705 ethyl alcohol and 0.1% sodium hypochlorite are sufficient to disinfect most surfaces.it is recommended that all individuals in charge of environmental cleaning laundry and dealing with soiled bedding, towels and clothes from patients should wear appropriate PPE. Soiled linen should be placed in appropriately labeled leak proof bags or containers after carefully removing any solid excreta.

It is recommended that utility gloves or heavy-duty reusable plastic aprons are cleaned with soap and water and decontaminated with 0.5% sodium hypochlorite each time they are used.

5. Management of dead bodies

The number of deaths in most healthcare emergencies can significantly increase. Management of dead bodies has to be considered from a cultural point view as different cultures view dead bodies in differently. Burial has to be done by the relatives of the deceased, but it can be dangerous in cases of death from an infectious disease that is transmitted by casual contact. Most cultural practices involve dressing dead bodies, and this can significantly lead to an increased transmission of diseases like Ebola (and other viral hemorrhagic fevers). Communities need to be educated on the dangers of handling dead bodies in these type of healthcare emergencies. There might need to train

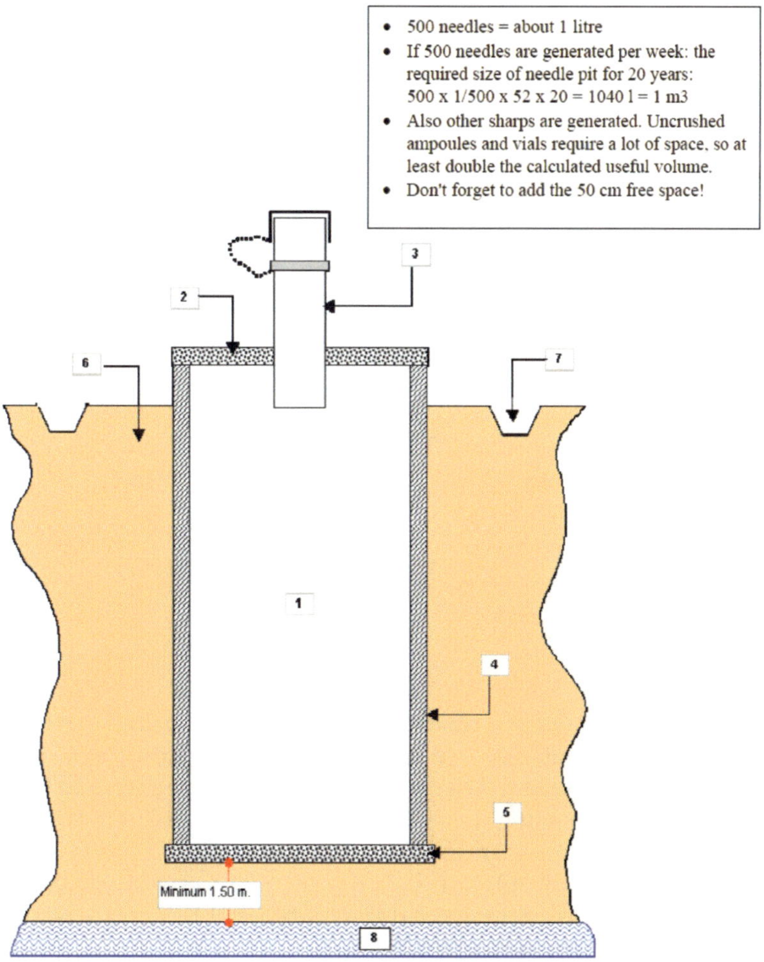

Key

1. Pit
2. Slab
3. Drop pipe with cover
4. Lining
5. Closed foundation
6. Soil
7. Drainage ditch
8. Water table

Inputs

- Shovels, picks, miner's bars
- Slab (concrete or wood in acute emergencies)
- Cover (for pipe in plastic or metal)
- Pipe (PVC, metal; diameter: 150 mm)
- Concrete or bricks
- Mason's tools
- Protective clothing for builders and operators

Figure 4.
Sharps disposal pit.

workers at morgues on how to handle dead bodies in cases of disease outbreaks. During the Ebola outbreak management of dead bodies became a significant source of spread and this management of dead bodies was taken over by health care professional up to burial. Traditional practices like body viewing were not practiced and the dead bodies were taken to the burial sites with minimal delay and no gatherings.

In case of natural disasters like earthquakes, volcanic eruptions and floods were there are mass deaths the need to identify the dead bodies before burial becomes a critical step. This has the potential of overwhelming mortuaries as pathology services are not usually decentralized in most countries. The delays in DNA analysis in most settings is due to a limited number of laboratories that offer this high specialty service. Culturally close families prefer to bury their families after accurate identification.

6. Management of chemical pharmaceutical waste

Chemical waste can be produced from increased laboratory testing. In managing chemical waste it is important to consider the risks associated with the chemicals which should be informed by the risk assessments. The chemical incompatibilities of the different chemicals involved together with their anticipated volumes to be produced. It might be necessary to have specific storage spaces for the chemical waste being produced. In most infectious disease outbreaks use of polymerase chain reaction (PCR) to confirm infections can lead to increased production of dangerous chemicals like ethidium bromide. However, the use of the chemical in medical laboratories is decreasing due to its mutagenic nature. Use of mercury-based measuring instruments can also lead to mercury waste which is dangerous. The impending ban on use of based thermometers and sphygmomanometers will great reduce the risk of having mercury as hazardous chemical waste in healthcare settings.

Pharmaceutical waste includes expired drugs, contaminated pharmaceutical products, drugs, vaccines and sera that is no longer needed. Items used in the handling of pharmaceuticals is also included in this class of waste and includes bottles gloves, masks, vials, and tubing contaminated with pharmaceutical residues.

7. Conclusion

Management of healthcare waste should be highly prioritized in healthcare emergencies. Recent healthcare emergencies like the Ebola outbreak in west Africa and now the covid 19 pandemic have improved awareness and need to invest in innovative ways of managing waste. The EBV outbreak also highlighted the risks associated with traditional/cultural norms of burying dead bodies. This was extended to covid 19 as people in full PPE gear could be seen burying dead bodies in most countries. Lessons learnt in the different types of healthcare emergencies are very important for the next emergency.

Risk assessment has become a very important concept in the management of biosafety issues (including waste management). It is important to have a formal way of anticipating for potential exposures and making sure that the potential risks of exposure are removed from the from the facility. If systematically done in different emergencies it can adequately prevent exposures. Involvement of everyone who has a role to play in waste management significantly improves its effectiveness.

Training of healthcare workers is of paramount importance. in some cases, due to the nature of the emergency it might be important to reorient people on how the waste is going to be managed. Different emergencies present different risks and it Is important to customize the training on order to make sure that it is effective. Consideration of the different levels of employees is key if there is to be prevention of exposures. The EBV out breaks restricted orderlies from doing many duties as the danger of exposure increased especially from dead bodies. This coupled with the expensive PPE meant that the healthcare professionals had to be heavily involved. Use of appropriate technical language is key to making use that there is transfer of usable skills. Additionally evaluation of the trainings in this case need to be done to make sure that people understand what they have been taught. A retraining can be organized in case people did not fully understand.

The sudden increase in healthcare waste generation or generation of healthcare waste in non-healthcare settings means there is need to mobile resources to manage the waste. In high income settings alternatives can include use of mobile incinerators to completement the onsite incinerators or to take care of healthcare waste in places where it is not possible to have incinerators like camps, quarantine centers and other non-healthcare settings. The reaction of the Chinese to the covid 19 pandemic has highlighted innovative ways of managing waste like the mobile incinerators that can be deployed to the places where the waste is being generated [8].

On the other hand, in low resource settings transitional methods can be applied as an interim measure as systems and resources are being put together to have more advanced technologies in place. The selection of the transitional methods needs to be made on the basis of adaptability to the setting. The methods should be readily available and adaptable with a known efficacy reducing the risk to public health by controlling the spread of infections and hazardous chemicals through healthcare waste. Technical options on the management of healthcare waste need be presented in the process of making a choice based on the resources that are available.

Expired drugs need to be disposed of as per the regulations of the country but incineration is the most common practice in most countries. Other classes of drugs are described as high risk and their disposal need to be monitored.

Proper healthcare waste management is imperative to preventing further infections that might not be part of the original healthcare emergency. Planning to manage waste is a process that requires information before implementation. Resource availability is key as some of the waster might require specific ways to manage it. The impending ban on mercury-based measuring instruments in healthcare will reduce the risks involved with their breakage in instruments like thermometers and sphygmomanometers. Risk assessments should inform all the waste management activities and should be carried out with everyone in mind.

Author details

Julius Manjengwa
University of Johannesburg, Harare, Zimbabwe

*Address all correspondence to: manjengwajt@gmail.com

References

[1] WHO, Solid Waste Management in emergencies. 2013

[2] The Global Fund 2020 Technical brief: Sustainable healthcare waste management. 2020

[3] WHO, Overview of technologies for the treatment of infectious and sharp waste from health care facilities. 2019

[4] UNEP, Compendium of technologies for treatment/ destruction of healthcare waste. 2012

[5] WHO Safe Management of Wastes from Health-care activities, A Summary. 2017

[6] United Nations Office for the Coordination of Humanitarian Affairs, Environmental emergencies section (2011, Disaster waste management guidelines. 2011

[7] Government of Nepal. Healthcare waste management in the context of COVID-19 emergency. 2020

[8] Lie Yang, Xiao Yu, Xiaolong Wu, Jia Wang, Xiaoke Yan, Shen Jiang, Zhuqi Chen, Emergency response to the explosive growth of health care wastes during COVID-19 pandemic in Wuhan, China, Conservation and Recycling, Volume 164, 2021

Chapter 13

Evidence-Based Preparedness for Post COVID-19

Yayehyirad Kitaw and Mirgissa Kaba

Abstract

In spite of skepticisms at various levels, the COVID-19 pandemic posed unprecedented impact on global health and economy. Although projections have yet to materialize, African countries are not at their worst with COVID-19. Yet, the worst is probably in the making despite swift, progressive, and adaptable responses many African countries have taken based on lessons from countries affected by the pandemic earlier. While efforts are underway to contain the current pandemic, the almost certain hit by another pandemic may call for appropriate preparation. This review aims to shade light on the need to align current COVID-19 prevention and management with preparation for the potential next one. A rapid review of available evidence was undertaken using clearly defined inclusion criteria and data analysis methods. The immediate focus of preparedness is coordination of interventions where evidence generation, policy making, public and private sector as well as community engagement is required to contain the current COVID-19 pandemic. Improved/adapted mathematical projections to guide decisions; improved/adapted methods for risk communication and community engagement; improved methods/technologies for surveillance, case detection and containment; optimal use of all the limited available resources; and strengthening partnerships at all levels need to be strengthened. Current endeavors should pay attention to strengthen the surveillance system for early detection; provision of adequate health care infrastructure; strong and capable health workforce and financing. Furthermore, strengthen research capacity to play its role to shape the post-COVID-19 is critical by strengthening inter and intra-disciplinary research capacities; forging partnerships at all levels. Evidently COVID-19 has posed unprecedented challenge to the globe at large. Yet, it also offered opportunities to reassess existing health system vis-à-vis the pandemics. Besides, useful lessons from COVID-19 are that it does not discriminate human beings across the globe by economy, political system and socio-cultural backgrounds. This is a useful lesson for global solidarity and align efforts to contain post COVID-19 implications as well as to prevent and manage similar such pandemics in the future.

Keywords: post COVID-19, responses to COVID-19, next pandemic, preparedness

1. Introduction

"This is like a world war, except in this case, we're all on the same side" (Gates 2020)

In spite of skepticisms at various levels including by scientists, the COVID-19 pandemic is spreading at unprecedented speed across borders severely impacting global health and economy [1–3]. Globalization, which has often been celebrated for interconnecting countries, has now offered much more space and opportunity for the pandemic to easily cross boundaries and has seemingly 'tipped the scales in favor of pathogens' [4, 5]. The pandemic is still unchecked with thousands of life lost every day. Although the highly severe projections have yet to materialize [6, 7], COVID-19 is now well established in Africa [8, 9]. Estimates of future deaths projected to be in millions, in Africa, because of general poverty, malnutrition, prevalence of diseases such as HIV and TB, constrained health services etc. [6, 10]. While the potential role of climate, demography, BCG and other vaccines, and weakness in the reporting system including low rate of testing could not be ruled out [10–16], the relatively low number of cases seem to be in part because many African countries have taken swift, progressive, and adaptable responses despite resource limitations. Some studies indicate that, having garnered experience from several recent epidemics, Africa might have got it right after all [17] even though there is 'no room for complacency' [15, 18, 19].

Lockdown and social/physical distancing has been imposed in several countries. These and pandemic related pressures on the health system could have potentially unintended consequences including disruption of routine health services; wide-spread economic challenge and hunger; worsening food insecurity; and increased violence with major impact on health/mortality [20, 21]. Even though the basic principles of infection control are universal, their concrete applications should be context specific [22]. Decisions must be based on risk sciences and as thorough risk and cost–benefit analyses [23, 24]. There are indications that early interventions could avert substantial number of infections and deaths [25, 26]. Thus, governments and public health authorities must play a balancing role as the evidence does not indicate a simple trade-off between lives lost to the pandemic and economic recession related to response [27]. The bottom line is policies must be internationally coordinated, as WHO has called for since the disease has first appeared, and must recognize that neither abandoning control nor eternal lockdown are healthy options [10, 28, 29].

The Director General of the World Health Organization (WHO) indicated that the outbreak is a test of political, financial and scientific solidarity for the world to fight a common enemy that does not respect borders... what matters now is stopping the outbreak and saving lives [30]. However, this solidarity has failed to materialize to date because the pandemic has highlighted weaknesses in both 'authoritarian' and 'democratic' states with all trying to trade blames or downplay the danger for various reasons [4, 31, 32]. As compared to the previous pandemics, the current one shock the fabrics of society and threatens to change the course of history. As in previous pandemics, 'public hysteria, fear, and conspiracy theories tend to derail public health responses' [5]. 'We Are Living in a Failed State' – for USA no less [33] but also the world order is being seriously tested [34], with some predicting revolutions 're-inventing Communism' or 'a new barbarian capitalism' [35]. The post-pandemic is going to be tough although it is considered as an opportunity to re-evaluate what we want to prioritize as a civilization [36]. Therefore, it is imperative that we prepare for it as we struggle through the current one.

Most predictions of the next pandemic had influenza in mind, even though other catastrophe such as asteroids, mega volcanic eruptions or coronal mass ejection (CME) cannot be ruled out. Influenza is a truly universal disease. No virus poses a greater threat to more people [37, 38]. It is only good fortune that we haven't seen another pandemic as severe as 1918 [39]. It is almost a certainty that there will be another influenza or other (of the some hundreds of new coronavirus species and the 10,000 potentially zoonotic mammalian viruses) [40] pandemic of one magnitude/type or another [30, 37]. The world is more interconnected. Global travel, internal migration; and large-scale population displacement following natural disasters or conflicts has increased tremendously [41]; humans have seemingly 'tipped the scales in favor of pathogens' [5]. Ethiopian Airlines alone transported more than 10 million passengers in 2018, 21% more as compared to 2017 [42].

Bearing in mind that rarely has scientific provisions been as challenged as it is now even in the most developed countries, it is advisable to remember that medical scientists in general and tropical medicine specialists in particular ignore history at their peril [35, 39, 43]. So we should, as we struggle to control the current one, do so with preparation for the future in mind and hopefully break 'the cycle of panic then forget' since the first recorded pandemic [5, 44].

To date we have more tools at our disposal: better surveillance and diagnostic systems, stronger frameworks and regulations, such as the Global Health Security Agenda and Joint External Evaluations (JEE), and a deeper understanding of how diseases spread and what is needed to stop the spread of the virus [38, 41, 45]. So, what led to the near global chaos in the current pandemic was that, in spite of repeated warnings, the global community was ill prepared including the fact that lifesaving innovations are not reaching those who need them [29, 38, 41]. If the virus continues to spread throughout 2020, it will demonstrate in a very cruel way how well the public health systems of individual countries are functioning. These will be very important lessons in preparation for a future pandemic, which could be even more dangerous [46]. Already, attempts are being made to draw lessons from the various country experiences [47, 48]. Evidently, there is a political/economic dimension to pandemic preparedness. Epidemic preparedness is not beyond any country's capacity although take proactive action remains a matter of political choice [38]. Uncannily, the COVID-19 pandemic began a few weeks after the end of PREDICT-2, the last-standing United States Agency for International Development (USAID) Emerging Pandemic Threats funding program, which supported a decade of virology, ecology, and epidemiology around the world [40].

As all low-income countries (LIC), Ethiopia is predicted to be heavily impacted by the current pandemic [49]. However, the force and united action garnered to fight the virus to recover from the COVID-19 economic losses and address the plethora of challenges that are impeding progress and sustainable development [50].

A global 'governance crisis is unfolding' [18]. While adjustments to the Public Health Emergency of International Concern (PHEIC) declaration process might be warranted [51], the rule, as advised globally, should be to follow World Health Organization's advice, end secrecy in decision-making and cooperate globally [24, 29, 52].

This should be done while resisting undue biologicalization/biomedical tunnel vision" (Thorp HH, 2020) of the disease or seeing the goal of containing COVID-19 as a purely technocratic or law-and-order problem and developing context-specific, ethical approach to physical distancing [8, 22].

This rapid review was undertaken to articulate ways to support the current efforts to mitigate COVID-19 pandemic, leverage current efforts to strengthen the health system including monitoring and surveillance systems for early detection, management of future such pandemic and leverage current effort to strengthen research and evidence generation.

2. Materials and methods

We employed a rapid review of evidences in the forms of publications and reports on coronaviruses and associated policy and management. Although numerous evidences are available, some are to date non-conclusive and others were not relevant to the theme in question. The rapid review thus helps to scope fragmented, opinion-based, large scale and sometimes-contradictory resources for easy use.

2.1 Search strategy

We searched through reports as well research outcomes on PubMed, and Google Scholar databases employing the key terms: "COVID-19", "SARS-CoV-2", "corona virus", and "viral infections", post "COVID-19". Additional resources from the databases and dashboards on the websites of relevant institutions and guidelines of international organizations such as the World Health Organization (WHO), Center for Disease Control and Prevention (CDC) and the Ethiopian Public Health Institute (EPHI) were include as we saw it fit. The search period went as far back as 2016 to July 15, 2020.

2.2 Inclusion criteria

Considering the broad scope of the theme under discussion, we maintained flexibility in terms of the documents that were eligible. Publications ranging from observational to experimental studies and from grey literatures to editorials and perspectives were included.

2.3 Data extraction and analysis

Data extraction and analysis included bringing together the evidences generated from different sources under current interventions and improving, leveraging the pandemic response to strengthen health systems, research and education. The research team comprising of four senior public health experts reviewed the contents of evidences separately to align them under defined categories.

3. Results and discussion

The findings is presented following specific themes in line with the objectives of the review. As such, articulation of ways to support current effort to contain the pandemic, strengthening the health system including monitoring and surveillance systems for early detection and management of future such pandemic and research interest were the major themes under which the findings are summarized.

3.1 Articulate ways to support current effort

The immediate focus of all concerned should, understandably, be to support the country articulate better ways to move out of the current crisis with as limited damage as possible. Moving out of the current crisis will clearly be a whole-society/ multi-sectoral effort as the pandemic will have major impact on the economic and social determinants of health [2, 49, 53]. Depending on measures taken, various outcomes are possible [54]. Experience show that pandemics hold several surprises and their control will require highly coordinated effort from all, scientists and policy makers in particular. WHO could strengthen the global effort by focusing on providing regularly updated recommendations from independent expert committees on preventive strategies and potential treatments for COVID-19; proposing universal and standardized ways of epidemiological data collection and reporting from countries. It could seek for ways of accelerating the evaluation, selection, and prequalification of diagnostic tests; consolidate information on COVID-19 vaccine research progress and work upstream with partners to ensure equitable access and affordability of therapeutics and vaccines as they become available. It could facilitate logistical coordination and supply of reagents, personal protective equipment, and potential treatments. Finally, it could support countries with fragile health systems to maintain continuity of routine health care, particularly for chronic diseases, and primary health care [29]. Since we currently have only non-pharmaceutical response measures, the involvement of social and behavioral scientists is critical [55]. Success in the science with strong political and social leadership determine which scenarios unfold, so it is time to focus on what we can all do to help [56].

In the health sector, this implies strengthening the primary health care (PHC) approach i.e. empowering people and communities; developing multisectoral policy and action for health; and strengthening and integrating health services, with good-quality primary care supported by essential public health functions at the core [22]. The aim should be to 'crush the curve' of the pandemic [57].

3.1.1 *Improved/adapted mathematical projections/outbreak science to help guide decisions*

Mathematical projections/outbreak science has become the driving force behind the pandemic responses with growing calls to follow science including potential lessons from other risk science experiences [23]. However, we should bear in mind that mathematical models are useful exploration of questions are also dangerous way to assert answers. Various teams, primarily comprised of academic modelers, organized by, for example, the World Health Organization, the US Centers for Disease Control and Prevention have been involved [58, 59]. Obviously, research does not get much more policy-relevant since governments across the globe relying on these projections [59]. However, there is yet a lot to be learned about how the virus spreads that the models should be constantly updated with increasing knowledge and information; a formidable task even with the best surveillance systems [60]. Because any single data type is likely to yield under- or over- estimate of the extent and spread of the disease, it is important to consider multiple data types and be cautious in relying on estimates without considering sources of bias [41]. Models (equation-based, agent-based ...) are, at best, simplified representations of reality based on assumptions on the behaviors of the virus (reproductive rate, incubation period, death rate ...), environmental/climate and individuals/societies including demographic composition and mobility [61, 62]. Even the best systems need regular updating and improvement based more on real data derived from epidemiologic investigations rather than assumptions [41, 63, 64]. In short, models should be used with prudence and we should ensure that modelling should not be considered with certainty than the models deserve; and politicians must not be allowed to offload accountability to models of their choosing.

In the Ethiopian context, the situation is compounded by the weak health management information system, diverse population and limited experience at modeling [65]. A recent modeling, for example (**Figure 1**), seems to clearly underestimate deaths by their won assumptions, leaving out possible deaths among those not hospitalized [66]. However, evidences reveal that majority of confirmed cases and deaths are from Addis Ababa.

Countries are expected to develop their own estimates based on demographic and epidemiological characteristics and update them periodically as data/info improves while networking and learning from the various efforts elsewhere. Typically, repeated runs with varying inputs and assumptions are undertaken on

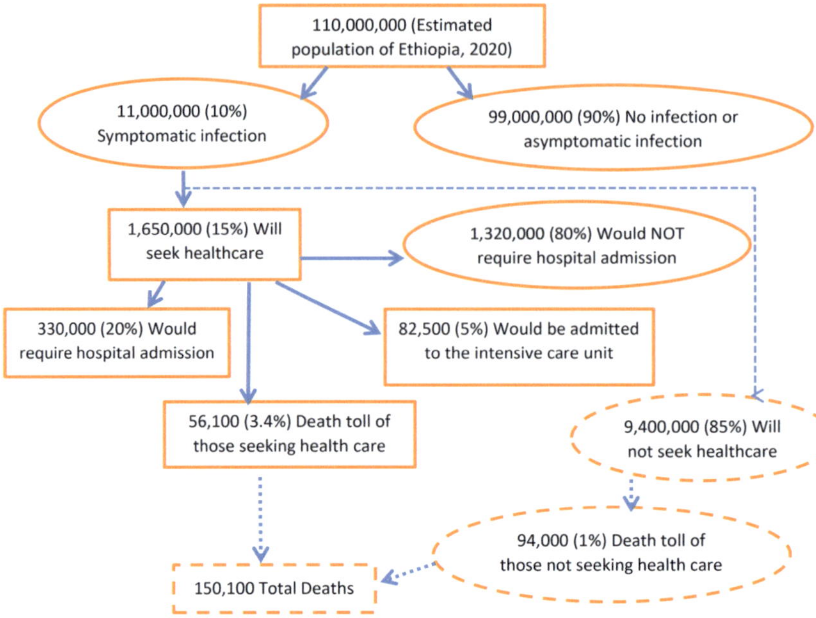

Figure 1.
Attempt at Modeling the COVID Pandemic for Ethiopia. (Source: Adapted from [66], --- authors additions)

several modes to avoid too much reliance on one mode [58]. The need, to develop the capacity to generate real-time, reliable, accessible and actionable data to empower leaders to act faster [42].

Based on experiences from the US, we should aim to change the health system by accelerating use of telemedicine; move away from traditional models of employer-based health insurance; move away from nursing homes; address health disparities and the social determinants of health; improve drugs affordability; increase local production of drugs; enhance epidemic preparedness with more task shifting and improved financial management [57].

Organizational structures vary from country to country [58] but, in the Ethiopian context, the Federal Ministry of Health (FMOH), the Ethiopian Public Health Institute (EPHI), Regional Health Bureaus (RHB) etc. are destined to play the major role. It seems advisable to create a multi/interdisciplinary (epidemiologists, clinicians, health managers, social scientists, mathematicians ...) team in 2–3 universities and establish network or even a National Infectious Disease Forecasting Center or revamp EPHI to play this role [42]. The network/center should have a direct link with policy makers, adequate funding and access to data during outbreaks. Models are only as robust as the data used to build them. In many settings, the infrastructure for collecting, collating, and cleaning high-quality data is underdeveloped [58]. The network/center could attempt to create one data bank; the aim being to achieve precision public health which requires robust primary surveillance data, rapid application of sophisticated analytics to track the geographical distribution of disease, and the capacity to act on such information. It could also join the WHO Global Research and Innovation Forum [30, 62]. Its term of reference (TOR) could include other non-epidemic issues see, for example, BARDA, CDC Health Economics and Modeling Unit; The Research and Policy for Infectious Disease Dynamics (RAPIDD) group in the Fogarty International Center at the National Institutes of Health (NIH), The International Initiative on Spatial Life course Epidemiology (ISLE) which could serve as possible contacts. Collaboration with other (neighboring) African countries should be promoted [42, 62]. It is also important to consolidate training in field epidemiology and outbreak science methodologies [58] and, remember that no public-health research is complete until the key findings are effectively communicated and, ideally, implemented [67].

3.1.2 Improved/adapted methods for communication

The experience to date has, if need be, taught us the importance of timely, honest, credible, empathetic, informative and balanced information as lack of information can become misinformation and lead to untowardly consequences [23, 27, 32]. Even ensuring clear and effective communication with staff and students in higher education systems could prove challenging [68]. Credible sources such as religious or community leaders should be identified and engaged as appropriate. Attention should be paid to 'infodemic', the misinformation type – i.e., conspiracy theories, fake news etc. - in particular, on messenger apps and social media which could harm public health and put millions of lives at risk [55, 69].

The information should be conveyed using local context and vernacular languages and as jargon free as possible, making science accessible [67]. It should avoid language [that] creates a public health discourse that seems reactive rather than proactive, reductive rather than holistic, disempowering rather than empowering [70]. This has proved a slippery ground even under seemingly more auspicious circumstances that leads to increasing erosion of trust in science [71, 72]. There is, therefore, need to be especially careful to communicate transparent information about our capabilities, uncertainties, disagreements or agreements and being trustworthy including on vaccines indicated areas for improvement [73, 74]. A study in a major town, after less than two weeks of the outbreak in Ethiopia shows widespread misconceptions about the pandemic [75]. There have also been calls to make full use of digital technologies but their limitations in deprived areas, where access to the internet is relatively scarce, patients have little digital literacy, and language barriers abound should be factored [9, 76, 77].

3.1.3 Improved methods/technologies for surveillance, identification and containment

Innovations are required in testing, contact tracing, treatments, vaccines, policies for opening up since no single system can capture all parameters of the pandemic, multiple, complementary surveillance systems should be implemented [78].

Testing - for diagnosis and clinical management or for surveillance and outbreak control - is critical but countries such as Ethiopia are facing a daunting task because of limited facilities, testing kits, reagents etc. The case reports are likely to be an underestimate as, by mid-March, Ethiopia has carried out only about 11,000 tests/10 for every 100,000 people compared to, for example, about 280 for South Africa, 2,000 for Australia and 1,560 for the United States [42]. Ethiopia has, thus, a long way to go to reach testing levels recommended by WHO. There are indications that global solidarity has faltered as market restrictions are being imposed by a number of countries [32]. Ethiopia, as for other African countries, should plan for its own quality assurance of diagnostic tests, drugs, and vaccines production, including antibody and nano-technology based testing [79, 80]. These could be along the lines of the Africa CDC initiative of Partnership to Accelerate COVID-19 Testing (PACT) and the Ethiopian Food and Drug Authority (EFDA) Digital Health Activity (DHA) system. It should also explore the potentials of pooled testing in the Ethiopian context [42, 81].

For contact tracing, Ethiopia should bolster its relatively strong community level services by mobilizing health extension workers (HEW), health development army (HDA), model families etc. [65, 82] using tested epidemic models and experiences in other settings [77, 83]. It could enhance this by using digital technology, 'coronavirus apps' – with due attention to privacy and other pitfalls [84, 85] not only for contact tracing but also for testing, isolation and physical/social distancing [86]. Overall, control of the pandemic will require action at the individual, community, and population levels as recent data show that asymptomatic cases could play a major role in transmission.

Evidence shows that strict implementation of physical distancing, optimum use of face masks, respirators, and eye protection in public and health-care settings provide, in spite of some contextual challenges, high levels of protection against transmission [26, 87]. A systematic review and meta-analysis [88]. Mobility/lockdown restrictions could have variable results depending on areas – high for retail and recreational areas and transit stations but could be challenged by lockdown fatigue or the practicalities of daily living [89].

The development of safe and effective vaccine, including the potential use of vaccines for other diseases such as BCG and polio, is a priority [12, 14]. In terms of personal protection equipment (PPE) for care providers in particular, treatments – which seem to be a long shot, country specific guideline should be developed as well as strengthen inter-African collaboration policies for opening up etc. [87]. Access pool and to categorize Covid-19 vaccines as 'global good' and GAVI's Covax Advance Market Commitment and other initiatives, the temptation to prioritize producer countries will be high. As often seen, the potential of selfish gain trumping over collective good is high [39].

Vaccine hesitancy has, to date, been low in Ethiopia [90], but measures should be taken to ward off the global trend of vaccine hesitancy and politicization [73, 91]. Measures should also be taken to strengthen the vaccine delivery system as whether new or already in use, is only as effective as the system that provides it.

3.1.4 Optimal use of all the limited available resources

Ethiopia's health care system, already highly limited, will be extremely strained by the response to the pandemic [65]. As in other LIC, there are already signs that essential services such as immunizations, reproductive health etc. could be sidelined for various reasons with dire consequences [15, 22, 92, 93].

There are also indications that the pandemic could affect pregnancy outcomes and, in general, exacerbate social inequalities in health [94]. Therefore, ensuring access to basic support water, sanitation, and hygiene to most vulnerable ones is important [15, 56, 95–98]. The system should also improve quality of care including improved supply chain, adopt improved technology for delivery of health care for new therapies and roll out vaccines as soon as they become available including mitigating potential hesitancies based on already mounting misinformation [99, 100].

3.1.5 Forging partnerships at all levels

COVID-19 is menacing the whole of humanity and so the whole of humanity must fight back. Individual country responses are not going to be enough [9]. As Bill Gates put it some 3 years ago, 'What the world needs – and what our safety, if not survival, demands – is a coordinated global approach. Specifically, we need better tools, an early detection system, and a global response system' [101]. UN agencies at all levels (local, national, continental and international) and across all disciplines and sectors, WHO in particular, should lead in forging partnerships.

All stakeholders in Africa, the AU and CDC Africa in particular, should contribute towards a unified continent-wide anti-COVID-19 Strategy [10].

3.2 Leverage current effort to strengthen the health system including monitoring and surveillance systems

The post-pandemic demands on the health care, because of increases in chronic mental or physical health conditions, are bound to exacerbate the burden on the system – the solution of which may benefit future such challenges [36, 102]. The resources mobilized to control the current pandemic and others could contribute to strengthen the health system in general and in preparation of future pandemics in particular [9, 49]. We should always have in mind the adage that when it comes to fighting infectious diseases, the best offense is a strong defense [103]. Strengthening implies helping the country 'prepare for pandemics the way the military prepares for war'. This includes simulations and other preparedness exercises so we can better understand how diseases will spread and how to deal with things like quarantine and communications to minimize panic [101]. Various forms of health system for outbreaks preparedness are critical for considerations.

3.2.1 Strong monitoring and surveillance systems for early detection

Strong monitoring and surveillance system implies adequate number of contact tracers, adoption of the one health approach and improved laboratory and technical capacities including digital technology [9, 104]. The country's laboratory and technical capacities are highly limited even for routine health care provision calling for major effort will be required to ensure universal access [65].

3.2.2 Adequate and accessible health care infrastructure

As mentioned above Ethiopia's health system is, as for Africa in general, under-resourced and unprepared to withstand the onslaught of pandemics [105]. Investing in strong health systems is our best bet to protect ourselves and stop local outbreaks before they turn into global pandemics [103]. This would mean improving availability, access and quality of services i.e. progress towards UHC which could face challenges in the post pandemic period [106]. Experiences from similar events, developing Community Care Centers (CCC) within Health Posts could be attempted [107]. Besides, remote shared care delivery' such as shared medical appointments (SMAs) could be adapted to the Ethiopian context [108].

3.2.3 Strong and capable health workforce

A strong and capable health workforce, including sufficient numbers of adequately trained critical-care physicians is required for appropriate response [87]. As compared to most African countries, Ethiopia has major health workforce crisis and, even though dented by recent 'flooding strategy', the workforce remains inadequate and of dubious quality.

3.2.4 Adequate financing

The health care system is highly underfunded and heavily dependent on foreign financing [65]. Pandemic preparedness will require dedicated and adequate financing bearing in mind that the amount of financing preparedness is minuscule compared to pandemic costs [109].

3.3 Leverage current effort to strengthen research and evidence generation

'The challenge for humans is to learn as much about influenza viruses as these viruses have already learned about us'. Higher education and research institutions should play a major role in this learning process and in helping to shape the post-COVID-19 world [110]. In conjunction with health research institutions, it should make meaningful contribution to this as all countries need to develop strong and sustainable core capacities at the intersection of health systems and research i.e., pro-active, empowered and coordinated research committed to fair and equitable access [30]. Hence, there is good reason to support priority research agenda that leads to the development of sustainable global research platforms pre-prepared for the next disease X epidemic. This will allow for accelerated research, innovative solutions and Research and Development of diagnostics, therapeutics and vaccines, as well as the timely and equitable access to these life-saving tools for those at highest risk [38]. Even before the pandemic, universities, 'sinking ships'?, were facing several challenges. These could be exacerbated by the post-pandemic situation. Thus, as indicated for US public universities, universities must not just adapt but lead with new models to resolve/mitigate current and future challenges and optimally use opportunities [68, 111, 112]. But, to date, in spite of the national commitment to evidence based development, the Ethiopian higher education and research institutions have contributed little and the prospects could be grim if, as projected and in line with historical trends during economic downturns universities come out of the pandemic weakened [90, 113–116]. One way to avert this could be to leverage the national and international/global solidarity that will be galvanized in response to the pandemic to strengthen university labs, develop research universities, forge partnerships and garner sustainable funding. In line with this, it is important to strengthen the labs in the universities and create strong coordination with other labs in the country to enhance tests and participate in sero-epidemiological studies [116, 117].

3.3.1 Develop a number of 'research universities'

'Research universities'[1] would serve as resource centers for prioritizing and effective translation of science into both operational and policy action with the objective is to make a difference [38, 118, 119]. In short, paraphrasing what has been indicated in a different context, universities with 'civic values, openness, and societal relevance', where financing is [no longer] the leading factor, but one where contributing to the world beyond forms a leitmotif for actions [111]. They would guide policy decision including mathematical projections; developing surveillance, diagnostics, primary health care, and effective health security measures; assessing and promoting the potential role of traditional medicine/control measures and other essential topics [2, 59, 120].

Educators, policy-makers, employers and investors must urgently give thought to what a post-COVID world should look like and what role higher education institutions must play to make that world a reality. In short, they should serve as resource centers to inform policy in general and on how to maintain a cohesive and good-quality learning environment if and when the next pandemic, recession or natural disaster occurs [121].

[1] Only AAU, as member of The African Research Universities Alliance (ARUA), currently approaches this status ranking 16th among African best universities in *Times Higher Education ranking*. For some background material and the debate on the teaching versus research role of the university see NRC 2012, Barron 2015, Shapira 2015, van der Zwaan 2017, Cloete et al. 2020, Kraemer-Mbula et al. 2020.

They will also contribute to strengthening, in particular, the staff of the growing number of (new) higher education institutions thus promoting beneficial interactions with senior peers and mitigating the impact on the quality of an already highly challenged education system [45]. Projections in other settings indicate that the post pandemic period will generally need greater access to higher education and vocational training programs, probably including a more online experience with blended learning [121, 122]. All these will require thought-through solutions ensuring meaningful research impact and 'reconciling the needs of scientists and society at large.

3.3.2 Forge partnerships

As is the case for health services, 'research universities' in particular, should forge partnerships at all levels (local, national, continental and international), and across all disciplines and sectors. There are indications that the pandemic may foster good, even though limited in Africa, relation between the higher education community and governments [68]. In the short term, this could mean tapping into the relatively high reactive research funding [112]. Partnerships could include the Coalition for Epidemic Preparedness Innovations (CEPI), the African Research Universities Alliance (ARUA), the African CDC, the Guild of European Research-Intensive Universities (the Guild), Diaspora scientists etc. This implies applying 'the all-of-government and all-of-society approaches' recommended by WHO [7, 123, 124]. The potential of S-N-S/South–North–South triangulation should be explored [125]. The establishment of a scientific coordinating committee incorporating health/medicine, social sciences, mathematics/technology, One Health/human-animal-environment interface [38] etc. with focus on the multi-inter and trans-disciplinary, applied and context/country specific health policy and systems research (HPSR) for which Ethiopia is among leaders in LIC should also be explored [126].

3.3.3 Ensure sustainable financing

'Innovation does not happen by chance. It has to be nurtured and funded' [127]. Efforts to raise research grants from various sources are left to individual staff members instead of the institutions as a whole. Sustainable success will only be achieved if these efforts are supplemented and scaled up by the state and industry and are duly documented and synergized.

4. Conclusion

The unique feature of the current pandemic is its unprecedented global coverage as compared to several other flu-like outbreaks. Although case fatality is still incomparable to the Spanish flu of 1918, this pandemic could yet to cost human life and jeopardize global economies as well as impact the social and political landscape of individual countries. Although the pandemic has posed so much challenge, it could also offer opportunities to reassess the health system and improve on how it could readily respond to such pandemics, improve research and education in health sciences to develop competencies and evidences to respond to outbreaks of different size. While countries are to align their effort to contain the pandemic, commensurate measure should be taken to prevent and manage potential similar pandemics in the future. Globally, COVID-19 offered an opportunity for human beings across the world to recognize such outbreaks do not discriminate by geography, economy, political system and socio-cultural backgrounds. As such, human beings across the world are expected to see for mechanisms to strengthen global solidarity, align efforts to contain post COVID-19 implications as well as to prevent and manage similar pandemics in the future. Such lessons are particularly outstanding for Africa and Ethiopia where the health system is not as strong and prepared to such unexpected pandemic. African leaders may have drawn as much lesson to better articulate plans on how to respond to emerging pandemics, review its health system to preposition for such pandemic and improved mechanisms put in place to generate evidence use for planning to respond.

Role of funding source

Funding was not available for this undertaking.

Conflict of interest statement

There was no conflict of interest.

Ethical approval

There was no ethical implication of this activity and no informed consent was sought.

Author details

Yayehyirad Kitaw[1] and Mirgissa Kaba[2]*

1 Senior Public Health Consultant, Addis Ababa, Ethiopia

2 Department of Preventive Medicine, School of Public Health, Addis Ababa University, Ethiopia

*Address all correspondence to: mirgissa.kaba@aau.edu.et

References

[1] Raoult D. Épidémies, vrais dangers et fausse alertes. Éditions Michel Lafon, 2020.

[2] ElHani CN and V Machado. COVID19: The need of an integrated and critical view. Ethnobio Conserv, May 2020; 9:18(18). doi:10.15451/ec2020-05-9.18-1-20.

[3] Committee for the Coordination of Statistical Activities (CCSA). How COVID-19 is changing the world: a statistical perspective. 2020.

[4] **Strauss-Kahn D.** L'être, l'avoir et le pouvoir dans la crise. **Politique Internationale, Preprint May 2020.**

[5] M'ikanatha NM. Book Review: Mark Honigsbaum, The Pandemic Century: One Hundred Years of Panic, Hysteria and Hubris. Emerging Infectious Diseases, 2020; 26(6): 1349DOI: https://doi.org/10.3201/eid2606.191739.

[6] Gilbert M, Pullano G, Pinotti F, Valdano E, Poletto C, Boëlle P-Y, et al. Preparedness and vulnerability of African countries against importations of COVID-19: A modelling study. Lancet, February, 2020. https://doi.org/10.1016/S0140-6736(20)30411-6.

[7] Kaba M and Y Kitaw. Novel coronavirus (2019-nCoV) – reminiscent of Spanish flu: A challenge to global public health systems. Ethiop. J. Health Dev (editorial). 2020;34(1): 68-71.

[8] Divala T, RM Burke, L Ndeketa, EL Corbett and P MacPherson. Africa faces difficult choices in responding to COVID-19. The Lancet, May 12, 2020 https://doi.org/10.1016/S0140-6736(20)31056-4.

[9] UN Ethiopia. Novel Corona Virus (COVID-19) UPDATE # 107. 8 June 2020.

[10] Dupoux P, J Larson, S Unnikrishnan, and W Woods. Fighting COVID-19 in Africa will be different. Boston Consulting Group, 2020.

[11] Kathleen M O'Reilly, Megan Auzenbergs,Yalda Jafari, Yang Liu,Stefan Flasche, Rachel Lowe. Effective transmission across the globe: the role of climate in COVID-19 mitigation strategies. The Lancet Published online May 6, 2020 https://doi.org/10.1016/S2542-5196(20)30106-6.

[12] Curtis N, A Sparrow, TA Ghebreyesus, MG Netea. Considering BCG vaccination to reduce the impact of COVID-19. The Lancet, Published Online April 30, 2020 https://doi.org/10.1016/ S0140-6736(20)31025-4.

[13] WHO. The use of oral polio vaccine (OPV) to prevent SARS-CoV2. WHO Polio Global Elimination Initiative (PGEI), 2020a. Geneva

[14] WHO. Bacille Calmette-Guérin (BCG) vaccination and COVID-19: Scientific Brief. 12.April 2020b, Geneva.

[15] Editorial. COVID-19 in Africa: no room for complacency. The Lancet 2020a, 395: 1669.

[16] Ntoumi F and T Velavan. COVID-19 in Africa: between hope and reality. Lancet Infect Dis, 2020 Published online June 15, 2020 https://doi.org/10.1016/S1473-3099(20)30465-5.

[17] Moore J. What African Nations Are Teaching the West About Fighting the Coronavirus. The Newyorker, May 15, 2020

[18] Matthew M Kavanagh, Ngozi A Erondu, Oyewale Tomori, Victor J Dzau, Emelda A Okiro, Allan Maleche et.al. Access to lifesaving medical resources for African countries: COVID-19 testing and response, ethics, and

politics. The Lancet, Published online May 7, 2020 https://doi.org/10.1016/S0140-6736(20)31093-X.

[19] Gibney E. Whose coronavirus strategy worked best? Scientists hunt most effective policies. Nature 2020; 581: 15-16.

[20] Timothy Roberton, Emily D Carter, Victoria B Chou, Angela R Stegmuller, Bianca D Jackson, Yvonne Tam et.al et al. Early estimates of the indirect effects of the COVID-19 pandemic on maternal and child mortality in low-income and middle-income countries: a modelling study. The Lancet Global Health, Published online May 12, 2020 https://doi.org/10.1016/S2214-109X(20)30229-1

[21] Menendez C, R Gonzalez, F Donnay and R F Leke. Avoiding indirect effects of COVID-19 on maternal and child health. Lancet, Published online May 12, 2020 https://doi.org/10.1016/S2214-109X(20)30239-4.

[22] Cash R & V Patel. The art of medicine: Has COVID-19 subverted global health?. The Lancet, Published online May 5, 2020 https://doi.org/10.1016/S0140-6736(20)31089-8.

[23] Bostrom A, G Böhm, RE O'Connor, D Hanss, O Bodi-Fernandez & P Halder. Comparative risk science for the coronavirus pandemic. Journal of Risk Research, 2020, DOI: 10.1080/13669877.2020.1756384. https://doi.org/10.1080/13669877.2020.1756384.

[24] WHO. Novel Coronavirus (2019-nCoV): Strategic Preparedness and Response Plan. 2020c, Geneva.

[25] Pei S, S Kandula and J Shaman. Differential Effects of Intervention Timing on COVID-19 Spread in the United States. medRxiv preprint, 2020. doi: https://doi.org/10.1101/2020.05.15.20103655.

[26] MacIntyre CR. Case isolation, contact tracing, and physical distancing are pillars of COVID-19 pandemic control, not optional choices. Lancet Infect Dis, Published online June 16, 2020 https://doi.org/10.1016/S1473-3099(20)30512-0.

[27] Editorial. Post-COVID-19 spending. The Lancet Planetary-Health, 2020b; 4: e168.

[28] The *PLOS Medicine* Editors. Pandemic preparedness and responses: WHO to turn to in a crisis? PLoS Med, 2020: 17(5): e1003167. https://doi.org/10.1371/journal.pmed.1003167

[29] Nay O, MP Kieny, L Marmora and M Kazatchkine. The WHO we want. The Lancet, Published online June 5, 2020 https://doi.org/10.1016/S0140-6736(20)31298-8.

[30] WHO. A coordinated global research roadmap: 2019 novel coronavirus. World Health Organization, March 2020d, Geneva.

[31] Fukuyama F. The Thing that Determines a Country's Resistance to the Coronavirus. The Atlantic March 30, 2020

[32] Kavanagh MM. Authoritarianism, outbreaks, and information politics. The Lancet Public Health, 2020; 5: e135-e136.

[33] Packer G. We Are Living in a Failed State. The Atlantic, June 2020.

[34] Harari YN. The world after coronavirus. March 20, 2020.

[35] Horton R. Offline: After COVID-19—is an "alternate society" possible? The Lancet, 2020a;395: 1682.

[36] Editorial. The future belongs to the globalists. EClinicalMedicine 22, 2020c 100406 https://doi.org/10.1016/j.eclinm.2020.100406.

[37] Morens DM & AS Fauci. The 1918 Influenza Pandemic: Insights for the

21st Century. The Journal of Infectious Diseases, 2007;195:1018-1028.

[38] WHO. Pandemic influenza preparedness in WHO Member States: report of a Member States survey. Geneva: World Health Organization; 2019a. Licence: CC BY-NC-SA 3.0 IGO.

[39] Dunavan CP. Uncomfortable Truths about Modern Epidemics: A Review of The Pandemic Century and Interview with Author Mark Honigsbaum. Am. J. Trop. Med. Hyg., 2019: 101(3): 724-725. doi:10.4269/ajtmh.19-0388.

[40] Carlson CJ. From PREDICT to prevention, one pandemic later. The Lancet Microbiology, 2020: 1: e6-e7. https://doi.org/10.1016/S2666-5247(20)30002-1.

[41] National Academies of Sciences, Engineering, and Medicine (NASEM). Exploring the Frontiers of Innovation to Tackle Microbial Threats: Proceedings of a Workshop, 2020. Washington, DC: The National Academies Press. https://doi.org/10.17226/25746.

[42] John N. Nkengason. How Africa can quell the next disease outbreaks: A personal take on event. Nature, 2019: vol 567:14; 14

[43] Madrigal AC and R Meyer. 'How Could the CDC Make That Mistake?' The Atlantic May 2020.

[44] Jacobsen KH. Will COVID-19 generate global preparedness? The Lancet, Published online March 18, 2020 https://doi.org/10.1016/S0140-6736(20)30559-6.

[45] Kandel M, S Chungong, A Omaar, J Xing. Health security capacities in the context of COVID-19 outbreak: an analysis of International Health Regulations annual report data from 182 countries. The Lancet, Published online March 18, 2020 https://doi.org/10.1016/S0140-6736(20)30553-5

[46] Rudan I. A cascade of causes that led to the COVID-19 tragedy in Italy and in other European Union countries. Journal of Global Health, 2020: 10(1): 1-10.

[47] Moatti JP. The French response to COVID-19: intrinsic difficulties at the interface of science, public health, and policy. Lancet Public Health 2020 Published Online April 7, 2020 https://doi.org/10.1016/S2468-2667(20)30087-6.

[48] Editorial(a). How to be ready for the next influenza pandemic. The Lancet Infectious Disease 2018; 18: 697.

[49] Geda A. The Macroeconomic and Social Impact of COVID-19 in Ethiopia and Suggested Directions for Policy Response. Preprint · April 2020, https://www.researchgate.net/publication/340938630.

[50] Tezazu B, F Fullas and M Muchie. Leap Through COVID-19 With Full Action Towards A Better Life. NES Commentary 47, 2020

[51] Durrheim DN, LO Gostin and K Moodley. When does a major outbreak become a Public Health Emergency of International Concern? Lancet Infect Dis, Published Online May 19, 2020 https://doi.org/10.1016/S1473-3099(20)30401-1.

[52] Editorial (b). Make universal health care a priority. Nature 2020e: 578: 191.

[53] Maureen Kelley, Rashida A Ferrand, Kui Muraya, Simukai Chigudu, Sassy Molyneux, Madhukar Pai et.al. An appeal for practical social justice in the COVID-19 global response in low-income and middle-income countries. The Lancet Published online May 14, 2020 https://doi.org/10.1016/S2214-109X(20)30249-7.

[54] Kelley M, RA Ferrand, K Muraya, S Chigudu et al. An appeal for practical

social justice in the COVID-19 global response in low-income and middle-income countries. The Lancet Published online May 14, 2020 https://doi.org/10.1016/S2214-109X(20)30249-7.

[55] Jay J Van Bavel, Katherine Baicker, Paulo S. Boggio, Valerio Capraro, Aleksandra Cichocka, Mina Cikara et.al. Using social and behavioural science to support COVID-19 pandemic response. Nature Human Behaviour, 2020; 4: 460-471.

[56] Thorp HH. Time to pull together. Science. Published online 16 March 2020; 10.1126/science.abb7518.

[57] Fineberg HV. Ten Weeks to Crush the Curve. N Engl J Med. 2020;382(17):e37. doi:10.1056/NEJMe2007263

[58] Caitlin Rivers, Elena Martin, Diane Meyer, Thomas V. Inglesby, Anita J. Cicero, Julia Cizek. Modernizing and Expanding Outbreak Science to Support Better Decision Making During Public Health Crises: Lessons for COVID-19 and Beyond. The Open Philanthropy Project, Johns Hopkins University, 2020.

[59] Adam D. Modelling the pandemic: The simulations driving the world's response to COVID-19. Nature, 2020: 580: 316-318.

[60] Jordan RE and P Adab. Who is most likely to be infected with SARS-CoV-2?. The Lancet Published online May 15, 2020 https://doi.org/10.1016/S1473-3099(20)30395-9.

[61] O'Reilly KM, M Auzenbergs, Y Jafari, Y Liu et al. Effective transmission across the globe: the role of climate in COVID-19 mitigation strategies. The Lancet Published online May 6, 2020 https://doi.org/10.1016/S2542-5196(20)30106-6.

[62] Layne SP, JM Hyman, DM Morens, JK Taubenberger, New coronavirus outbreak: Framing questions for pandemic prevention. Sci. Transl. Med. 2020, 12, eabb1469

[63] Rybniker J and G Fätkenheuer. Importance of precise data on SARS-CoV-2 transmission dynamics control. The Lancet, Published online May 15, 2020 https://doi.org/10.1016/S1473-3099(20)30359-5.

[64] Anastassopoulou C, Russo L, Tsakris A, Siettos C. Data-based analysis, modelling and forecasting of the COVID-19 outbreak. PLoS ONE, 2020: 15(3): e0230405. https://doi.org/10.1371/ journal.pone.0230405.

[65] Kitaw, Y., Teka, GE. & Meche, H., Damen HM and Mesganaw F. 'Evolution of Public Health in Ethiopia', 1941-2015 (3rd Edition). Ethiopian Public Health Association (EPHA), Addis Ababa, Ethiopia. 2017.

[66] Zelalem K, Sabit A, Firmaye B, Dagmawit S, Ermias W, Samson M, Desalegn A, Emana A, Yosef G. Rapid Evidence synthesis on COVID19 Pandemic to Inform Ethiopian Ministry of Health: Knowledge Translation Directorate, Ethiopian Public Health Institute, Addis Ababa, Ethiopia, April 2020

[67] Yammine S. Fight Coronavirus Misinformation: Use social media to spread good pandemic science. Nature, 2020; 581: 345-346.

[68] Marinoni G., van't Land H., and Jensen T. The Impact of COVID-19 on Global Higher Education. International Association of Universities (IAU), May 2020, Paris.

[69] Priyadarshini S. Fighting the coronavirus misinformation epidemic. Nature India, 2020.36. doi:10.1038/nindia. Published online 23 February 2020.

[70] Brandt AM & A Botelho. Not a Perfect Storm-Covid-19 and the Importance of Language. N Engl J Med, 2020: 382(16): 1493-1495.

[71] Cowper A. Covid-19: Are we getting the communications right? BMJ, 2020;368:m919 doi: 10.1136/bmj.m919.

[72] Editorial (c). COVID-19: learning from experience. Lancet 2020f:395: 1011.

[73] Cardew G. People will not trust unkind science. Nature 2020; 578: 9.

[74] The COCONEL Group. A future vaccination campaign against COVID-19 at risk of vaccine hesitancy and politicization. Lancet Infect Dis, Published Online May 20, 2020 https://doi.org/10.1016/S1473-3099(20)30426-6.

[75] Kebede Y, Yitayih Y, Birhanu Z, Mekonen S, Ambelu A. Knowledge, perceptions and preventive practices towards COVID-19 early in the outbreak among Jimma university medical center visitors, Southwest Ethiopia. PLoS ONE, 2020: 15(5): e0233744. https://doi.org/10.1371/journal. pone.0233744.

[76] JSI. Ethiopia's Digital Health Response to COVID-19. May 14th, 2020a, John Snow, Inc..

[77] Julia C, Saynac Y, Le Joubioux C, Cailhol J, Lombrail P, Bouchaud O. Organising community primary care in the age of COVID-19: challenges in disadvantaged areas. Lancet Public Health. 2020 May 13. doi: 10.1016/S2468-2667(20)30115-8. Epub ahead of print. PMID: 32411922; PMCID: PMC7220164.

[78] Adam J Kucharski, Petra Klepac, Andrew J K Conlan, Stephen M Kissler, Maria L Tang, Hannah Fry, et.al. Effectiveness of isolation, testing, contact tracing, and physical distancing on reducing transmission of SARS-CoV-2 in different settings: a mathematical modelling study. Lancet Infect Dis, Published online June 16, 2020 https://doi.org/10.1016/S1473-3099(20)30457-6

[79] Abbasi J. The Promise and Peril of Antibody Testing for COVID-19. JAMA, Published online April 17, 2020. doi:10.1001/jama.2020.6170.

[80] Kotz D. Researchers develop experimental rapid COVID-19 test using nanoparticle technique. May 29, 2020 https://phys.org/news/2020-05-experimental-rapid-covidnanoparticle-technique.html.

[81] Majid F, SB Omer and AI Khwaja. Optimising SARS-CoV-2 pooled testing for low-resource settings. Lancet Microbe, Published online June 8, 2020 https://doi.org/10.1016/S2666-5247(20)30056-2.

[82] MOH. National Assessment of the Ethiopian Health Extension Program: Abridged Report. November 2019. Addis Ababa.

[83] Jinnong Zhang, Luqian Zhou, Yuqiong Yang, Wei Peng, Wenjing Wang, Xuelin Chen. Therapeutic and triage strategies for 2019 novel coronavirus disease in fever clinics. Lancet Respir Med 2020 Published online February 13, 2020 https://doi.org/10.1016/S2213-2600(20)30071-0.

[84] Editorial (d). COVID-19: Fighting panic with information. Lancet. Vol 395 February 22, 2020g. www.thelancet.com/journals /lancet/article/PIIS0140-6736(20)30379-2/fulltext

[85] Sinha P and AE Paterson. Contact tracing: Can 'Big tech' come to the rescue, and if so, at what cost?, Clinical Medicine, 2020, https://doi.org/10.1016/j.eclinm.2020.100412.

[86] Editorial (e). Technology in the COVID-19 era: pushing the boundaries. Lancet Diabetes Endocrinol, Published online June 8, 2020h https://doi.org/10.1016/S2213-8587(20)30191-1

[87] Zhongjie Li, Qiulan Chen, Luzhao Feng, Lance Rodewald, Yinyin Xia, Hailiang Yu, et.al. Active case finding with case management: the key to tackling the COVID-19 pandemic. The Lancet, Published online June 4, 2020:396, 63-70, https://doi.org/10.1016/S0140-6736(20)31278-2

[88] Derek K Chu, Elie A Akl, Stephanie Duda, Karla Solo, Sally Yaacoub, Holger J Schünemann. Physical distancing, face masks, and eye protection to prevent person-to-person transmission of SARS-CoV-2 and COVID-19: a systematic review and meta-analysis. Lancet 2020; 395: 1973-87 Published online June 1, 2020 https://doi.org/10.1016/S0140-6736(20)31142-9

[89] Thomas M Drake, Annemarie B Docherty, Thomas G Weiser, Steven Yule, Aziz Sheikh, Ewen M Harrison. The effects of physical distancing on population mobility during the COVID-19 pandemic in the UK. Lancet Digital Health, Published online June 12, 2020 https://doi.org/10.1016/S2589-7500(20)30134-5 Published online June 12, 2020 https://doi.org/10.1016/S2589-7500(20)30134-5.

[90] Ethiopian Academy of Sciences (EAS). Report on Mapping the Health Research Landscape in Ethiopia. EAS, Addis Ababa pp. 147. 2013

[91] Luis Alberto Martinez-Juarez, Ana Cristina Sedas, Miriam Orcutt, Raj Bhop.Governments and international institutions should urgently attend to the unjust disparities that COVID-19 is exposing and causing, EClinicalMedicine, 2020:12,7, https://doi.org/10.1016/j.eclinm.2020.100376.

[92] Ball P. Anti-vaccine Movement Might Undermine Pandemic Efforts. Nature 2020; 581: 251.

[93] Editorial (f). Pandemic versus pandemonium: fighting on two fronts. The Lancet Digital Health, June 2020i: 2: e268.

[94] Roberton T, ED Carter, VB Chou, AR Stegmuller et al. Early estimates of the indirect effects of the COVID-19 pandemic on maternal and child mortality in low-income and middle-income countries: a modelling study. The Lancet Published online May 12, 2020 https://doi.org/10.1016/S2214-109X(20)30229-1.

[95] Smith V, Seo D, Warty R, Payne O, Salih M, Chin KL, et al. Maternal and neonatal outcomes associated with COVID-19 infection: A systematic review. PLoS ONE, 20202: 15(6): e0234187. https://doi.org/10.1371/journal.pone.0234187.

[96] Ranscombe P. Rural areas at risk during COVID-19 pandemic. Lancet, Published online April 17, 2020 https://doi.org/10.1016/S1473-3099(20)30301-7.

[97] Ezekiel J. Emanuel, Govind Persad, Ross Upshur, Beatriz Thome, Michael Parker, Aaron Glickman, et.al. N Engl J Med 2020; 382:2049-2055, DOI: 10.1056/NEJMsb2005114

[98] Fore HH. A wake-up call: COVID-19 and its impact on children's health and wellbeing. Lancet GH, Published online May 12, 2020 https://doi.org/10.1016/S2214-109X(20)30238-2.

[99] Roder-DeWan S. Health system quality in the time of COVID-19. The Lancet, Published online May 6, 2020 https://doi.org/10.1016/S2214-109X(20)30223-0.

[100] Ledford H. Dozens of coronavirus drugs are in development — what

happens next? Nature, 2020; 581: 247-248.

[101] Gates B. Ring the alarm: The next epidemic is coming. Here's how we can make sure we're ready. **Shattuck Lecture, April 27, 2018, Boston, MA.**

[102] Andrew Clark, Mark Jit, Charlotte Warren-Gash, Bruce Guthrie, Harry H X Wang, Stewart W Mercer, et.al. Global, regional, and national estimates of the population at increased risk of severe COVID-19 due to underlying health conditions in 2020: a modelling study. Lancet Glob Health 2020; 8: e1003-17 Published Online June 15, 2020 https://doi.org/10.1016/S2214-109X(20)30264-3.

[103] Dhaliwal M. Opinion: Strong health systems are our best defense against pandemics. www.devex.com/news/opinion-strong-health-systems-are-our-best-defense-against-pandemics-92023, 2018.

[104] John H Amuasi, Christian Walzer, David Heymann, Hélène Carabin, Le Thi Huong, Andrew Haines et.al. Calling for a COVID-19 One Health Research Coalition. The Lancet 2020; 395: 1543-1544.

[105] Anna C. Africa Dangerously Behind in Global Race for Medical Equipment Amid Coronavirus. University World News, April 24, 2020.

[106] Khan M and S Shanks. Decolonising COVID-19: delaying external debt repayments. Lancet, Global Health Published online June 1, 2020 https://doi.org/10.1016/S2214-109X(20)30253-9.

[107] Mokuwa EY, Maat H. Rural populations exposed to Ebola Virus Disease respond positively to localised case handling: Evidence from Sierra Leone. PLoS Negl Trop Dis, 2020: 14(1): e0007666. https://doi.org/10.1371/journal. pntd.0007666.

[108] Ramdas K, F Ahmed and A Darzi. Remote shared care delivery: a virtual response to COVID-19. Lancet Digital Health, Published Online April 30, 2020 https://doi.org/10.1016/S2589-7500(20)30101-1.

[109] Kitaw Yand Aseffa A. Teaching article: Preparing a policy brief: review of the basics In the Ethiopian context. Ethiop Med J, 2017, 55(4): 299-311.

[110] Vernon J Lee, Marc Ho, Chen Wen Kai, Ximena Aguilera, David Heymann, Annelies Wilder-Smith. Epidemic preparedness in urban settings: new challenges and opportunities. Lancet Glob Health, Published Online March 27, 2020 https://doi.org/10.1016/S1473-3099(20)30249-8.

[111] Senghore M, MK Savi, B Gnangnon, WP Hanage and IN Okeke. Leveraging Africa's preparedness towards the next phase of the COVID-19 pandemic. The Lancet, Published online May 14, 2020 https://doi.org/10.1016/S2214-109X(20)30234-5.

[112] van der Zwaan B. Higher Education in 2040: A Global Approach. Amsterdam University Press, 2017.

[113] Brown RJ and MG Head. Monitoring investments in coronavirus research and development. Lancet Microbe, 2020; 1: e61.

[114] Nega M and M Kassaye. Research and PhD capacities in Sub-Saharan Africa: Ethiopia report. British Council, 2018.

[115] Burki TH. COVID-19: consequences for higher education. Lancet Oncol, Published online May 21, 2020 https://doi.org/10.1016/S1470-2045(20)30287-4.

[116] Abbey E, E Adu-Danso and E Aryeetey. Research universities' multiple responses to COVID-19. University World News, 23 April 2020.

[117] Weston Struwe, Edward Emmott, Melanie Bailey, Michal Sharon, Andrea Sinz, Fernando J Corrales et.al. The COVID-19 MS Coalition—accelerating diagnostics, prognostics, and treatment. The Lancet, Published online May 27, 2020 https://doi.org/10.1016/S0140-6736(20)31211-3.

[118] African Academy of Sciences. Research and Development goals for COVID-19 in Africa: The African Academy of Sciences Priority Setting Exercise. 2020, Nairobi.

[119] Graeden E, C Carlson and R Katz. Answering the right questions for policymakers on COVID-19. Lancet Glob Health, published online April 20, 2020 https://doi.org/10.1016/S2214-109X(20)30191-1.

[120] Larson HJ. A lack of information can become misinformation. Nature 2020; 580: 306.

[121] Perris K and R Mohee. Quality assurance is key to sustainable blended learning. University World News, 18 June 2020.

[122] Douglass JA. Higher education is key for the post-COVID recovery. University World News, 25 April 2020.

[123] Editorial (g). Riding the coronacoaster of uncertainty. The Lancet, Published online May 15, 2020j https://doi.org/10.1016/S1473-3099(20)30378-9.

[124] Cash-Gibson L, G Guerra and VN Salgado-de-Snyder. SDH-NET: a South–North-South collaboration to build sustainable research capacities on social determinants of health in low- and middle-income countries. Health Research Policy and Systems (2015) 13:45 DOI 10.1186/s12961-015-0048-1.

[125] Edward-Ekpu U. African scientists sense a once-in-a-life opportunity to push for research funding. Quartz Africa May 11, 2020.

[126] English KM and B Pourbohloul. Increasing health policy and systems research capacity in low- and middle income countries: results from a bibliometric analysis. Health Research Policy and Systems, 2017:15:64. DOI 10.1186/s12961-017-0229-1.

[127] Bekoe R. Pandemic spotlights need for greater R&D investment. University World News, 23 April 2020.